Trauma Across the Continuum

Editor

MARCIE FEINMAN

SURGICAL CLINICS
OF NORTH AMERICA

www.surgical.theclinics.com

Consulting Editor
RONALD F. MARTIN

April 2024 • Volume 104 • Number 2

ELSEVIER

1600 John F. Kennedy Boulevard • Suite 1800 • Philadelphia, Pennsylvania, 19103-2899

http://www.surgical.theclinics.com

SURGICAL CLINICS OF NORTH AMERICA Volume 104, Number 2
April 2024 ISSN 0039–6109, ISBN-13: 978-0-443-13103-5

Editor: John Vassallo (j.vassallo@elsevier.com)
Developmental Editor: Anita Chamoli

Surgical Clinics of North America (ISSN 0039–6109) is published bimonthly by Elsevier Inc., 360 Park Avenue South, New York, NY 10010-1710. Months of publication are February, April, June, August, October, and December. Business and Editorial Offices: 1600 John F. Kennedy Blvd., Suite 1800, Philadelphia, PA 19103-2899. Periodicals postage paid at New York, NY and additional mailing offices. Subscription prices are $503.00 per year for US individuals, $100.00 per year for US & Canadian students and residents, $592.00 per year for Canadian individuals, $597.00 for international individuals, and $250.00 per year for foreign students/residents. For institutional access pricing please contact Customer Service via the contact information below. To receive student/resident rate, orders must be accompanied by name of affiliated institution, date of term, and the *signature* of program/residency coordinator on institution letterhead. Orders will be billed at individual rate until proof of status is received. Foreign air speed delivery is included in all *Clinics* subscription prices. All prices are subject to change without notice. POSTMASTER: Send address changes to *Surgical Clinics*, Elsevier Health Sciences Division, Subscription Customer Service, 3251 Riverport Lane, Maryland Heights, MO 63043. **Customer Service (orders, claims, online, change of address): Telephone: 1-800-654-2452 (U.S. and Canada); 314-447-8871 (outside U.S. and Canada). Fax: 314-447-8029. E-mail: journalscustomerservice-usa@elsevier.com (for print support); journalsonlinesupport-usa@elsevier.com (for online support).**

Reprints. For copies of 100 or more, of articles in this publication, please contact the Commercial Reprints Department, Elsevier Inc., 360 Park Avenue South, New York, New York 10010-1710. Tel. 212-633-3874, Fax: 212-633-3820, E-mail: reprints@elsevier.com.

Surgical Clinics of North America is also published in Spanish by McGraw-Hill Interamericana Editores S.A., P.O. Box 5-237 06500 Mexico D.F. Mexico; and in Portuguese by Interlivros Edicoes Ltda., Rua Comandante Coelho 1085, CEP 21250, Rio de Janeiro, Brazil; and in Greek by Paschalidis Medical Publications, Athens Greece.

Surgical Clinics of North America is covered in *MEDLINE/PubMed (Index Medicus)*, *EMBASE/Excerpta Medica*, *Current Contents/Clinical Medicine*, *Current Contents/Life Sciences*, *Science Citation Index*, and *ISI/BIOMED*.

Contributors

CONSULTING EDITOR

RONALD F. MARTIN, MD, FACS
Colonel (Retired), United States Army Reserve, Department of General Surgery, Pullman Regional Hospital and Clinic Network, Pullman, Washington, USA

EDITOR

MARCIE FEINMAN, MD, MEHP, FACS
Vice Chairperson, Division Chief-Acute Care Surgery, Program Director, General Surgery Residency, Department of Surgery, Sinai Hospital of Baltimore, Baltimore, Maryland, USA

AUTHORS

REN J. ABRAHAM, MD
Research Assistant, Department of Surgery, School of Medicine, Creighton University, Omaha, Nebraska, USA

JENNIFER E. BAKER, MD
Acute Care Surgery Fellow, Division of GI, Trauma, and Endocrine Surgery, Department of Surgery, University of Colorado Anschutz Medical Campus, Aurora, Colorado, USA

MEGAN BRENNER, MD, MS, FACS
Professor, UCLA Department of Surgery, UCLA David Geffen School of Medicine, Los Angeles, California, USA

MEAGHAN BRODERICK, MD
Clinical Instructor, Department of Surgery, R Adams Cowley Shock Trauma Center, Baltimore, Maryland, USA

CLAY COTHREN BURLEW, MD
Professor, Division of GI, Trauma, and Endocrine Surgery, Department of Surgery, University of Colorado Anschutz Medical Campus, Aurora, Colorado, USA

THOMAS W. CLEMENTS, MD, FRCSC
Fellow, Trauma Surgery and Abdominal Wall Reconstruction, The Red Duke Trauma Institute, Memorial Hermann Hospital, McGovern Medical School, University of Texas Health Science Center-Houston, Houston, Texas, USA

BRYAN A. COTTON, MD, MPH
The John B Holmes Endowed Chair of Clinical Sciences, The John B Holmes Distinguished Professor of Clinical Sciences Surgery, Trauma Surgeon, The Red Duke Trauma Institute, Memorial Hermann Hospital, McGovern Medical School, University of Texas Health Science Center-Houston; Senior Researcher, Center for Translational Injury Research, Houston, Texas, USA

CHRISTOPHER DAI, DO
General Surgery Resident, Good Samaritan Regional Medical Center, Corvallis, Oregon, USA

MICHAEL DITILLO, DO
Associate Professor of Surgery, Division of Trauma, Surgical Critical Care, Burns, and Acute Care Surgery, University of Arizona, Tucson, Arizona, USA

ERIN FARRELLY, MD
Orthopedic Surgeon, Department of Orthopaedic Surgery, MedStar Orthopaedic Institute, Union Memorial Hospital, Baltimore, Maryland, USA

RYAN B. FRANSMAN, MD
Assistant Professor of Surgery, Department of Trauma, Acute Care Surgery, and Surgical Critical Care, Emory University School of Medicine, Grady Memorial Hospital, Atlanta, Georgia, USA

SABRINA D. GODDARD, MD
Assistant Professor, Division of Trauma and Acute Care Surgery, Department of Surgery, University of Alabama at Birmingham, Birmingham, Alabama, USA

JARED GRIFFARD, MD, FACS
Clinical Fellow, Division of General Surgery, Trauma and Surgical Critical Care, Department of Surgery, Yale School of Medicine, New Haven, Connecticut, USA

JEREMEY GRUSHKA, MD, MSc, MPH, FRCSC, FACS
Assistant Professor, Division of General Surgery, Department of Surgery, McGill University, Montreal, Quebec, Canada

JAMES REECE HARRIS, DO
General Surgery Resident, Good Samaritan Regional Medical Center, Corvallis, Oregon, USA

ZAIN G. HASHMI, MD
Assistant Professor, Division of Trauma and Acute Care Surgery, Department of Surgery, University of Alabama at Birmingham, Birmingham, Alabama, USA

ELLIOTT R. HAUT, MD, PhD, FACS
Professor of Surgery, Anesthesiology/ Critical Care Medicine (ACCM) and Emergency Medicine, Division of Acute Care Surgery, Department of Surgery, The Johns Hopkins University School of Medicine, Baltimore, Maryland, USA

NICHOLAS JAMES, MD, MSc
Research Student, Division of Vascular Surgery, Schulich School of Medicine and Dentistry, Western University, London, Ontario, Canada

MOLLY P. JARMAN, PhD
Assistant Professor, Department of Surgery, Center for Surgery and Public Health, Harvard Medical School, Harvard T.H. Chan School of Public Health, Brigham and Women's Hospital, Boston, Massachusetts, USA

ATIF JASTANIAH, MD, MHSc, FRCSC
Affiliated Staff, Division of General Surgery, Department of Surgery, McGill University, Montreal, Quebec, Canada

LISA M. KODADEK, MD, FACS
Assistant Professor, Division of General Surgery, Trauma and Surgical Critical Care, Department of Surgery, Yale School of Medicine, New Haven, Connecticut, USA

WILLIAM ROBERT LEEPER, MD, MEd, FRCSC, FACS
Associate Professor, Department of Surgery, Trauma and Critical Care, Western University; Program Director, Royal College Surgical Foundations, Victoria Hospital, London Health Sciences Centre, London, Ontario, Canada

SIERRA LINDSEY, MD
Resident Physician, Department of Orthopaedic Surgery, MedStar Orthopaedic Institute, Union Memorial Hospital, Baltimore, Maryland, USA

NICOLE LUNARDI, MD, MSPH
Surgical Resident, Department of General Surgery, University of Texas Southwestern, Dallas, Texas, USA

MEGAN ELIZABETH LUNDY, MD
Acute Care Surgery Fellow, Division of Trauma, Surgical Critical Care, Burns, and Acute Care Surgery, University of Arizona, Tucson, Arizona, USA

GEORGE PHILIP, MD
Assistant Professor, Department of Surgery, School of Medicine, Creighton University, Omaha, Nebraska, USA

JOSEPH V. SAKRAN, MD, MPH, MPA
Executive Vice Chair of Surgery, Director of Clinical Operations, Associate Professor of Surgery and Nursing, Department of Surgery, Johns Hopkins Hospital, Baltimore, Maryland, USA

ALEC J. SCARBOROUGH, MD
General Surgery Resident Physician, Department of Surgery, School of Medicine, Creighton University, Omaha, Nebraska, USA

PAUL J. SCHENARTS, MD, FACS, MAMSE
Professor and Associate Dean, MAMSE Professor, Department of Surgery, School of Medicine, Creighton University, Omaha, Nebraska, USA

MARINDA SCRUSHY, MD
Surgical Resident, Department of General Surgery, University of Texas Southwestern, Dallas, Texas, USA

JENNIFER SERFIN, MD
Trauma Medical Director, Designated Institutional Official, Good Samaritan Regional Medical Center, Corvallis, Oregon, USA

NATHAN SMITH, DO
Program Director, Acute Care Surgeon, Good Samaritan Regional Medical Center, Corvallis, Oregon, USA

DEBRORAH STEIN, MD, MPH
Professor, Department of Surgery, R Adams Cowley Shock Trauma Center, Baltimore, Maryland, USA

RAE TARAPORE, MD
Orthopaedic Surgery Resident, Department of Orthopaedic Surgery, MedStar Orthopaedic Institute, Union Memorial Hospital, Baltimore, Maryland, USA

JAN-MICHAEL VAN GENT, DO
Fellow, Trauma Surgery and Surgical Critical Care, The Red Duke Trauma Institute, Memorial Hermann Hospital, McGovern Medical School, University of Texas Health Science Center-Houston, Houston, Texas, USA

CHRISTOPHER M. WEND, MD
Resident Physician, Department of Emergency Medicine, The Johns Hopkins University School of Medicine, Baltimore, Maryland, USA

NICOLE L. WERNER, MD, MS
Assistant Professor, Division of Acute Care and Regional General Surgery, Department of Surgery, University of Wisconsin School of Medicine and Public Health, Madison, Wisconsin, USA

MARK D. WIELAND, MD
Resident Physician, Department of Orthopaedic Surgery, MedStar Orthopaedic Institute, Union Memorial Hospital, Baltimore, Maryland, USA

RENALDO WILLIAMS, MD
Interim Trauma Medical Director, Associate SICU Director, Surgical ECMO Director, Assistant Professor, Department of Surgery, Denver Health Medical Center, University of Colorado, Ernest E. Moore Shock Trauma Center, Denver, Colorado, USA

DANIEL DANTE YEH, MD, MHPE
Chief of Emergency General Surgery, Professor, Department of Surgery, Denver Health Medical Center, University of Colorado, Ernest E. Moore Shock Trauma Center, Denver, Colorado, USA

BO ZHANG, MD
Acute Care Surgery Fellow, Division of Trauma, Surgical Critical Care, Burns, and Acute Care Surgery, University of Arizona Tucson, Arizona, USA

Contents

Traumatic injury is a leading cause of death in the United States. Risk of traumatic injury varies by sex, age, geography, and race/ethnicity. Understanding the nuances of risk for a particular population is essential in designing, implementing, and evaluating injury prevention initiatives.

Trauma imposes a significant societal burden, with injury being a leading cause of mortality worldwide. While numerical data reveal that trauma accounts for millions of deaths annually, its true impact goes beyond these figures. The toll extends to non-fatal injuries, resulting in long-term physical and mental health consequences. Moreover, injury-related health care costs and lost productivity place substantial strain on a nation's economy. Disparities in trauma care further exacerbate this burden, affecting access to timely and appropriate care across various patient populations. These disparities manifest across the entire continuum of trauma care, from prehospital to in-hospital and post-acute phases. Addressing these disparities and improving access to quality trauma care are crucial steps toward alleviating the societal burden of trauma and enhancing equitable patient outcomes.

Prehospital trauma evaluation begins with the primary assessment of airway, breathing, circulation, disability, and exposure. This is closely followed by vital signs and a secondary assessment. Key prehospital interventions include management and resuscitation according to the aforementioned principles with a focus on major hemorrhage control, airway compromise, and invasive management of tension pneumothorax. Determining the appropriate time and method for transportation (eg, ground ambulance, helicopter, police, private vehicle) to the hospital or when to terminate resuscitation are also important decisions to be made by emergency medical services clinicians.

Start balanced resuscitation early (pre-hospital if possible), either in the form of whole blood or 1:1:1 ratio. Minimize resuscitation with crystalloid to minimize patient morbidity and mortality. Trauma-induced coagulopathy can be largely avoided with the use of balanced resuscitation, permissive hypotension, and minimized time to hemostasis. Using protocolized "triggers" for massive and ultramassive transfusion will assist in minimizing delays in transfusion of products, achieving balanced ratios, and avoiding trauma induced coagulopathy. Once "audible" bleeding has been addressed, further blood product resuscitation and adjunct replacement should be guided by viscoelastic testing. Early transfusion of whole blood can reduce patient morbidity, mortality, decreases donor exposure, and reduces nursing logistics during transfusions. Adjuncts to resuscitation should be guided by laboratory testing and carefully developed, institution-specific guidelines. These include empiric calcium replacement, tranexamic acid (or other anti-fibrinolytics), and fibrinogen supplementation.

The reader of this article will now have the ability to reflect on all aspects of high-quality trauma bay care, from resuscitation to diagnosis and from leadership to debriefing. Although there is no replacement for experience, both clinically and in a simulation environment, trauma clinicians are encouraged to make use of this article both as a primer at the beginning of a trauma rotation and as a reference text to revisit after difficult cases in the trauma bay.

Resuscitative endovascular balloon occlusion of the aorta (REBOA) has been utilized by trauma surgeons at the bedside for over a decade in both civilian and military settings. Both translational and clinical research suggest it is superior to resuscitative thoracotomy for specific patient populations. Technological advancements in recent years have significantly enhanced the safety profile of REBOA. Resuscitative balloon occlusion of the aorta has also swiftly found implementation in patients in shock from non-traumatic hemorrhage.

Traumatic brain injury (TBI) represents a heterogenous spectrum of disease. It is essential to rapidly assess a patient's neurologic status and implement measures to prevent secondary brain injury. Intracranial hypertension, a common sequela of TBI, is managed in a tiered and systematic fashion, starting with the least invasive and moving toward the most invasive. TBI has long-lasting effects on patients and their families and represents a substantial financial and social influence on society. Research regarding the prognosis and treatment of TBI is essential to limit the influence of this widespread disease.

achieved. The modified Nutritional Risk in the Critically Ill score can help identify patients who will benefit most from aggressive and early nutritional intervention. In the first week of critical illness, the patient should receive only 70% to 80% of estimated calories and protein should be targeted to 1.5 to 2 g/kg. Parenteral nutrition can be provided safely without increased adverse events. Peri-operative (and intra-operative) feeding has been shown to be safe in selected patients.

With a rapidly aging worldwide population, the care of geriatric trauma patients will be at the forefront of every career in Trauma and Acute Care Surgery. The unique intersection of advanced age, comorbidities, frailty, and physiologic changes presents a challenge in the care of elderly injured patients. It is well established that increasing age is associated with higher mortality and worse outcomes after injury, but it is also clear that there is room for improvement in the management of this special patient population.

This article delves into the role of minimally invasive surgeries in trauma, specifically laparoscopy and video-assisted thoracic surgery (VATS). It discusses the benefits of laparoscopy over traditional laparotomy, including its accuracy in detecting peritoneal violation and intraperitoneal injuries caused by penetrating trauma. The article also explores the use of laparoscopy as an adjunct to nonoperative management of abdominal injuries and in cases of blunt trauma with unclear abdominal injuries. Furthermore, it highlights the benefits of VATS in diagnosing and treating thoracic injuries, such as traumatic diaphragmatic injuries, retained hematomas, and persistent pneumothorax.

Teaching during a surgical resuscitation can be difficult due to the infrequency of these events. Furthermore, when these events do occur, the trainee can experience cognitive overload and an overwhelming amount of stress, thereby impairing the learning process. The emergent nature of these scenarios can make it difficult for the surgical educator to adequately teach. Repeated exposure through simulation, role play, and "war games" are great adjuncts to teaching and preparation before crisis. However, surgical educators can further enhance the knowledge of their trainees during these scenarios by using tactics such as talking out loud, targeted teaching, and debriefing.

SURGICAL CLINICS
OF NORTH AMERICA

SERIES OF RELATED INTEREST

Advances in Surgery
https://www.advancessurgery.com/
Surgical Oncology Clinics
https://www.surgonc.theclinics.com/
Thoracic Surgery Clinics
https://www.thoracic.theclinics.com/

THE CLINICS ARE AVAILABLE ONLINE!
Access your subscription at:
www.theclinics.com

Foreword

Trauma Across the Continuum

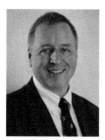

Ronald F. Martin, MD, FACS
Consulting Editor

The phrase, "life is nasty, brutish, and short," is attributed to Thomas Hobbes and taken from his work *Leviathan.* To be more correct, though, the sentiment above was prefaced to reflect the nature of man's (sic) life should it be lived "outside of society." That distinction, inside or outside of *society*, makes all the difference. The condensed and perhaps more oft-quoted shorter statement implies that our lives are simply predetermined to be a challenging affair with a high likelihood of dismal outcome, while the somewhat more extended phrase reflects the potential conditionality of that outcome. While I cannot confirm that Hobbes, a well-known pessimist, would agree, I would suggest that we can all improve our individual outcomes through participation in society—whatever that might mean. To Hobbes, that participation in society may have implied "arts and letters," though to me, as more a simple-minded surgeon rather than a philosopher, I suggest it implies collectivism of action and responsibility over individual action alone on a broader scale.

In our world of surgery, the promise of collective action over individual (spelled disjointed) action is most apparent in our treatment of the traumatized patient. Since before my time in this profession, the major impetus on the "big surgery" scale for trauma care has been the development of systems-based thinking and system-based standards. ATLS (Advance Trauma Life Support) and trauma verification schemes lie at the heart of this progression toward systematic care. Yet, multiple forces are at play that frequently frustrate the realization of those goals.

I posit that a "true" trauma system would include prevention (in all its forms), prehospital response, hospital care and interhospital patient movement (based on levels of care available), posthospital care (ranging from home care to rehabilitation to long-term acute care), and posttraumatic support. At first glance, none of these items are under single control. Certainly, they all influence one another, but they are quite separated. Prevention largely falls under the purviews of government and other regulatory agencies—usually state or federal. Prehospital care largely falls under smaller governmental control, such

Surg Clin N Am 104 (2024) xiii–xv
https://doi.org/10.1016/j.suc.2024.01.004
0039-6109/24/© 2024 Published by Elsevier Inc.

municipalities or counties. Hospital care is largely up to whatever current financial structure has evolved within regions but is supported by patient reimbursement, which relies on insurance status primarily as well as various grants and other public support, when available. Interhospital care coordination and transport are, at best, quasi-regulated through the Emergency Medical Treatment and Active Labor Act (EMTALA). The rules of EMTALA are such that they are not equally applicable to all patients' situations (such as inpatient vs patients in emergency room settings), and they cannot address facility constraints that hinder the smooth transfer of patients at times. Posthospital care again is largely available based on patient insurance status and personal resources, which for many present a serious barrier to more full recovery.

I have tried during my tenure as the Consulting Editor of this series to stay out of politics, and I will again try as I write this foreword. That said, if one believes even a smattering of what is described above, one must at least consider the possibility that the most efficient solution to the above problem, as regards system evolution, is to consider a single source of rules, regulations, revenues, risk-distribution (including cost distribution), and oversight. How that "oneness" could be achieved could be accomplished in many ways: single-payor health care overall, public utilities models, funding based on taxes (personal, corporate, and on commercial products) with processes to earmark monies to cover costs of trauma care, large regional systems that have substanital enough financial and personnel capacities to be self-sustaining, and so forth. We could treat trauma the way we treat organ transplantation. There are lots of way to bridge the system funding gaps independent of one's baseline ideology.

As with any other problem we consider, we must have a firm grasp on the nature of the dilemma we face. Dr Feinman and her colleagues have provided us with an excellent collection of articles that guides us through the care of the individual patient as well as gives us the basic building blocks of system requirements. In addition, we are given information on how the current system is working, and sometimes not working, as well as guidance for how to learn and teach based on our experiences. These writings give us a sound foundation to understand our concerns and how to convey these concerns to our colleagues and our communities. I urge you to dive deeply into each of these articles.

We need leadership, true leadership. There is a difference between those who simply want to be in charge for their own aggrandizement and power and those who choose to lead to make the world a better place for now and in the future. We as a nation, and perhaps even more globally, are divided in ways now that are difficult to comprehend. I have been around long enough to remember Vietnam, Watergate, and any number of any divisive topics within the United States. I remember the Cold War well, and I remember the years following the collapse of the Soviet Bloc. I spent years abroad in Iraq, Afghanistan, Kuwait, and other places under war conditions. I have never seen anything similar to what we see now in terms of division amongst us on almost every level.

One of the most lasting things I learned during my various adventures was that every person I met, without fail, wanted a better and safer place for their families and their children to live and grow up in. They wanted safety and freedom from hunger. They wanted their children to learn and grow. They wanted to help and be helped in times of difficulty. Individually, everyone I met wanted an end to strife in their world. However, when they got together in groups—sometimes the simple desires fell apart and darker, usually more tribal, desires rose in prominence. Invariably, the leaders of those groups—many of whom were far away and had never met these people—were who made the difference—for better or worse.

In my opinion, trauma care in the United States continues to stand in the middle of an intersection, which is a dangerous place to mill about. We as surgeons need to coordinate and advocate for transition to something more efficient, more reliable, and more stable. Either we do that or we see where the winds will blow us next—whether that wind is another pandemic, financial peril, escalation of global hostilities, or just plain apathy and failure to prepare for changing requirements. I am hoping that those of you who read this issue will take it to heart and help us improve our professional relationship with society such that we can make life for all of us less nasty, brutish, and short.

Ronald F. Martin, MD, FACS
Colonel (Retired), United States Army Reserve
Department of General Surgery
Pullman Surgical Associates
Pullman Regional Hospital and Clinic Network
825 Southeast Bishop Boulevard, Suite 130
Pullman, WA 99163, USA

E-mail address:
rfmcescna@gmail.com

Preface

Trauma Across the Continuum: New Challenges for a New Era

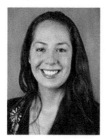

Marcie Feinman, MD, MEHP, FACS
Editor

In our post-COVID-19 world, a lot has changed. Masks are commonplace, staying home from work when sick is accepted, and virtual meetings are here to stay. While there was a decrease in trauma volume during the height of COVID-19, the rebound in cases has reached prepandemic numbers and then some. Gun violence is on the rise with more deaths from gun-related injuries in 2021 than any time prior. Physicians and other health care providers have had to adapt to this new reality by finding innovative ways to take care of the influx of trauma patients while continuing to focus on their own well-being.

This issue of *Surgical Clinics* focuses on modern care of the trauma patient from insult to result. While the principles of trauma care have remained much the same over the years, advances in prehospital interventions, transfusion medicine, hemorrhage control, and minimally invasive surgical techniques have shaped the specifics of how we care for patients today. Throughout this issue, you will find both long-standing standards of care and cutting-edge practices that are just being incorporated into traumatology. I would like to encourage the reader to remain open-minded to emerging practices. If the past few years of pandemic life have taught us nothing else, it is clear that the only constant is change.

I would like to thank Ron Martin, the Consulting Editor of *Surgical Clinics*, for the opportunity to host this issue. The article authors represent academic and community trauma centers in both the United States and Canada, and their wide-ranging expertise elevates the caliber of this text. They have done a fantastic job of capturing current issues in the care of the traumatically injured patient and have provided a look into the future. I thank them for their contributions both to this issue and to the field of traumatology.

Surg Clin N Am 104 (2024) xvii–xviii
https://doi.org/10.1016/j.suc.2024.01.001
0039-6109/24/© 2024 Published by Elsevier Inc.

surgical.theclinics.com

It was my honor to edit this issue of *Surgical Clinics*. I learned an incredible amount from reading each article, and I know you will, too.

Marcie Feinman, MD, MEHP, FACS
Department of Surgery
Acute Care Surgery
Sinai Hospital of Baltimore
2435 West Belvedere Avenue, Suite 42
Baltimore, MD 21215, USA

E-mail address:
mfeinman@lifebridgehealth.org

Trauma Demographics and Injury Prevention

Marinda Scrushy, MD[a], Nicole Lunardi, MD, MSPH[a],
Joseph V. Sakran, MD, MPH, MPA[b],*

KEYWORDS

- Traumatic injury • Demographics • Injury prevention

KEY POINTS

- Intentional and unintentional traumatic injury are leading causes of death in the United States.
- Injury patterns vary by key demographic factors including biologic sex, age, and geography.
- Injury prevention initiatives should be tailored to a particular population's risk, exposure, outcomes, and access to trauma care. These initiatives should be the subject of ongoing monitoring and evaluation.

INTRODUCTION

Traumatic injury is a leading cause of mortality in the United States, with as many as 278,345 injury-related deaths in 2020 and 306,086 in 2021.[1,2] The Centers for Disease Control and Prevention (CDC) fatal and nonfatal injury reports distinguish between unintentional and intentional injury. Unintentional injuries are not inflicted by deliberate means while intentional injuries are those carried out with intent to injure oneself or another person. Both intentional and unintentional injuries remain on the list of top 5 leading causes of death in the United States, irrespective of sex or race. This is why unintentional injury accounts for the highest number of years of potential life lost, followed closely by both suicide and homicide.[1] The burden of trauma care continues to rise, with 181,194,431 trauma admissions between 2006 and 2012.[3] Increasing admissions has resulted in inpatient hospital costs doubling between 2001 and 2011. Estimates in the overall cost of injury have risen from $693 billion in 2010 to $4.6 trillion in 2020.[1,4] Trauma-related hospital care has been estimated to account for 6% of total inpatient hospital costs in the United States.[5]

---

[a] Department of General Surgery, University of Texas Southwestern, Dallas, TX, USA;
[b] Department of Surgery, Johns Hopkins Hospital, 1800 Orleans Street, Sheikh Zayed Tower / Suite 6107A, Baltimore, MD 21287, USA
* Corresponding author.
E-mail address: jsakran1@jhmi.edu

Surg Clin N Am 104 (2024) 243–254
https://doi.org/10.1016/j.suc.2023.11.013
0039-6109/24/© 2023 Elsevier Inc. All rights reserved.
surgical.theclinics.com

Despite significant growth and interest in the field of injury prevention, the risk of injury and burden of trauma care in the United States remain high. Targeted injury prevention efforts must be tailored to a population's injury risk, exposure, and outcomes as well as access to trauma care. As such, current epidemiologic trends in mechanism, sex, age, race/ethnicity, and geography must be understood.

EPIDEMIOLOGY

Sex

Unintentional injury is the leading cause of nonfatal injury for both males and females. Compared to females, males have a higher overall rate of traumatic injury and higher mortality rates for both unintentional and intentional injuries in 2020.
[1,6] However, the rate of overall injuries in female patients has been increasing over the last 10 years with a particular increase in penetrating, blunt, and fall mechanisms.[6]

Race/Ethnicity

Unintentional injury remains the leading cause of traumatic death across all racial and ethnic groups. Over the last 10 years, the Hispanic and Latino population has seen a significant increase in overall injury rates while the white population has seen an overall decrease. Violent firearm injury remains predominantly high among racial and ethnic minorities, particularly in young black males.[1,6]

Age

Life expectancy in the United States is increasing due to improved medical care with a large amount of the elderly population now living with multiple comorbidities. It is projected that 73.1 million people will be over the age of 65 by 2030 and over 90 million by 2060.[7,8] Trauma demographics are following this trend with geriatric adults quickly becoming the largest group of trauma patients presenting to trauma centers. The average age of patients discharged from a US hospital with a traumatic injury increased from 56 to 65 between 2000 and 2011 and data from the National Trauma Database have shown an increase in traumatic injury over time in patients aged greater than 65.[5,6] This subset of patients requires specialized care as polypharmacy, increased comorbidities, and physiologic changes put them at high risk of both morbidity and mortality.[7]

Common mechanisms of injury in the geriatric population include falls, MVC (motor vehicle collision), pedestrian injuries, suicide, and elder abuse.[9] Currently, the most common injuries are orthopedic in nature including both hip and femur fractures, likely due to the high prevalence of falls in this population.[5,6] Traumatic brain injury (TBI) rate is more common in older adults > age 85 with an incidence rate of 29% in 2006 to 2012.[3] These observations have incited a particular interest in geriatric trauma with implementation of specific geriatric trauma guidelines, protocols, and triage criteria leading to decreases in in-hospital mortality.[10]

Although the overall age of the traumatic population in the United States is increasing, patients aged 18 to 44 are still more likely to experience severe traumatic injuries. Unintentional injury remains the leading cause of death in ages 1 to 44.[1,2,5,6] Common mechanisms in this age group include firearm, motor vehicle, and pedestrian injuries.[6]

Traumatic injury remains a leading cause of death in the pediatric population as well. Unintentional injury is the most common cause of death for children aged less than 1 year. It is estimated that over 8.7 million children are treated in the US emergency departments due to traumatic injury and that over 7,000 pediatric deaths are attributable to trauma each year.[11] Motor vehicle collisions remain the top mechanism in all pediatric age groups; however, penetrating injuries including stab wounds and gunshot wounds are the second most common mechanism in ages 15 to 19 years. Falls are more common in children aged < 5 subsequently leading to an increase in rates of TBI in this age group.[12,13] Orthopedic injury remains the most common injury requiring admission.[12]

Geography

The relationship between geographic location and overall physical health in the United States has been well described.[14,15] The field of trauma is no exception, as geography affects injury risk and clinical outcomes. Geographic injury patterns vary by region of the country, urban versus rural, and poverty levels. The relative proportion of risk factors, high-risk populations, and access to trauma systems vary geographically.

In general, rural areas have higher rates of death from unintentional injury and urban areas demonstrate higher rates of interpersonal violence leading to injury, while rates of suicide are equal for both.[16–18] Neighborhoods with higher poverty rates have a higher proportion of traumatic injury regardless of urban or rural location.[5,19–21] In 2018 to 2019, the mortality for unintentional injury in children was higher in rural areas with higher rates of burns and MVC-related mortality.[17]

Access to trauma care contributes to the geographic difference in outcomes. Trauma deserts defined as areas located more than 8.0 km from a trauma center, lead to higher transport times and associated increased mortality. Rural areas in the United States have been shown to have less access to a trauma center, and, as such, have higher risk of pre-hospital death.[19,22,23] Conversely, greater access to trauma centers, defined by living within 45 minutes by ground transport, in pediatric populations is associated with lower rates of crude injury-related pediatric mortality.[24] Trauma center access is not only a problem for rural populations. Despite living in major US cities with high-level trauma centers, black majority neighborhoods are often located in "trauma deserts" with distance to the closest trauma center greater than 8 km.[25]

Tools like the CDC fatal injury mapping application and the American College of Surgeons Needs Based Assessment of Trauma Systems aim to incorporate geospatial location in order to aid in policy decisions regarding injury prevention and trauma system optimization. Defining geographic access to trauma centers in both urban and rural areas can have implications for survival after both intentional and unintentional injury.

Mechanism and Intent

Cause of injury can be described based on intent and mechanism. Intent refers to whether an injury was carried out intentionally either by oneself or by another party. Categories of intent include unintentional, homicide/assault, suicide/intentional self-harm and legal intervention. Mechanism refers to the way in which the injury occurred. Common mechanisms of injury in the United States include penetrating injuries (firearm, cut/pierce), blunt injury (crush, fall, struck), transportation injuries (motor vehicle injuries, pedestrian, motorcycle, bicycle), suffocation, drowning, poisoning, and burns.[26,27]

Firearm injuries remain a leading cause of injury in the United States with 44,364 reported deaths related to gun violence in 2022.[28] Unintentional firearm injuries encompass mechanisms such as accidental discharge and intentional injuries include homicide, suicide, and mass shootings. Unintentional injuries are more common in children less than age 10 while injuries of violent intent are more common in adolescents and young adults.[29] In the United States, firearm injuries were responsible for 75% of all homicides and 91% of homicides in ages 10 to 19 from 2018 to 2019.[20,29] Although mass shootings represent the minority (<2%) of firearm injuries, between 2015 and 2021, there were 2423 reported mass shootings with an increase in number over time from 335 in 2015 to 693 in 2021. Based on location, the largest number of mass shootings occurred in southern states.[30]

Suicide remains the 10th leading cause of death in the United States with over 187,000 emergency room (ER) visits in 2020 for self-harm injury and 48,183 reported deaths in 2021. The most common mechanism is firearm suicide followed by suffocation and poisoning.[31] After an initial decline in 2019 to 2020, suicide rates increased in 2021 with an age-adjusted rate of 14.1 suicides per 100,000 persons. Those at highest risk have been reported to be young black persons aged 10 to 24 with an increased risk in ages 25 to 44 regardless of sex or race.[32]

Intimate partner violence (IPV) refers to abuse occurring in a romantic relationship and encompasses stalking, psychological aggression, and both physical and sexual violence. In the 2016 to 2017 CDC's National Intimate Partner and Violence Survey, more than 2 in 5 women and men reported some form of physical violence–related IPV during their lifetime. In addition, 40.5 million women and 29 million men reported an episode of severe physical violence. The majority of men and women reported becoming victims to IPV prior to age 25 with 1 in 4 female and 1 in 5 males reporting abuse starting before age 18.[33]

Child abuse encompasses physical, sexual, and emotional abuse as well as neglect. In the year 2020, there were 1750 deaths reported due to child abuse and 1 in 7 children in the United States are likely to experience abuse or neglect.[26] Abuse also affects older adults with elder abuse defined as abuse occurring in a patient over age 60. This is most commonly at the hands of a caregiver. In adults over age 70, 1 in 10 have reported some form of abuse within the last year with up to 1.7% reported as physical abuse. There were over 643,000 ER visits for abuse in older adults from 2002 to 2016 with higher rates for men than women. Risk factors for elder abuse include lack of access to health care, high levels of dependence on a caregiver, lack of social support, as well as poor physical and mental health and current or past abuse of drugs or alcohol[1,34]

Common causes of unintentional injury in the United States include falls and transportation injuries. In 2018, there were an estimated 3 million ER visits for fall-related injury. This mechanism is becoming increasingly more common, with a 46% increase in fall-related mortality noted from 2002 to 2010.[35,36] However, the majority of falls are non-fatal and are a leading cause of preventable injury.[6] Falls are most common in the extremes of age-in pediatric patients less than 5 years and in geriatric patients greater than 85.[36] In the geriatric population, falls are more likely to be ground level and account for increased morbidity with loss of ability to perform activities of daily living and higher likelihood of discharge to an acute care facility or nursing home.[37]

Despite a rapid increase in fall-related injury, transportation injuries remain the most common unintentional injury in the United States. An average of 2.1 million emergency department visits for motor vehicle crashes occurred during 2020, with almost 41,000 mortalities. Of these, over 7000 were pedestrians. The highest rates of death after motor-pedestrian crash are in adults aged greater than 65 and children under the age of 15. Although this remains a leading cause of death in the United States, MVC injury mortality rates have decreased over time due to improvements in car safety and restraints.[1,12,35,38] Motorcycle crash injuries account for more than 180,000 ER visits per year with a reported 5500 deaths in 2020. Although much lower, bicycle crash mortality rates still reach 1000 per year and account for over 130,000 injuries annually.

Although injury rates are higher for youths aged 10 to 24, the mortality rate is higher for older adults.[1]

INJURY PREVENTION
History of Injury Prevention

Early public health efforts to address injury included the development of the National Safety Council in 1913 which was chartered to store safety information. However, early approaches to injury prevention were hindered by the thought that accidents were random, inevitable acts without a causal relationship.[39,40] The scientific study of injury prevention was first introduced in the 1940s to 1960s, with basic principles described by an experimental psychologist, James J. Gibson. He described the scientific principle of how an "accident" leads to injury by concluding that energy exchange causes tissue damage leading to functional impairment.[41] In 1949, John E. Godfrey published "The Epidemiology of Accidents" which classified injury as a public health problem by equating the study and prevention of injuries to infectious disease.[39,42] In 1953, the first accident prevention conference was held at the University of Michigan aiding in the development of an accident prevention program through the Public Health Services (PHS). PHS was later dismantled and funding was redirected to organizations known now as the Food and Drug Administration, Health Services and Mental Health Administration, and the CDC.[39,43]

From the 1960s to present, injury prevention and control has experienced rapid growth. Early policy was directed toward traffic and road safety with the first National Conference on Street and Highway Safety developed by President Hoover in 1924. This paved the way for the eventual development of the National Traffic and Motor Vehicle Safety Act and the Highway Safety Act in 1966. These laws spearheaded the start of the development of modern Emergency Medical Services (EMS), including the EMS Systems Act of 1973 that led to the regional development of both emergency and trauma systems.[39,44,45] It was in this period that William Haddon developed the "Haddon Matrix," a framework to identify the injury origin and measures of prevention. It was first applied to traffic and road injury prevention strategies.[46]

Federal interest in injury prevention continued to grow in the 1960s to 1970s with developments including the beginning of recognition of child maltreatment and intimate partner violence by President Johnson in 1968 and the signing of the Occupational Safety and Health Act in 1970 by President Nixon.[39] However, the greatest overall growth came in the 1980s to 1990s when congress tasked the CDC with the development of a national injury and violence prevention sector supported by government funding. This led to rapid growth in the scientific study of injury prevention and eventually led to the establishment of the National Center for Injury Prevention and Control (NCIPC) in 1992 whose mission is to "provide leadership in preventing and controlling injuries by reducing the incidence, severity, and adverse outcomes of injury which is achieved through research, surveillance, implementation of programs, and communications."[39,47]

In the 30 years since the establishment of the NCIPC, there has been an increase in injury prevention funding and research, much of which has focused on violent injury. The first major charter for violent injury prevention came in 1993 when the CDC published its research findings in "Youth Violence Prevention: A Framework for Community Action." This publication supported the conceptual reframing of violence as a problem that could be targeted by preventative efforts. From 1994 to 1996, research efforts were expanded to both IPV and school -related violence. In 2000, following the Columbine High School mass shooting, the CDC established the National Academic

Centers of Excellence on Youth Violence and expanded the field of injury prevention by providing funding for state-specific programs. The web-based statistics query and reporting system online CDC database was also established in 2000 to aid in providing injury data to the public.

It is important to recognize that progress in firearm injury prevention was stalled for many years by a ban on federal funding for firearm research. In 2018, CDC updates provided funding for gun violence research, specifically on injury prevention. From 2001 to 2020, efforts were made to understand and prevent violence and injury toward vulnerable populations with a focus on violence against women, children, and the elderly. In addition, injury prevention was encouraged at both the state and local level with increased funding to city, country, and state health departments to address violent injury.[48]

Fundamentals of Injury Prevention

The public health approach

The public health approach to injury uses the same standardized scientific method as the study and prevention of disease. There are 4 main steps to this approach that include (1) defining the problem, (2) identifying both protective factors and risk factors, (3) the development and testing of prevention strategies, and (4) widespread adoption of these strategies. Defining the problem relies on epidemiologic data collection that often includes retrospective analysis and surveillance studies. This step provides data on demographics, trends in injury patterns over time, and the extent of injury burden. In addition, research can provide information on the impact of current injury prevention programs. Once these parameters have been defined, risk factors for and protective factors of injury can be determined. This key step allows for the identification of specific targets for injury prevention programs and policies that seek to reduce risk and increase protection. The third step involves developing interventions and subsequent evaluation of their impact. Lastly, adoption includes knowledge sharing as well as funding and community outreach to replicate successful prevention strategies.[39,49–51]

Identifying risk factors and developing injury prevention strategies

Identifying risk factors for injury is the second step in the public health approach.

Major risk factors for disease or injury can be broadly divided into 3 categories: host, agent, and environment. The host is the person with risk of injury. The agent or vehicle refers to either the type of energy leading to injury or the vehicle through which injury is transmitted, such as a person or firearm. Physical environment includes injury setting. Social environment refers to cultural and legal practices that inform the societal setting in which the injury takes place.

First described in the 1970s by William Haddon, the "Haddon Matrix" describes a framework for identification of risk factors for injury using these causal factors and how they play a role in each phase of injury in order to identify preventative interventions.[46] Injury phases can be categorized as pre-event, event, and post-event and represent stages during which interventions could potentially be incorporated to reduce risk. These stages can also be interpreted as levels of prevention referred to as primary (pre-event), secondary (event), and tertiary (post-event). He described the formulation of a matrix, which describes the phases and factors each as dimensions. The phases are arranged in 3 rows and the factors in 4 columns. After identification of the injury to be addressed and identification of each row and column in the matrix, then intervention strategies can be discussed and identified. Stakeholders must then determine which intervention strategies will be the most beneficial and how to implement these strategies (**Table 1**).

Table 1
Haddon matrix for pedestrian struck

Phase	Host	Influencing Factors		
		Agent/Vehicle	Physical environment	Social environment
Preevent	Intoxicated driver Fatigued driver Pedestrian crossing street Intoxicated pedestrian Elderly pedestrian Pedestrian with osteoporosis Pedestrian wearing headphones Hearing-impaired pedestrian	Speeding automobile Worn tires Worn brakes Momentum of automobile	Poor street lighting Slick pavement Portholes Inadequate signage Nighttime	
Event	Part of pedestrian's body struck by vehicle	Impact of automobile with pedestrian Portion of vehicle impacting pedestrian	Hospitals nearby with specialty in trauma care Part of body impacting ground	Good samaritan laws
Postevent	Ability of victim to recover Postinjury care received Psychological coping of victim in aftermath of event	Severity of physical injuries Severity of postevent psychological impact	Rehabilitation facility	Health insurance Access to rehabilitation services Family and social support

Barnett, Daniel J, Ran D. Balicer, David W. Blodgett, Ayanna L. Fews, Cindy L. Parker and Jonathan M. Links. "The Application of the Haddon Matrix to Public Health Readiness and Response Planning." Environmental Health Perspectives 113 (2005): 561 - 566. Reproduced from Environmental Health Perspectives with permission from the authors.

System and community values can aid in the decision-making process for policy and program implementation. Suggested value criteria include characteristics like cost and feasibility, but also focus on community preferences and the overall effectiveness of the intervention. This addition of a value system is often referred to as the "third dimension" of the Haddon Matrix.[52–55]

Another model to aid in the determination of risk factors and intervention strategies includes the "Three E's" which refers to environment/engineering, education, and enforcement. Engineering refers to the modification of products or environment to increase safety. Enforcement refers to new policies including laws and regulations and education works to provide information to individuals and also includes skills development.[50] The interventions developed can be broadly referred to as active or passive. Passive interventions work to provide protection without any necessary action or work from the individual such as airbags to prevent injury from MVC while active approaches require an individual to put the intervention into action such as seatbelt use.[56]

Injury Prevention Effectiveness, Implementation, and Widespread Adoption

After careful injury intervention development, it must be implemented, evaluated, and disseminated. The "research practice gap" refers to the dissociation between the program development and successful implementation at the community level. This is often due to the knowledge gap between risk factors for injury and the effective implementation. Implementation or translational science is a method to aid in closing this gap by using scientific methods to describe the way in which science is transcribed into every day practice.[49,57–59] Strategies for successful adoption should focus on the specific process for that intervention's implementation as well as sustainability, cost effectiveness, and population impact.[59–61]

Barriers to injury prevention

Despite best efforts, barriers to the success of injury prevention strategies do exist and arise at multiple levels of development and delivery. At the individual level, differences in socioeconomic as well as cultural background, lack of resources, and misunderstanding or misinformation can hinder adherence. In addition, injury prevention strategies often require a behavioral change that can be difficult to follow if the injury is viewed as unlikely to happen. Lastly, larger systems level problems include economic, resource, and political barriers.[58,59,62,63]

CLINICS CARE POINTS

- Traumatic injury is a leading cause of mortality in the United States and the burden of trauma care continues to rise.
- Cause of injury can be described based on intent and mechanism.
- Trauma remains a public health problem and systematic intervention is needed.
- The Haddon Matrix is one conceptual framework that can provide a simplified visual of a traumatic event and allow for identification of targeted prevention strategies.
- Barriers continue to exist to the success of injury prevention strategies.

DISCLOSURE

The authors have nothing to disclose.

REFERENCES

1. System) NCfIPaCWW-bISQaR. Centers for disese control and prevention: injury prevention & control data and statistics. Secondary Centers for Disese Control and Prevention: Injury Prevention & Control Data and Statistics; 2020. https://www.cdc.gov/injury/wisqars/index.html.

2. Rhee P, Joseph B, Pandit V, et al. Increasing trauma deaths in the United States. Ann Surg 2014;260(1):13–21 [published Online First: Epub Date]|.

3. DiMaggio CJ, Avraham JB, Lee DC, et al. The epidemiology of emergency department trauma discharges in the United States. Acad Emerg Med 2017;24(10):1244–56 [published Online First: Epub Date]|.

4. Peterson C, Rice KL, Williams DD, et al. WISQARS Cost of Injury for public health research and practice. Inj Prev 2023;29(2):150–7 [published Online First: Epub Date]|.

5. DiMaggio C, Ayoung-Chee P, Shinseki M, et al. Traumatic injury in the United States: In-patient epidemiology 2000-2011. Injury 2016;47(7):1393–403 [published Online First: Epub Date]|.

6. Tomas C, Kallies K, Cronn S, et al. Mechanisms of traumatic injury by demographic characteristics: an 8-year review of temporal trends from the national trauma data bank. Inj Prev 2023. https://doi.org/10.1136/ip-2022-044817 [published Online First: Epub Date]|.

7. Nagassima Rodrigues Dos Reis K, McDonnell JM, Ahern DP, et al. Changing demographic trends in spine trauma: the presentation and outcome of major spine trauma in the elderly. Surgeon 2022;20(6):e410–5 [published Online First: Epub Date]|.

8. Statistics FIFoAR. Older Americans 2020: Population. Secondary Older Americans 2020: Population 2020. https://agingstats.gov/data.html.

9. Kozar RA, Arbabi S, Stein DM, et al. Injury in the aged: geriatric trauma care at the crossroads. J Trauma Acute Care Surg 2015;78(6):1197–209 [published Online First: Epub Date]|.

10. Karam BS, Patnaik R, Murphy P, et al. Improving mortality in older adult trauma patients: Are we doing better? J Trauma Acute Care Surg 2022;92(2):413–21 [published Online First: Epub Date]|.

11. Myers SR, Branas CC, French B, et al. A national analysis of pediatric trauma care utilization and outcomes in the United States. Pediatr Emerg Care 2019;35(1):1–7 [published Online First: Epub Date]|.

12. Oliver J, Avraham J, Frangos S, et al. The epidemiology of inpatient pediatric trauma in United States hospitals 2000 to 2011. J Pediatr Surg 2018;53(4):758–64 [published Online First: Epub Date]|.

13. Peterson AB, Thomas KE. Incidence of nonfatal traumatic brain injury-related hospitalizations - United States, 2018. MMWR Morb Mortal Wkly Rep 2021;70(48):1664–8 [published Online First: Epub Date]|.

14. Molnar BE, Gortmaker SL, Bull FC, et al. Unsafe to play? Neighborhood disorder and lack of safety predict reduced physical activity among urban children and adolescents. Am J Health Promot 2004;18(5):378–86 [published Online First: Epub Date]|.

15. Widener MJ, Metcalf SS, Bar-Yam Y. Dynamic urban food environments a temporal analysis of access to healthy foods. Am J Prev Med 2011;41(4):439–41 [published Online First: Epub Date]|.

16. Kegler SR, Dahlberg LL, Mercy JA. Firearm homicides and suicides in major metropolitan areas - united states, 2012-2013 and 2015-2016. MMWR Morb Mortal Wkly Rep 2018;67(44):1233–7 [published Online First: Epub Date]|.

17. Garnett MF, Spencer MR, Hedegaard H. Urban-rural differences in unintentional injury death rates among children aged 0-17 years: United States, 2018-2019. NCHS Data Brief 2021;421:1–8.

18. Rowhani-Rahbar A, Quistberg DA, Morgan ER, et al. Income inequality and firearm homicide in the US: a county-level cohort study. Inj Prev 2019;25(Suppl 1):i25–30 [published Online First: Epub Date]|.

19. Jarman MP, Hashmi Z, Zerhouni Y, et al. Quantifying geographic barriers to trauma care: Urban-rural variation in prehospital mortality. J Trauma Acute Care Surg 2019;87(1):173–80 [published Online First: Epub Date]|.

20. Carter PM, Cook LJ, Macy ML, et al. Individual and neighborhood characteristics of children seeking emergency department care for firearm injuries within the PECARN Network. Acad Emerg Med 2017;24(7):803–13 [published Online First: Epub Date]|.

21. Kegler SR, Dahlberg LL, Vivolo-Kantor AM. A descriptive exploration of the geographic and sociodemographic concentration of firearm homicide in the United States, 2004-2018. Prev Med 2021;153:106767 [published Online First: Epub Date]|.

22. Carr BG, Bowman AJ, Wolff CS, et al. Disparities in access to trauma care in the United States: A population-based analysis. Injury 2017;48(2):332–8 [published Online First: Epub Date]|.

23. Beiriger J, Silver D, Lu L, et al. The geography of injuries in trauma systems: using home as a proxy for incident location. J Surg Res 2023;290:36–44 [published Online First: Epub Date]|.

24. Pender TM, David AP, Dodson BK, et al. Pediatric trauma mortality: an ecological analysis evaluating correlation between injury-related mortality and geographic access to trauma care in the United States in 2010. J Public Health 2021;43(1):139–47 [published Online First: Epub Date]|.

25. Tung EL, Hampton DA, Kolak M, et al. Race/ethnicity and geographic access to urban trauma care. JAMA Netw Open 2019;2(3):e190138 [published Online First: Epub Date]|.

26. CfDCa Prevention. Definitions for leading causes of nonfatal injury reports, . Secondary definitions for leading causes of nonfatal injury reports. https://www.cdc.gov/injury/wisqars/nonfatal_help/definitions_leading.html.

27. Hedegaard H, Johnson RL, Garnett MF, et al. The 2020 international classification of diseases, 10th revision, clinical modification injury diagnosis framework for categorizing injuries by body region and nature of injury. Natl Health Stat Report 2020;150:1–27.

28. Gun Violence Archive. Gun Violence Archive. https://www.gun- violencearchive.org/. Published 2020 Accessed June 27, 2020.

29. Kegler SR, Stone DM, Mercy JA, et al. Firearm homicides and suicides in major metropolitan areas - united states, 2015-2016 and 2018-2019. MMWR Morb Mortal Wkly Rep 2022;71(1):14–8 [published Online First: Epub Date]|.

30. Newsome K, Sen-Crowe B, Autrey C, et al. A closer look at the rising epidemic of mass shootings in the united states and its association with gun legislation, laws, and sales. J Surg Res 2022;280:103–13 [published Online First: Epub Date]|.

31. Ehlman DC, Yard E, Stone DM, et al. Changes in suicide rates - United States, 2019 and 2020. MMWR Morb Mortal Wkly Rep 2022;71(8):306–12 [published Online First: Epub Date]|.

32. Stone DM, Mack KA, Qualters J. Notes from the field: recent changes in suicide rates, by race and ethnicity and age group - United States, 2021. MMWR Morb Mortal Wkly Rep 2023;72(6):160–2 [published Online First: Epub Date]|.

33. Leemis RW, Friar N, Khatiwada S, et al. The national intimate partner and sexual violence Survey: 2016/2017 report on intimate partner violence. Atlanta, GA: National Center for Injury Prevention and Control, Centers for Disease Control and Prevention; 2022.

34. Rosay ABP, Mulford CFP. Prevalence estimates and correlates of elder abuse in the United States: the national intimate partner and sexual violence survey. J Elder Abuse Negl 2017;29(1):1–14 [published Online First: Epub Date]|.

35. Sise RG, Calvo RY, Spain DA, et al. The epidemiology of trauma-related mortality in the United States from 2002 to 2010. J Trauma Acute Care Surg 2014;76(4): 913–9, discussion 20.

36. Burns E, Kakara R. Deaths from falls among persons aged ≥65 years - United States, 2007-2016. MMWR Morb Mortal Wkly Rep 2018;67(18):509–14 [published Online First: Epub Date]|.

37. Khurrum M, Chehab M, Ditillo M, et al. Trends in geriatric ground-level falls: report from the national trauma data bank. J Surg Res 2021;266:261–8 [published Online First: Epub Date]|.

38. Davis D, Cairns C. Emergency department visit rates for motor vehicle crashes by selected characteristics: united states, 2019-2020. NCHS Data Brief 2023; 466:1–8.

39. Sleet DA, Baldwin G, Marr A, et al. History of injury and violence as public health problems and emergence of the national center for injury prevention and control at CDC. J Safety Res 2012;43(4):233–47 [published Online First: Epub Date]|.

40. Langley JD. The need to discontinue the use of the term "accident" when referring to unintentional injury events. Accid Anal Prev 1988;20(1):1–8 [published Online First: Epub Date]|.

41. Gibson JJ. The contribution of experimental psychology to the formulation of the problem of safety–a brief for basic research. Behavioral approaches to accident research 1961;1(61):77–89.

42. Godfrey ES. Rôle of the health department in the prevention of accidents. Am J Public Health Nation's Health 1937;27(2):152–5 [published Online First: Epub Date]|.

43. Waller JA. Reflections on a half century of injury control. Am J Publ Health 1994; 84(4):664–70.

44. Mullner R, Goldberg J. Toward an outcome-oriented medical geography: an evaluation of the Illinois trauma/emergency medical services system. Soc Sci Med Part D Med Geogr 1978;12(2):103–10.

45. Shah MN. The formation of the emergency medical services system. Am J Publ Health 2006;96(3):414–23.

46. Haddon W Jr. A logical framework for categorizing highway safety phenomena and activity. J Trauma Acute Care Surg 1972;12(3):193–207.

47. Sleet D, Bonzo S, Branche C. An overview of the national center for injury prevention and control at the centers for disease control and prevention. Inj Prev 1998; 4(4):308–12 [published Online First: Epub Date]|.

48. Centers for Disease Control and Prevention NCfIPaC. Injury center timeline 1992-2022. secondary injury center timeline 1992-2022 2022. https://www.cdc.gov/injury/about/timeline.html.

49. Greenspan AI, Noonan RK. Twenty years of scientific progress in injury and violence research and the next public health frontier. J Safety Res 2012;43(4):249–55 [published Online First: Epub Date]|.

50. Jullien S. Prevention of unintentional injuries in children under five years. BMC Pediatr 2021;21(Suppl 1):311 [published Online First: Epub Date]|.

51. Prevention CfDCa. Injury Prevention & Control Secondary Injury Prevention & Control 2023. https://www.cdc.gov/injury/.

52. Runyan CW. Using the Haddon matrix: introducing the third dimension. Inj Prev 2015;21(2):126–30 [published Online First: Epub Date]|.

53. Susser M. Causal thinking in the health sciences: concepts and strategies of epidemiology. Causal thinking in the health sciences: concepts and strategies of epidemiology 1973;xii:181, xii.

54. Kleinbaum DG, Kupper LL, Morgenstern H. Epidemiologic research: principles and quantitative methods. Hoboken (NJ): John Wiley & Sons; 1991.

55. Haddon W Jr. Advances in the epidemiology of injuries as a basis for public policy. Publ Health Rep 1980;95(5):411–21.

56. Teitge BD, Francescutti LH. Time for lifestyle medicine to take injury prevention seriously. Am J Lifestyle Med 2016;10(1):4–9 [published Online First: Epub Date]|.

57. Newcomb AB, Zadnik M, Carlini AR, et al. Barriers and facilitators to the implementation of injury prevention programs: a qualitative exploration and model development. J Trauma Nurs 2020;27(6):335–45 [published Online First: Epub Date]|.

58. Ferlie EB, Shortell SM. Improving the quality of health care in the United Kingdom and the United States: a framework for change. Milbank Q 2001;79(2):281–315 [published Online First: Epub Date]|.

59. Mercy JA, Rosenberg ML, Powell KE, et al. Public health policy for preventing violence. Health Aff 1993;12(4):7–29 [published Online First: Epub Date]|.

60. Hanson DW, Finch CF, Allegrante JP, et al. Closing the gap between injury prevention research and community safety promotion practice: revisiting the public health model. Publ Health Rep 2012;127(2):147–55 [published Online First: Epub Date]|.

61. Wilkins N, McClure RJ, Mack K. Injury prevention: achieving population-level change. Inj Prev 2018;24(Suppl 1):i1–2 [published Online First: Epub Date]|.

62. Johnston CA, Vaughan E, Moreno JP. The difficulty of prevention: a behavioral perspective. Am J Lifestyle Med 2016;10(1):14–6 [published Online First: Epub Date]|.

63. Smithson J, Garside R, Pearson M. Barriers to, and facilitators of, the prevention of unintentional injury in children in the home: a systematic review and synthesis of qualitative research. Inj Prev 2011;17(2):119–26 [published Online First: Epub Date]|.

Societal Burden of Trauma and Disparities in Trauma Care

Sabrina D. Goddard, MD[a], Molly P. Jarman, PhD[b],
Zain G. Hashmi, MD[a],*

KEYWORDS

- Disparities • Trauma • Access • Social determinants of health

KEY POINTS

- Injury remains a leading cause of mortality worldwide, accounting for 4.4 million deaths each year and 8% of all deaths globally and places a tremendous burden on global economies.
- Evidence suggests that 20,000 to 30,000 injury-related deaths are potentially preventable each year in the United States, due to several gaps in the civilian trauma system contributing to this disparity.
- Disparities after injury exist across the continuum of trauma care from bystander and pre-hospital care through to long-term rehabilitation, encompassing factors such as race, gender, geographic location, socioeconomic status, and insurance coverage.
- Current mitigation strategies focus on improving access to trauma center care and improving the quality of trauma care.

SOCIETAL BURDEN OF TRAUMA

Injury remains a leading cause of mortality worldwide accounting for 4.4 million deaths each year and 8% of all deaths globally.[1] This burden is nearly 1.7 times the number of deaths due to human immunodeficiency virus (HIV)/acquired immunodeficiency syndrome (AIDS), tuberculosis, and malaria combined.[2] Injury disproportionately affects young people, with road traffic accidents being the leading cause of death among persons aged 15 to 29 years world-wide. Poverty is a known risk factor for injury mortality; 90% of injury-related deaths occur in low-income and middle-income countries—here injuries account for 12% of all deaths versus 6% in high-income countries.[3] Yet this

[a] Division of Trauma and Acute Care Surgery, Department of Surgery, University of Alabama at Birmingham, 1808 7th Avenue South, BDB 622, Birmingham, AL 35294, USA; [b] The Department of Surgery, Center for Surgery and Public Health, Harvard Medical School, Harvard T.H. Chan School of Public Health, Brigham and Women's Hospital, One Brigham Circle,1620 Tremont Street, Suite 2-016, Boston, MA 02120, USA
* Corresponding author.
E-mail address: mhashmi@uabmc.edu

Surg Clin N Am 104 (2024) 255–266
https://doi.org/10.1016/j.suc.2023.09.009
0039-6109/24/© 2023 Elsevier Inc. All rights reserved.

surgical.theclinics.com

injury-related death burden only constitutes the tip of the iceberg. For every injury-related death, thousands more suffer non-fatal, long-term consequences of physical and mental-health disorders leading to an estimated 8% of all years lived with disability. From a societal perspective, injury places an enormous burden on our nation's economy with billions of US dollars spent in direct health care–related costs and indirect costs due to lost productivity.

The United States represents a microcosm of the global injury burden. With more than 300,000 deaths each year, injury is the fourth leading cause of death among all ages and the leading cause of death among persons aged 1 to 44 years.[4] The majority of these deaths are due to unintentional injuries (72%), followed by intentional injuries including those by suicide (16.5%) and homicide (8.8%). Firearm injuries resulted in nearly 36,000 deaths in 2020, constituting more than half of all violent deaths nationwide.[5] In 2020, unintentional injury contributed to more years of potential life lost than cancer and heart disease combined. Similar to global estimates, nonfatal injuries far outnumber injury-related deaths in the United States. In 2020, nonfatal injuries resulted in nearly 23 million emergency department (ED) visits and 3.53 million hospital admissions resulting in combined medical, work loss, and quality of life loss costs of an estimated $1.92 trillion. This puts the total estimated cost burden of injury in the United States for 2020 at a staggering $4.61 trillion, nearly 22% of the US gross domestic product that year.[6] The significant societal burden of preventable traumatic deaths calls for a comprehensive approach to enhance injury prevention, treatment, and long-term rehabilitation.

One crucial aspect of this approach is recognizing and addressing health care disparities that impede the delivery of quality care. While significant strides have been made, data from 2 independently performed studies by Kwon and colleagues and Hashmi and colleagues suggest that between 20,000 to 30,000 injury-related deaths are potentially preventable each year in the United States.[7] The recent seminal report by the National Academies of Sciences, Engineering, and Medicine (NASEM) describes several knowledge and implementation gaps in the civilian trauma system as potentially contributing to this disparity.[8] These gaps include variability in emergency medical service systems, trauma system access, adoption of best trauma care practices, and implicit bias resulting in differential quality of care delivery across select conditions and patient populations. Only by acknowledging and mitigating these disparities can the goal of "Zero Preventable Death After Injury" set forth by NASEM be met.

In the next section, the authors review seminal works that highlight the presence of disparities across each link of the trauma chain of survival and describe some of the ongoing efforts at injury disparity mitigation.

DISPARITIES IN THE PREHOSPITAL PHASE OF INJURY CARE

Access to timely and appropriate trauma care is essential for improving patient outcomes and reducing morbidity and mortality associated with traumatic injuries. Studies have shown that states with poor trauma center access have more prehospital deaths, which contributes to a higher overall injury mortality rate.[9]

Emergency Medical Services (EMS) play a vital role in trauma care access, especially during prehospital transportation. Byrne and colleagues[10] examined the association between Emergency Medical Service (EMS) response time and motor vehicle crash mortality in the United States and found a 1.4% increase in odds of mortality among crash victims for each minute increase in EMS response time. This underscores the vital role of rapid EMS response in enhancing survival chances for individuals involved in motor vehicle crashes by ensuring quick access to definitive care. Studies highlight disparities in EMS use and response times based on race, socioeconomic status (SES), and rural-urban locations. Racial minorities, uninsured patients, and those in rural areas may have limited access to EMS services, potentially leading to delays in trauma care and poorer outcomes.

Despite the known benefits of timely trauma care, disparities in access exist and disproportionately affect certain patient populations. Concentration of trauma centers and specialized health care facilities in urban areas creates limited access for individuals residing in rural or remote regions. A significant proportion of the US population (representing 38.4 million people) does not have access to trauma care within 1 hour by ground or air ambulance.[11] Additionally, closures of trauma centers have been seen in communities with disproportionately high numbers of Black residents, uninsured people, and people living in poverty, further worsening disparities in access.[12]

These discrepancies in access to trauma care have far-reaching consequences, as delayed medical interventions contribute to higher morbidity and mortality. Addressing these disparities is imperative to ensure equitable access to life-saving trauma care for all patients, regardless of their geographic location or SES.

Prehospital Disparities by Age

Barriers to trauma center care impact both the geriatric and pediatric populations. Current trauma triage guidelines recommend most older trauma patients should be transported to a trauma center, out of an abundance of caution with respect to occult shock and higher risk of hemorrhage due to anticoagulant use.[13] Studies have shown a survival benefit for older adults treated at trauma centers.[14] Despite these recommendations, only half of older trauma patients reach designated trauma centers.[15] The cause of this disparity remains unknown.

Like older trauma patients, triage guidelines recommend trauma center care for pediatric patients, with the additional recommendation for treatment at a specialized pediatric trauma center when possible.[13] As of 2020, 26% of children in the United States lacked access to a pediatric trauma center within 1 hour by ground or air transport. Access to care was even worse for Native American and Native Hawaiian children.[16] These geographic barriers to care contribute to national under-triage rate >20% for pediatric trauma patients.[17]

Prehospital Disparities by Gender

Research has shed light on gender disparities in trauma care access.[18–21] These disparities may result from differences in symptom recognition and triage decisions leading to differential care delivery between genders. In these studies, female trauma patients were found to receive less aggressive care compared to male trauma patients. In a study by Wahlin and colleagues, male patients were more likely to be given higher priority and transported directly to a trauma center.[18] Similarly, Gomez and colleagues showed a smaller proportion of female patients received care at trauma centers (OR 0.87), were transported directly to trauma centers (OR 0.88), and underwent transfer to trauma centers (OR 0.85) compared to male patients. Gender disparities have also been observed in treatments, with studies suggesting that women are less likely to receive adequate pain relief compared to men in similar traumatic injury scenarios.[22,23] Consequently, consensus-based recommendations have urged further research into gender-specific injury patterns, sex-specific responses to treatment, hormonal influences, psychological and social aspects, as well as gender bias in trauma care.[19]

Prehospital Disparities by Race and Ethnicity

In recent years, significant investments have been made to train laypersons in rapidly identifying and controlling life-threatening hemorrhage through the American College of Surgeons' Stop the Bleed Program.[24] Despite this, racial disparities in bystander support after injury have been reported. Cornwell and colleagues performed a retrospective analysis of data reported by 33 states to National Emergency Services Information System . The authors reported that black patients were 57% less likely to receive bystander support compared to white patients.[25]

Racial and ethnic minority groups face obstacles in accessing trauma care due to various factors, including geographic location,[11] language barriers, cultural differences, and implicit bias within the health care system. Black and Hispanic patients may experience longer prehospital time intervals, less access to trauma centers, and higher rates of under-triage.[26–28] These disparities may be driven by both structural and interpersonal biases in the health care system.

Studies examining disparities in pain control for trauma patients have consistently highlighted the existence of differences in health care settings, including prehospital care. This is particularly true for across multiple races.[29] For instance, Lord and colleagues[30] found discrepancies in analgesia administration based on patient race in the prehospital setting. In simulated patients, the student paramedics were less likely to administer analgesia to Black patients compared to White patients with the same level of pain and clinical presentation. Similarly, Young and colleagues[31] revealed racial disparities in morphine administration for Black patients with blunt trauma. This has been confirmed in other studies.[23,32] Patients with limited English proficiency or belonging to different cultural backgrounds may face challenges in communicating their pain needs effectively, which can impact pain management. Schwartz and colleagues[33] found that patients with limited English proficiency (LEP) experienced disparities in pain control compared to English-speaking patients. LEP patients were less likely to receive appropriate pain medication and had longer wait times for pain management. The study highlights the importance of addressing language barriers to ensure equitable pain control for trauma patients from diverse linguistic backgrounds.

Prehospital Disparities by Rurality

Geographic location plays a crucial role in trauma care access, especially for patients residing in rural or remote areas. Studies[34–38] have highlighted the impact of geography on trauma center access and prehospital care. Patients in rural or remote regions may experience longer transport times to reach trauma centers, leading to delays in care. Jarman and colleagues showed that rural residents are significantly more likely than nonrural residents to die after traumatic injury.[39,40] The authors suggest that identification of geographic areas with the highest risk of injury mortality can aid in prevention and treatment efforts, including targeted efforts to reduce injury incidence, as well as identify regions in need of additional prehospital or trauma center resources.[41]

Prehospital Disparities by Socioeconomic and Insurance Status

SESsignificantly influences access to trauma care. Income has been identified as a predictor of trauma mortality, with the lowest quartile showing a more than 6-fold increase in mortality rates.[26] Patients from lower socioeconomic backgrounds may encounter financial barriers, lack of health insurance, or limited resources to afford transportation to distant trauma centers.[42] Social Vulnerability Indices can serve as predictors of trauma fatality rates.[43] Insurance status is a critical determinant of trauma care access.[44] Given that areas of lower income, higher uninsurance rates, and higher rates of Medicaid and Medicare-eligible individuals have less access to trauma care, implies that payer mix plays a role in the development and designation of trauma centers.[45] Individuals from lower socioeconomic backgrounds may encounter barriers in accessing trauma care due to financial constraints, lack of health insurance, or limited resources to afford transportation to distant health care facilities. Uninsured trauma patients experience higher mortality rates compared to insured patients, irrespective of age, injury type, or region.

In addition to race, disparities in pain control extend to SES and insurance coverage. Haider and colleagues investigated the association between insurance status and prehospital pain management for trauma patients.[26] The findings revealed that uninsured patients were less likely to receive adequate pain management compared to insured patients, highlighting the disparity in pain control based on insurance coverage.

Disparities in accessing trauma care based on age, gender, geographic location, SES/insurance status, and race are multifaceted and interconnected. These disparities have significant implications for patient outcomes and overall health care equity. Addressing these disparities requires targeted interventions, including improving access to trauma centers in underserved areas, enhancing EM services, providing financial support for uninsured patients, and promoting cultural competency within the health care system.

DISPARITIES IN THE INHOSPITAL PHASE OF INJURY CARE

Previous research has demonstrated that nonclinical factors are associated with differences in clinical care. Disparities in the quality of trauma care received have been reported based on factors such as race, ethnicity, and SES. These disparities manifest in several ways, including limited health care services, insufficient pain management, reduced post-discharge care, and higher mortality rates.

Inhospital Disparities by Race

Studies have shown variations in the type and timing of treatments and interventions received by different patient groups. Some research indicates that minority patients may be less likely to receive certain surgical procedures or timely interventions, potentially impacting outcomes. In a study by De Angelis and colleagues,[46] Black patients had a longer time to trauma consultation. Noteworthy differences exist in the management of splenic trauma patients based on race/ethnicity and SES.[47] Non-White race is associated with a decreased likelihood of rib fixation and/or epidural placement, while underinsurance is associated with higher mortality in patients with thoracic trauma.[48]

A systematic bias operates in the treatment of pain that is qualitatively different for certain groups and outcomes.[49] Multiple studies have shown that Black and Hispanic patients are less likely to receive adequate pain management. These disparities exist despite similar pain scores and severity of injuries between racial and ethnic groups. Studies by Todd and colleagues found that Black and Hispanic patients with isolated long-bone fractures were 66% more likely to receive no analgesics compared to White patients with similar fractures.[50,51] Another systematic review and meta-analysis by Lee and colleagues revealed that racial and ethnic minorities, especially Black and Hispanic patients, continue to be less likely to receive pain medications for acute pain management in the ED.[52] Additionally, Beaudoin and colleagues evaluated pain, pain-related characteristics, and analgesic treatment in Black and non-Hispanic White trauma patients after motor vehicle collisions. They found that Black patients were less likely to receive opioid analgesics and more likely to receive nonsteroidal anti-inflammatory drugs in the ED and at discharge, even though they reported similar levels of acute pain.[53]

A substantial body of literature describes disparities in in-hospital outcomes by race after injury.[28,44,54–57] A meta-analysis evaluating the impact of race on outcomes after injury demonstrated that Black patients were nearly 20% more likely to die compared to similarly injured white patients.[26] Explanatory studies have suggested several causes for this including structural reasons, such as hospital quality effects, and those rooted in behavioral patterns and/or implicit bias.[58–61]

Inhospital Disparities by Gender

Based on the findings from articles by Ingram[20] and de Angelis,[46] there is evidence of significant gender-based disparities in the delivery of trauma care within the hospital setting. Ingram and colleagues revealed that female trauma patients experienced an extended ED length of stay (LOS) compared to male patients, as well as delays in receiving timely interventions after sustaining traumatic injuries. Similarly, de Angelis and colleagues identified that females also faced longer time to trauma consultation compared to males, indicating potential delays in accessing specialized trauma care services. These findings suggest that females may encounter barriers in accessing prompt and efficient trauma care from the moment of arrival at the hospital, which could impact the overall quality of care and patient outcomes.

Inhospital Disparities by Socioeconomic and Insurance Status

Studies have indicated that uninsured patients were less likely to receive analgesia for acute pain compared to insured patients. Uninsured and Medicaid patients have more than twice the odds of leaving against medical advice (AMA). Leaving AMA results in higher readmission rates, in-hospital mortality, and costs up to 56% more than comparable patients.[62]

DISPARITIES IN THE POST-ACUTE PHASE OF INJURY CARE

Disparities also exist in the post-acute phase of injury care, with some patients facing challenges in accessing rehabilitation services and follow-up care. This is true based on socioeconomic/insurance status,[53–55] race,[57] and gender.[20] This can impact recovery and long-term outcomes after the initial trauma event.

Studies suggest that insurance status plays a significant role in determining the hospital LOS for trauma patients.[59,63] Englum and colleagues, in a study of the National Trauma Data Bank, showed an association between insurance status and hospital LOS among trauma patients, with publicly insured patients having longer LOS and uninsured patients having shorter LOS compared to privately insured patients. The authors showed that publicly insured patients tended to be older, racial minorities, with intentional and penetrating injuries, and were more likely to be discharged to a nursing facility while uninsured patients tended to be younger, racial minorities, with intentional and penetrating injuries, and were more likely to be discharged home. The study showed publicly insured patients have a significantly longer LOS by an overall risk-adjusted average of 0.9 days compared to privately insured patients. In contrast, uninsured patients had risk-adjusted mean LOS that were shorter than privately insured patients. Lee and colleagues investigated the impact of a health care reform mandate on hospital and ICU LOS, mortality, and discharge disposition among trauma patients. The authors found a significant decrease in hospital LOS of 2 days, from a median of 9.0 days to a median of 7.0 days.

Lumbard and colleagues highlight the impact of race and insurance on mortality and discharge disposition among firearm trauma patients.[64] The study finds that race and insurance status are influential factors in determining both mortality rates and the final destination for patients after their hospital stay. Chun and colleagues focus on racial disparities in post-discharge health care utilization after trauma. The study reveals that there are racial disparities in accessing health care services after leaving the hospital, suggesting potential inequalities in follow-up care based on race.[65] In a study by Englum and colleagues, the authors emphasize the importance of considering racial, ethnic, and insurance status factors in understanding variations in post-trauma care utilization.[66] The findings underscore the need for targeted interventions to address disparities and promote equitable access to health care services for trauma patients.

STRATEGIES TO MITIGATE DISPARITIES IN INJURY CARE

President Biden has identified the resolution of health disparities as a key focus, as evident in the Executive Order titled "Advancing Racial Equity and Support for Underserved Communities Through the Federal Government." The American Medical Association also prioritizes addressing health disparities in its mission, aiming to achieve health equity by addressing factors contributing to disparities within the patient population. It is essential for health care providers and policy makers to recognize that disparities exist in health care in order to implement interventions and policies to promote access to high-quality trauma care for all individuals. Trauma care has often been thought immune to these disparities given the perceived universal access; however, as outlined in this review, disparities in trauma care are widespread and persistent. Fortunately, there are multiple opportunities to mitigate disparities.

Improving Access to Care

There is an increasing body of evidence indicating barriers to timely trauma care are a substantial driver of racial, ethnic, geographic, and socioeconomic disparities. For example, greater distances and drive times to reach trauma centers contribute to a 22% increase in risk of death for Black trauma patients, and a 14% increase in risk of death for rural trauma patients.[39,67] While Black patients experience higher case fatality rates following traumatic injury in national studies, shorter drive times appear to reduce disparities for Black patients in Maryland,[67] but national efforts to reduce time to trauma care appear to benefit White patients more than Black patients.[27,68] The primary approach to improving access to trauma care is the establishment of new trauma centers in geographic regions without existing trauma care or where existing trauma centers do not have capacity to care for the volume of patients in their catchment area. Thoughtful, data-driven selection of new trauma center sites can increase the number of severely injured patients transported to advanced trauma centers, reduce total prehospital travel time, and balance patient loads across hospitals within a region.[69]

Adding new trauma centers is costly and time consuming. Recent analyses of the Georgia trauma system estimated readiness costs for level I, II, and III trauma centers to be $10 million, $4.9 million, and $1.7 million, respectively. Consequently, there have been no substantial improvements in access to trauma centers among geographically underserved regions in over 10 years.[45] In light of these findings, evaluation and implementation of alternative strategies, such as telehealth, to enhance the capacity of regional trauma systems should also be considered.[70,71]

Improving Quality of Care

In addition to barriers to timely trauma center care, there is evidence that hospital-level variation in quality of care contributes to injury disparities. Black and Hispanic trauma patients are more likely to be treated at trauma centers with higher-than-average patient mortality rates.[58] The exact causes of this phenomenon are unknown. One possible explanation is variation in resources available at trauma centers. For example, overcrowding at trauma centers where Black hip fracture patients tend to receive treatment appears to contribute to delays in surgical intervention and subsequently increases risk of complications.[72] Recommendations for improving quality of trauma care at the hospital level are extensive and well documented through the American College of Surgeons Trauma Quality Improvement Program and evidence-based clinical practice guidelines published by the Eastern Association for the Surgery of Trauma and the Western Trauma Association. Stakeholders seeking to mitigate disparities due to variation in quality of care can leverage these programs to standardize approaches to all patients.

Future Research

Disparities in access to trauma care and subsequent outcomes are well documented. Mitigation of trauma disparities is a critical component of any effort to achieve the NASEM goal of "Zero Preventable Death After Injury." Future research efforts should seek to identify modifiable causes of disparities, including structural factors that limit access to care, hospital-level interventions that facilitate equitable quality of care, and individual interventions to support long-term recovery for vulnerable patients.

CLINICS CARE POINTS

- Injury remains a leading cause of mortality worldwide, accounting for 4.4 million deaths each year and 8% of all deaths globally and placing a tremendous burden on global economies.
- Evidence suggests that 20,000 to 30,000 injury-related deaths are potentially preventable each year in the United States, due to several gaps in the civilian trauma system contributing to this disparity.
- Disparities after injury exist across the continuum of trauma care from bystander and prehospital care through long-term rehabilitation, encompassing factors such as race, gender, geographic location, SES, and insurance coverage.
- Current mitigation strategies focus on improving access to trauma center care and improving the quality of trauma care.

DISCLOSURE

The authors have nothing to disclose relevant to this work.

REFERENCES

1. World Health Organization. *Injuries and Violence: The Facts*; 2014. Available at: https://iris.who.int/handle/10665/149798. Accessed June 6, 2023.
2. Organization, W.H. Preventing Injuries and Violence: An Overview. 2020 cited 2023 August 1; Available from: apps.who.int/iris/bitstream/handle/10665/332070/9789240005105-eng.pdf.
3. Norton R, Kobusingye O. Injuries. N Engl J Med 2013;368(18):1723–30.

4. Centers for Disease Control and Prevention. National Center for Health Statistics Fast Stats Death and Mortality. Available at: https://www.cdc.gov/nchs/fastats/deaths.htm. Accessed June 6, 2023.
5. Centers for Disease Control and Prevention National Center for Injury Prevention and Control. Web-based Injury Statistics Query and Reporting System (WISQARS). Available at: http://www.cdc.gov/injury/wisqars. Accessed June 6, 2023.
6. WISQARS Cost Of Injury. Centers for Disease Control and Prevention. Available at: https://wisqars.cdc.gov/cost/. Accessed June 6, 2023.
7. Kwon AM, Garbett NC, Kloecker GH. Pooled preventable death rates in trauma patients : Meta analysis and systematic review since 1990. Eur J Trauma Emerg Surg 2014;40(3):279–85.
8. Berwick D, Downey A, Cornett E, editors. In A National Trauma Care System: Integrating military and civilian trauma systems to achieve zero preventable deaths after injury. 2016. Washington (DC).
9. Hashmi ZG, Jarman MP, Uribe-Leitz T, et al. Access Delayed Is Access Denied: Relationship Between Access to Trauma Center Care and Pre-Hospital Death. J Am Coll Surg 2019;228(1):9–20.
10. Byrne JP, Mann NC, Dai M, et al. Association Between Emergency Medical Service Response Time and Motor Vehicle Crash Mortality in the United States. JAMA Surg 2019;154(4):286–93.
11. Hsia R, Shen YC. Possible geographical barriers to trauma center access for vulnerable patients in the United States: an analysis of urban and rural communities. Arch Surg 2011;146(1):46–52.
12. Hsia RY, Shen YC. Rising closures of hospital trauma centers disproportionately burden vulnerable populations. Health Aff 2011;30(10):1912–20.
13. Newgard CD, Fischer PE, Gestring M, et al. National guideline for the field triage of injured patients: Recommendations of the National Expert Panel on Field Triage, 2021. J Trauma Acute Care Surg 2022;93(2):e49–60.
14. Garwe T, Stewart KE, Newgard CD, et al. Survival Benefit of Treatment at or Transfer to a Tertiary Trauma Center among Injured Older Adults. Prehosp Emerg Care 2020;24(2):245–56.
15. Uribe-Leitz T, Jarman MP, Sturgeon DJ, et al. National Study of Triage and Access to Trauma Centers for Older Adults. Ann Emerg Med 2020;75(2):125–35.
16. Burdick KJ, Lee LK, Mannix R, et al. Racial and Ethnic Disparities in Access to Pediatric Trauma Centers in the United States: A Geographic Information Systems Analysis. Ann Emerg Med 2023;81(3):325–33.
17. Peng J, Wheeler K, Groner JI, et al. Undertriage of Pediatric Major Trauma Patients in the United States. Clin Pediatr (Phila) 2017;56(9):845–53.
18. Rubenson Wahlin R, Ponzer S, Lövbrand H, et al. Do male and female trauma patients receive the same prehospital care?: an observational follow-up study. BMC Emerg Med 2016;16:6.
19. Sethuraman KN, Marcolini EG, McCunn M, et al. Gender-specific issues in traumatic injury and resuscitation: consensus-based recommendations for future research. Acad Emerg Med 2014;21(12):1386–94.
20. Ingram ME, Nagalla M, Shan Y, et al. Sex-Based Disparities in Timeliness of Trauma Care and Discharge Disposition. JAMA Surg 2022;157(7):609–16.
21. Gomez D, Haas B, de Mestral C, et al. Gender-associated differences in access to trauma center care: A population-based analysis. Surgery 2012;152(2):179–85.
22. Hoffmann DE, Tarzian AJ. The girl who cried pain: a bias against women in the treatment of pain. J Law Med Ethics 2001;29(1):13–27.

23. Supples MW, Vaizer J, Liao M, et al. Patient Demographics Are Associated with Differences in Prehospital Pain Management among Trauma Patients. Prehosp Emerg Care 2022;1–6.

24. Jacobs L, Keating JJ, Hunt RC, et al. Stop the Bleed. Curr Probl Surg 2022; 59(10):101193.

25. York Cornwell E, Currit A. Racial and Social Disparities in Bystander Support During Medical Emergencies on US Streets. Am J Public Health 2016;106(6): 1049–51.

26. Haider AH, Weygandt PL, Bentley JM, et al. Disparities in trauma care and outcomes in the United States: a systematic review and meta-analysis. J Trauma Acute Care Surg 2013;74(5):1195–205.

27. Alber DA, Dalton MK, Uribe-Leitz T, et al. A Multistate Study of Race and Ethnic Disparities in Access to Trauma Care. J Surg Res 2021;257:486–92.

28. Haider AH, Chang DC, Efron DT, et al. Race and insurance status as risk factors for trauma mortality. Arch Surg 2008;143(10):945–9.

29. Kennel J, Withers E, Parsons N, et al. Racial/Ethnic Disparities in Pain Treatment: Evidence From Oregon Emergency Medical Services Agencies. Med Care 2019; 57(12):924–9.

30. Lord B, Khalsa S. Influence of patient race on administration of analgesia by student paramedics. BMC Emerg Med 2019;19(1):32.

31. Young MF, Hern HG, Alter HJ, et al. Racial differences in receiving morphine among prehospital patients with blunt trauma. J Emerg Med 2013;45(1):46–52.

32. Hewes HA, Dai M, Mann NC, et al. Prehospital Pain Management: Disparity By Age and Race. Prehosp Emerg Care 2018;22(2):189–97.

33. Castro MRH, Schwartz H, Hernandez S, et al. The Association of Limited English Proficiency With Morbidity and Mortality After Trauma. J Surg Res 2022;280: 326–32.

34. Morgan JM, Calleja P. Emergency trauma care in rural and remote settings: Challenges and patient outcomes. Int Emerg Nurs 2020;51:100880.

35. Beiriger J, Silver D, Lu L, et al. The Geography of Injuries in Trauma Systems: Using Home as a Proxy for Incident Location. J Surg Res 2023;290:36–44.

36. Gonzalez RP, Cummings G, Mulekar M, et al. Increased mortality in rural vehicular trauma: identifying contributing factors through data linkage. J Trauma 2006;61(2):404–9.

37. Sampalis JS, Denis R, Lavoie A, et al. Trauma care regionalization: a process-outcome evaluation. J Trauma 1999;46(4):565–79 ; discussion 579-81.

38. Newgard CD, Schmicker RH, Hedges JR, et al. Emergency medical services intervals and survival in trauma: assessment of the "golden hour" in a North American prospective cohort. Ann Emerg Med 2010;55(3):235–46.e4.

39. Jarman MP, Castillo RC, Carlini AR, et al. Rural risk: Geographic disparities in trauma mortality. Surgery 2016;160(6):1551–9.

40. Jarman MP, Hashmi Z, Zerhouni Y, et al. Quantifying geographic barriers to trauma care: Urban-rural variation in prehospital mortality. J Trauma Acute Care Surg 2019;87(1):173–80.

41. Jarman MP, Haut ER, Curriero FC, et al. Mapping areas with concentrated risk of trauma mortality: A first step toward mitigating geographic and socioeconomic disparities in trauma. J Trauma Acute Care Surg 2018;85(1):54–61.

42. Maybury RS, Bolorunduro OB, Villegas C, et al. Pedestrians struck by motor vehicles further worsen race- and insurance-based disparities in trauma outcomes: the case for inner-city pedestrian injury prevention programs. Surgery 2010; 148(2):202–8.

43. Phelos HM, Deeb AP, Brown JB. Can social vulnerability indices predict county trauma fatality rates? J Trauma Acute Care Surg 2021;91(2):399–405.

44. Greene WR, Oyetunji TA, Bowers U, et al. Insurance status is a potent predictor of outcomes in both blunt and penetrating trauma. Am J Surg 2010;199(4):554–7.

45. Carr BG, Bowman AJ, Wolff CS, et al. Disparities in access to trauma care in the United States: A population-based analysis. Injury 2017;48(2):332–8.

46. de Angelis P, Kaufman EJ, Barie PS, et al. Disparities in Timing of Trauma Consultation: A Trauma Registry Analysis of Patient and Injury Factors. J Surg Res 2019; 242:357–62.

47. Haines KL, Woldanski LM, Zens T, et al. The Impact of Race and Socioeconomic Status on Treatment and Outcomes of Blunt Splenic Injury. J Surg Res 2019; 240:60–9.

48. Rebollo Salazar D, Velez-Rosborough A, DiMaggio C, et al. Race and Insurance Status are Associated With Different Management Strategies After Thoracic Trauma. J Surg Res 2021;261:18–25.

49. Meghani SH, Byun E, Gallagher RM. Time to take stock: a meta-analysis and systematic review of analgesic treatment disparities for pain in the United States. Pain Med 2012;13(2):150–74.

50. Todd KH, Deaton C, D'Adamo AP, et al. Ethnicity and analgesic practice. Ann Emerg Med 2000;35(1):11–6.

51. Todd KH, Samaroo N, Hoffman JR. Ethnicity as a risk factor for inadequate emergency department analgesia. JAMA 1993;269(12):1537–9.

52. Lee P, Le Saux M, Siegel R, et al. Racial and ethnic disparities in the management of acute pain in US emergency departments: Meta-analysis and systematic review. Am J Emerg Med 2019;37(9):1770–7.

53. Beaudoin FL, Gutman R, Zhai W, et al. Racial differences in presentations and predictors of acute pain after motor vehicle collision. Pain 2018;159(6):1056–63.

54. Arthur M, Hedges JR, Newgard CD, et al. Racial disparities in mortality among adults hospitalized after injury. Med Care 2008;46(2):192–9.

55. Falcone RA Jr, Brown RL, Garcia VF. Disparities in child abuse mortality are not explained by injury severity. J Pediatr Surg 2007;42(6):1031–6, discussion 1036-7.

56. Hicks CW, Hashmi ZG, Velopulos C, et al. Association between race and age in survival after trauma. JAMA Surg 2014;149(7):642–7.

57. Martin CA, Care M, Rangel EL, et al. Severity of head computed tomography scan findings fail to explain racial differences in mortality following child abuse. Am J Surg 2010;199(2):210–5.

58. Haider AH, Hashmi ZG, Zafar SN, et al. Minority trauma patients tend to cluster at trauma centers with worse-than-expected mortality: can this phenomenon help explain racial disparities in trauma outcomes? Ann Surg 2013;258(4):572–9, discussion 579-81.

59. Englum BR, Hui X, Zogg CK, et al. Association Between Insurance Status and Hospital Length of Stay Following Trauma. Am Surg 2016;82(3):281–8.

60. Haider AH, Schneider EB, Sriram N, et al. Unconscious race and class bias: its association with decision making by trauma and acute care surgeons. J Trauma Acute Care Surg 2014;77(3):409–16.

61. Haider AH, Sexton J, Sriram N, et al. Association of unconscious race and social class bias with vignette-based clinical assessments by medical students. JAMA 2011;306(9):942–51.

62. Haines K, Freeman J, Vastaas C, et al. I'm Leaving": Factors That Impact Against Medical Advice Disposition Post-Trauma. J Emerg Med 2020;58(4):691–7.

63. Lee J, Sudarshan M, Kurth T, et al. Mandatory health care insurance is associated with shorter hospital length of stay among critically injured trauma patients. J Trauma Acute Care Surg 2014;77(2):298–303.

64. Lumbard DC, Freese RL, Marek AP, et al. Firearm trauma: Race and insurance influence mortality and discharge disposition. J Trauma Acute Care Surg 2022; 92(6):1005–11.

65. Chun Fat S, Herrera-Escobar JP, Seshadri AJ, et al. Racial disparities in post-discharge healthcare utilization after trauma. Am J Surg 2019;218(5):842–6.

66. Englum BR, Villegas C, Bolorunduro O, et al. Racial, ethnic, and insurance status disparities in use of posthospitalization care after trauma. J Am Coll Surg 2011; 213(6):699–708.

67. Jarman MP, Pollack Porter K, Curriero FC, et al. Factors mediating demographic determinants of injury mortality. Ann Epidemiol 2019;34:58–64.e2.

68. Jarman MP, Dalton MK, Askari R, et al. Accessibility of Level III trauma centers for underserved populations: A cross-sectional study. J Trauma Acute Care Surg 2022;93(5):664–71.

69. Dooley JH, Ozdenerol E, Sharpe JP, et al. Location, location, location: Utilizing Needs-Based Assessment of Trauma Systems-2 in trauma system planning. J Trauma Acute Care Surg 2020;88(1):94–100.

70. Ashley DW, Mullins RF, Dente CJ, et al. How much green does it take to be orange? Determining the cost associated with trauma center readiness. J Trauma Acute Care Surg 2019;86(5):765–73.

71. Atkins EV, Vaughn KA, Medeiros RS, et al. Assessing trauma readiness costs in level III and level IV trauma centers. J Trauma Acute Care Surg 2023;94(2): 258–63.

72. Jarman MP, Sokas C, Dalton MK, et al. The impact of delayed management of fall-related hip fracture management on health outcomes for African American older adults. J Trauma Acute Care Surg 2021;90(6):942–50.

Prehospital Trauma Care

Christopher M. Wend, MD[a], Ryan B. Fransman, MD[b],
Elliott R. Haut, MD, PhD[a,c,d,e],*

KEYWORDS

- Prehospital • Ambulance • Emergency medical services • Trauma • Resuscitation
- Paramedic • Helicopter

KEY POINTS

- Prehospital trauma evaluations should begin with a primary survey, followed by vital signs and a secondary assessment.
- During trauma resuscitation, clinicians should minimize the use of crystalloids and, ideally, administer blood products targeting a permissive hypotension goal.
- Transport to the appropriate level trauma center should occur by whichever method will deliver patients to definitive care in the shortest amount of time safely.
- Bystanders are a critical component of the trauma system and can deliver care (ie, Stop the Bleed) before the arrival of prehospital clinicians.

EMERGENCY MEDICAL SERVICES SYSTEMS

Emergency medical services (EMS) in the United States are primarily provided by nonphysician clinicians with varying levels of certification, scope of practice, and education.[1] The National Registry of Emergency Medical Technicians currently identifies 4 main levels of certification in increasing education and scope of practice: emergency medical responder, emergency medical technician, advanced emergency medical technician, and paramedic.[2] Scope of practice and treatment protocols are also determined at different levels of oversight whether at the state, regional, or local/agency level. Jurisdictions vary widely in their amount of staffing, dispatch protocols, and resources. Some states formally or informally involve registered nurses, physician

a Department of Emergency Medicine, Johns Hopkins University School of Medicine, 1830 East Monument Street Suite 6-100, Baltimore, MD 21287, USA; b Department of Trauma, Acute Care Surgery, and Surgical Critical Care, Emory University School of Medicine, Grady Memorial Hospital, 80 Jesse Hill Jr. Drive, SE, Atlanta, GA 30303, USA; c Department of Surgery, Division of Acute Care Surgery, Johns Hopkins University School of Medicine, Sheikh Zayed 6107C, 1800 Orleans Street, Baltimore, MD 21287, USA; d Department of Anesthesiology and Critical Care Medicine, Johns Hopkins University School of Medicine, Baltimore, MD, USA; e Department of Health Policy and Management, The Johns Hopkins Bloomberg School of Public Health, Baltimore, MD, USA
* Corresponding author.
E-mail address: ehaut1@jhmi.edu

Surg Clin N Am 104 (2024) 267–277
https://doi.org/10.1016/j.suc.2023.10.005
0039-6109/24/© 2023 Elsevier Inc. All rights reserved.

assistants, and nurse practitioners in the practice of EMS care. On-scene physician involvement in EMS within the US has grown in recent years since the designation of EMS as a subspeciality of emergency medicine in 2010 with formal fellowship training opportunities and board certification.[3,4] While the US or "Anglo-American" model of EMS involves primarily nonphysician clinicians, internationally, the "Franco-German" model utilizes more field physicians, with varying backgrounds and specialization, most often from emergency medicine or anesthesiology.[5] Globally, nonphysicians are often limited in their scope of practice for prehospital trauma care.

PREHOSPITAL EVALUATION
Initial Evaluation and Vital Signs

The initial evaluation of the trauma patient should begin with a primary survey which is an overall assessment of (1) the airway patency and protection, (2) breathing mechanics and efficiency, (3) circulation with hemorrhage control, vascular access, and appropriate volume replacement, (4) disability (neurologic examination) and exposure, being sure to also identify any life-threatening hemorrhage.[6] Traditionally, the ABC (airway, breathing, and circulation) approach has been taught in both advanced trauma life support (ATLS) and prehospital trauma life support (PHTLS) for decades. However, there is now a more recent push toward the circulation first approach (CAB; circulation, airway, and breathing) with a focus on early hemorrhage control (Ferrada P, Dissanaike S. Circulation First for the Rapidly Bleeding Trauma Patient-It Is Time to Reconsider the ABCs of Trauma Care. JAMA Surg 2023;158(8):884–885.). After initial life-threatening pathology is managed and vital signs are obtained, a secondary head-to-toe evaluation can be performed, ideally during transport.

The vital signs (ie, heart rate, blood pressure, pulse oximetry, end-tidal carbon dioxide) EMS clinicians obtain are critically important in the identification of a trauma patient's hemodynamic stability or degree of shock. These data points can be combined into the Shock Index (SI), the ratio of heart rate to systolic blood pressure, to serve as a rapid guide to indicate future need for massive transfusion.[7] SI values>0.6 indicate shock but the index can become inaccurate due to numerous factors, notably chronic hypertension and the use of heart rate–lowering medications such as beta-blocking agents.[8,9] End-tidal carbon dioxide ($ETCO_2$) is an additional vital sign that has future potential to identify hypoperfusion in the prehospital setting and may also be a more sensitive and specific predictor of mortality than lactate, blood pressure, or venous pH.[10] Nasal $ETCO_2$ values of<27 to 30 mm Hg have been shown to predict the need for transfusion, but further research will need to assess the utility of adding $ETCO_2$ values to prehospital triage decision tools.[11]

Ultrasound

Ultrasound is an invaluable evaluation tool that is routinely used in trauma centers and has become increasingly more common outside of the hospital. The use of point of care ultrasound in the prehospital trauma patient primarily includes focused assessment with sonography for trauma (FAST) and thoracic exams (Extended or E-FAST), as well as evaluation for vascular access. Ultrasound can identify pathology necessitating prehospital intervention, such as evaluating for the presence of a pneumothorax with associated physiologic disturbances, and guide disposition with the identification of injury patterns requiring a trauma center evaluation (ie, pericardial effusion, hemoperitoneum).[12] While ultrasound has some promise in guiding prehospital decision-making, more evidence is needed to identify its ideal role. Given that there is strong evidence that prolonged scene times are associated with worse outcomes in trauma, it is important that clinicians do not delay pretransport times for performing ultrasound examinations.

PREHOSPITAL INTERVENTIONS
Airway Management

As the classic first step of the primary survey, airway assessment and management are integrally important in the treatment of trauma patients. Clinicians should focus initially on basic life support interventions, such as airway positioning, oropharyngeal or nasopharyngeal airway placement, and/or bag valve mask ventilation. These initial approaches are frequently sufficient to facilitate transport to the hospital in the most expeditious and safe way. In some cases, altered mental status, airway trauma, oropharyngeal trauma, airway obstruction, or overall physiologic complexity will require advanced intervention utilizing a host of techniques.[13–15] Intubation in the prehospital setting should only be done by skilled clinicians who remain broadly focused on all aspects of trauma care, including resuscitation, hemorrhage control, and rapid transport.

Chest Decompression

Tension pneumothorax is a life-threatening complication of chest trauma that must be treated with urgent decompression. It is identified by absence of unilateral lung sounds, lack of lung sliding on ultrasound, respiratory distress, hypoxia, and potentially hemodynamic instability in the event of tension physiologic changes. According to the latest ATLS guidelines, needle decompression should be performed in the 4th to 5th intercostal space along the anterior axillary line.[16] An appropriate length and diameter catheter, ideally 8 cm and at least 14 gauge, is found to improve the chances of success.[17] Finger thoracostomy is becoming a more popular intervention among EMS, given that needle decompression is associated with relatively high rates of complication.[17,18] Finger thoracostomy can be safely performed by paramedics in the field in the same location as the needle decompression and may be the preferred method of pleural decompression.[19]

Intravenous and Intraosseous Access

Rapid vascular access allows timely trauma resuscitation and medication delivery in the field. Multiple large bore (16 gauge or larger) intravenous (IV) catheters should be placed in patients with significant trauma, but if these cannot rapidly be obtained, intraosseous (IO) access is a viable and safe alternative that can often be performed faster than peripheral IVs.[20] When utilizing pressure bags, 15G IO access in the humerus or proximal tibia has flow rates comparable with 18G IV catheters.[21] Given these flow rates are not as large as 14G or 16G catheters, additional sites of access may be needed to match resuscitation requirements. With the addition of advanced providers in the prehospital setting, central venous access can also be established when necessary.

Volume Resuscitation

Prehospital volume resuscitation is a critical intervention for the hemorrhaging trauma patient. Until relatively recently, the only option for civilian prehospital clinicians has been crystalloid solutions such as normal saline or lactated ringers.[22] Crystalloids have been shown in numerous studies to have no benefit and may be harmful to patients with traumatic bleeding.[23,24] EMS clinicians should minimize the amount of crystalloids administered and allow for permissive hypotension until definitive bleeding control can be achieved at a trauma center.[25]

Blood administration programs are becoming more common within US EMS systems despite their significant logistical requirements.[26,27] However, randomized controlled trials (RCTs) comparing blood products and crystalloids in the prehospital setting have had mixed results.[28–30] Plasma appears to be superior to crystalloids primarily when transport times are prolonged (>20 minutes), but a recent trial showed no difference in mortality when randomizing patients to packed red blood cells and lyophilized plasma or up to 1L of normal saline.[28–31] In the civilian prehospital setting, particularly due to its simplicity in administration compared to component therapy, cold-stored, low titer O$^+$ whole blood has become increasingly popular. Recent, prospective, observational studies have supported the benefit of cold stored whole blood over component therapy, but RCTs are needed to truly compare these 2 therapies.[32,33]

Mechanical Hemorrhage Control

Hemorrhage remains a leading cause of preventable deaths in trauma.[34] Direct pressure is the first mainstay of hemorrhage control, but with large injuries or vascular injury, this may not be enough. Commercial windlass tourniquets remain the next option to manage limb hemorrhage in the field and have been associated with markedly improved survival.[35] Tourniquets are extremely safe when application times are less than 2 hours but services providing prolonged field care in remote settings should have protocols to attempt conversion of tourniquets after this time.[36,37] For injuries not amenable to tourniquet application, such as in the groin, axilla, and neck, wound packing remains the next intervention to stop bleeding.[38] Packing is ideally performed with hemostatic impregnated gauze, but regular sterile gauze may be equally efficacious.[39] Junctional tourniquets may be used to address groin hemorrhage, which have shown some success in military theaters, but likely require stronger evidence before implementation in the civilian prehospital setting.[40] Resuscitative endovascular balloon occlusion of the aorta (REBOA) is a technique to temporally occlude blood flow in the aorta and stop bleeding. While most studies of REBOA are performed inside trauma centers, there are some case reports and case series of prehospital REBOA use.

Pharmacologic Hemorrhage Control

Multiple studies have shown that administration of tranexamic acid (TXA) in patients with traumatic hemorrhage has a survival benefit with a relative risk reduction in all-cause mortality, a reduction in hemorrhage-associated complications such as hypoperfusion and organ failure, as well as a total reduction in blood product usage.[41,42] A common concern, hypercoagulability, has been extensively studied and found to be similar to that of the non-TXA groups.[42] Early administration of TXA within the first hour of hemorrhage onset and no later than 3 hours after injury is critical for its effectiveness.[41] Current protocols suggest a loading dose of 1 g IV over 10 minutes with a second dose (1 g) to be infused over the subsequent 8 hours, but IO or intramuscular administration may be reasonable alternatives if IV access cannot be obtained.[43] Other options such as a single 2 g dose have also been suggested.

Spinal Immobilization or Spinal Motion Restriction

If cervical spine injury is suspected, clinicians should place a cervical collar, as recommended by PHTLS guidelines.[6] EMS protocols should guide clinicians to identify which patients do not require cervical collars with the assistance of validated tools such as the National Emergency X-Radiography Utilization Study criteria.[44] It is important to note that minimal evidence exists that collars prevent morbidity or mortality.[45] There is, however, evidence that cervical collars can cause harm such as worsening intubating conditions and increasing intracranial pressure (ICP).[46,47] Backboards should not be universally used by EMS clinicians given their well-documented association with pressure ulcers and restricted ventilation, without benefit of improved neurologic outcome.[48] In the setting of penetrating trauma specifically, spinal motion restriction has been associated with increased mortality and is strongly not recommended.[49,50]

Pelvic Binders

Pelvic ring fractures can be associated with severe hemorrhage in trauma patients. Pelvic circumferential compression devices (PCCDs), also known as pelvic binders, can be a prehospital attempt to slow bleeding prior to definitive intervention. EMS clinicians should have a high index of suspicion for pelvic ring fractures in hemodynamically unstable patients with polytrauma and/or suspected pelvic injuries. In these cases, they should consider early empiric pelvic binder placement, as numerous studies have shown that rates of placement in appropriate patients are low often due to unsuspected fractures.[51] To date, no clinical benefit has been shown by prehospital PCCD placement in retrospective studies.[51,52] In 1 retrospective emergency department study, PCCD placement was associated with a significant decrease in mortality and transfusion requirement, which indicates that there may be benefit in some patients.[53] In light of conflicting evidence, the Eastern Association for the Surgery of Trauma, PHTLS, and ATLS continue to recommend PCCD use in unstable patients with suspected pelvic injuries given the potential for benefit with a low cost and complication rate.[6,16,54]

Traumatic Brain Injury Management

Traumatic brain injury (TBI) remains the number one cause of overall mortality in trauma patients.[34] Prehospital clinicians should aggressively treat secondary causes of brain injury, including hypotension, hypoxemia, and hypothermia, which have all been independently associated with increased mortality.[55,56] Clinicians should target normal $ETCO_2$ values of 35 to 40 mm Hg, working to avoid prophylactic hyperventilation which is associated with worse neurologic outcomes.[57] Patients with true herniation physiology can be hyperventilated to $ETCO_2$ of 28 to 35 mm Hg, but this should only be temporary to facilitate additional treatments for herniation.[58] Additional treatments to lower ICP include avoiding tight cervical collars, maintaining head of bed at>30°, providing appropriate sedation or analgesia, hyperosmolar therapy, and, eventually, neurosurgical intervention.[59] Empiric prehospital administration of hyperosmolar therapy to patients with TBI does not appear to have benefit.[60]

Physician-Level Interventions

Physicians that provide care out of the hospital can bring an additional skillset above the scope of practice of paramedics. There are numerous potential interventions in the care of injured patients that physicians can perform, notably including REBOA, thoracotomy, advanced vascular access, and field amputations. REBOA is a technique to control abdominal and pelvic exsanguination, which in the prehospital setting could, in theory, provide temporary hemostasis during transport to a hospital that can provide definitive surgical care and hemostasis. Prehospital placement has been shown to be a feasible intervention by highly trained physicians outside of the United States, but more study is needed to evaluate its effect on clinical outcomes and to recommend routine use within the United States.[61] Thoracotomy is another prehospital intervention that could be performed by physicians to manage patients in peri-arrest or full cardiac arrest. The first documented case report of prehospital thoracotomy was in the United States in 1994 and resulted in the patient surviving neurologically intact.[62] While rare in the United States, some European countries have established protocols for prehospital thoracotomy in traumatic arrest and have shown comparable, or better, survival than in-hospital thoracotomy.[63,64] Prehospital amputations can allow needed extrication of patients with limb entrapment or those with anticipated prolonged extrication and hemodynamic compromise requiring more rapid transport. Apart from specific procedural skills, physicians also bring a wealth of knowledge and experience, the ability to provide in-person medical control, and medications that may be outside of an EMS clinician's protocol.[4]

TERMINATION OF RESUSCITATION

In the prehospital setting, termination of resuscitation (TOR) is the cessation of resuscitative efforts by clinicians on the patient in arrest that has failed to regain spontaneous circulation after a period of on-scene care.[65] Within an organized prehospital system, algorithmic protocols based on local, state, and national guidelines and strong operational support should exist to allow for the appropriate decision-making of resuscitation termination by EMS clinicians. Clinicians should also be able to decide not to terminate resuscitation and instead transport the patient, in case they feel termination would place them at risk of harm from bystanders. TOR guidelines take into account multiple factors.[65] For pediatrics, TOR has similar indications as in adults. The American Academy of Pediatrics recommends termination for patients with obvious signs of death or 30 minutes of unsuccessful resuscitation with medical direction consultation.[66] They also recommend immediate transport for patients with cardiac arrest and signs of life prior to CPR, who received CPR within 5 minutes of arrest, as well as transport for any patient where the cause of arrest is uncertain.

MODES OF TRANSPORTATION

There are numerous transportation options to get injured patients to trauma centers. Patients can be transported via ground ambulance or helicopter, but often patients are transported via private vehicles or law enforcement vehicles. EMS destination decisions should be made by regional protocols and guided by national field triage guidelines.[67] In those patients that are transported via ground ambulance, it is integral to keep scene times to a minimum as prolonged scene times are associated with worse survival.[68] Clinicians should focus on performing only time-sensitive, immediately lifesaving interventions on scene. When ground transport times will be markedly long, helicopter EMS (HEMS) can provide more rapid transport, additional interventions, and often a higher level of care. The evidence of HEMS benefit on trauma patients is mixed, and there are no definitive recommendations on how these resources should be utilized.[67,69]

Transport via ambulance or HEMS may not be the most rapid transportation option to get patients to definitive care. A large retrospective study of the National Trauma Databank associated private vehicle transport with 2-fold lower in-hospital mortality compared to EMS transport for patients with gunshot wounds.[70] The association of lower mortality in all penetrating trauma patients transported by private vehicle has also been shown.[71] Similar studies have evaluated transport to the hospital by law enforcement, but these demonstrated no difference in mortality compared to EMS.[71,72] Especially when there are delays to EMS arrival or when trauma centers are in close proximity, systems should not discourage private or law enforcement transport to the hospital, especially in patients with penetrating trauma.

BYSTANDER ENGAGEMENT

Bystanders and other nonmedical first responders, such as law enforcement officers, have significant opportunity to administer lifesaving interventions to trauma patients before EMS arrives. Akin to cardiopulmonary resuscitation training, public health interventions have attempted to provide necessary trauma skills to civilians, namely education on hemorrhage control. The Stop the Bleed campaign (https://www.stopthebleed. org), led by the American College of Surgeons, is one such intervention which has led to widespread training of the public and placement of bleeding control kits in public areas.[73] EMS systems should facilitate similar training to prepare their public to assist in the response to traumatic injuries.

CLINICS CARE POINTS

- Hemorrhage control (ie, tourniquet, wound packing) should come before airway and breathing in the primary survey in the evaluation and management of injured patients.
- Minimize crystalloid infusion; preferentially transfuse blood and blood products.
- Use TXA for injured patients with hemorrhage.
- Not every injured patient needs spinal motion restriction.
- Place a pelvic binder for injured patients with known or suspected pelvic ring injury.
- Avoid hypotension, hypoxemia, and hypothermia to prevent secondary brain injury after trauma.
- Consider when to terminate prehospital resuscitation based on local jurisdictional guidelines.
- Weigh the pros and cons of alternate transportation modes for injured patients including EMS (via ground or air) and private vehicle options.
- Teach the Stop the Bleed course to engage the lay public to improve outcomes after injury.

DISCLOSURE

Dr Haut reports research funding from the Patient-Centered Outcomes Research Institute, the Agency for Healthcare Research and Quality, the National Institutes of Health National Heart, Lung, and Blood Institute.

REFERENCES

1. Wilson MH, Habig K, Wright C, et al. Pre-hospital emergency medicine. Lancet Lond Engl 2015;386(10012):2526–34.
2. About The National Registry | National Registry of Emergency Medical Technicians. Accessed April 16, 2023. https://nremt.org.
3. EMS Examination Task Force, American Board of Emergency Medicine, Perina DG, Pons PT, Blackwell TH, et al. The core content of emergency medical services medicine. Prehosp Emerg Care 2012;16(3):309–22.
4. Rosenblum AJ, Wend CM, Ide RA, et al. Descriptive analysis of clinical encounters by emergency medical services physicians using the RE-AIM framework. J Public Health Manag Pract JPHMP 2023;29(2):E58–64.
5. Seblova J, Cimpoesu D, Khoury A, et al. Prehospital emergency care systems in Europe - EuSEM prehospital section survey 2016. Eur J Emerg Med 2018;25(6): 446–7.

6. PHTLS. Prehospital trauma life support. 9th edition. Burlington, MA: Jones & Bartlett Learning; 2020.

7. Mutschler M, Nienaber U, Münzberg M, et al. The shock index revisited - a fast guide to transfusion requirement? A retrospective analysis on 21,853 patients derived from the TraumaRegister DGU. Crit Care Lond Engl 2013;17(4):R172.

8. McNab A, Burns B, Bhullar I, et al. An analysis of shock index as a correlate for outcomes in trauma by age group. Surgery 2013;154(2):384–7.

9. Rau CS, Wu SC, Kuo SCH, et al. Prediction of massive transfusion in trauma patients with shock index, modified shock index, and age shock index. Int J Environ Res Public Health 2016;13(7):683.

10. Willis RG, Cunningham KW, Troia PA, et al. Prehospital end-tidal CO2: a superior marker for mortality risk in the acutely injured patient. Am Surg 2022;88(8): 2011–6.

11. Wilson BR, Bruno J, Duckwitz M, et al. Prehospital end-tidal CO2 as an early marker for transfusion requirement in trauma patients. Am J Emerg Med 2021; 45:254–7.

12. Mercer CB, Ball M, Cash RE, et al. Ultrasound use in the prehospital setting for trauma: a systematic review. Prehosp Emerg Care 2021;25(4):566–82.

13. Kovacs G, Sowers N. Airway management in trauma. Emerg Med Clin North Am 2018;36(1):61–84.

14. Carney N, Totten AM, Cheney T, et al. Prehospital airway management: a systematic review. Prehosp Emerg Care 2022;26(5):716–27.

15. Mayglothling J, Duane TM, Gibbs M, et al. Emergency tracheal intubation immediately following traumatic injury: an Eastern Association for the Surgery of Trauma practice management guideline. J Trauma Acute Care Surg 2012;73(5 Suppl 4):S333–40.

16. Advanced trauma life support 10th edition student course manual. 10th edition. Chicago, IL: American College of Surgeons; 2018.

17. Laan DV, Vu TDN, Thiels CA, et al. Chest wall thickness and decompression failure: A systematic review and meta-analysis comparing anatomic locations in needle thoracostomy. Injury 2016;47(4):797–804.

18. Sharrock MK, Shannon B, Garcia Gonzalez C, et al. Prehospital paramedic pleural decompression: A systematic review. Injury 2021;52(10):2778–86.

19. Hannon L, St Clair T, Smith K, et al. Finger thoracostomy in patients with chest trauma performed by paramedics on a helicopter emergency medical service. Emerg Med Australas EMA 2020;32(4):650–6.

20. Leidel BA, Kirchhoff C, Bogner V, et al. Is the intraosseous access route fast and efficacious compared to conventional central venous catheterization in adult patients under resuscitation in the emergency department? A prospective observational pilot study. Patient Saf Surg 2009;3(1):24.

21. Wang D, Deng L, Zhang R, et al. Efficacy of intraosseous access for trauma resuscitation: a systematic review and meta-analysis. World J Emerg Surg WJES 2023;18(1):17.

22. Dadoo S, Grover JM, Keil LG, et al. Prehospital fluid administration in trauma patients: a survey of state protocols. Prehosp Emerg Care 2017;21(5):605–9.

23. Haut ER, Kalish BT, Cotton BA, et al. Prehospital intravenous fluid administration is associated with higher mortality in trauma patients: a national trauma data bank analysis. Ann Surg 2011;253(2):371–7.

24. Sung CW, Sun JT, Huang EPC, et al. Association between prehospital fluid resuscitation with crystalloids and outcome of trauma patients in Asia by a cross-national multicenter cohort study. Sci Rep 2022;12(1):4100.

25. Tran A, Yates J, Lau A, et al. Permissive hypotension versus conventional resuscitation strategies in adult trauma patients with hemorrhagic shock: a systematic review and meta-analysis of randomized controlled trials. J Trauma Acute Care Surg 2018;84(5):802–8.

26. Bullock W, Schaefer R, Wampler D, et al. Stewardship of prehospital low titer O-positive whole blood in a large urban fire-based EMS system. Prehosp Emerg Care 2022;26(6):848–54.

27. Guyette FX, Zenati M, Triulzi DJ, et al. Prehospital low titer group O whole blood is feasible and safe: Results of a prospective randomized pilot trial. J Trauma Acute Care Surg 2022;92(5):839–47.

28. Sperry JL, Guyette FX, Brown JB, et al. Prehospital Plasma during Air Medical Transport in Trauma Patients at Risk for Hemorrhagic Shock. N Engl J Med 2018;379(4):315–26.

29. Moore HB, Moore EE, Chapman MP, et al. Plasma-first resuscitation to treat haemorrhagic shock during emergency ground transportation in an urban area: a randomised trial. Lancet Lond Engl 2018;392(10144):283–91.

30. Crombie N, Doughty HA, Bishop JRB, et al. Resuscitation with blood products in patients with trauma-related haemorrhagic shock receiving prehospital care (RePHILL): a multicentre, open-label, randomised, controlled, phase 3 trial. Lancet Haematol 2022;9(4):e250–61.

31. Guyette FX, Sperry JL, Peitzman AB, et al. Prehospital Blood Product and Crystalloid Resuscitation in the Severely Injured Patient: A Secondary Analysis of the Prehospital Air Medical Plasma Trial. Ann Surg 2021;273(2):358–64.

32. Siletz AE, Blair KJ, Cooper RJ, et al. A pilot study of stored low titer group O whole blood + component therapy versus component therapy only for civilian trauma patients. J Trauma Acute Care Surg 2021;91(4):655–62.

33. Shea SM, Staudt AM, Thomas KA, et al. The use of low-titer group O whole blood is independently associated with improved survival compared to component therapy in adults with severe traumatic hemorrhage. Transfusion (Paris) 2020; 60(Suppl 3):S2–9.

34. Oyeniyi BT, Fox EE, Scerbo M, et al. Trends in 1029 trauma deaths at a level 1 trauma center: Impact of a bleeding control bundle of care. Injury 2017; 48(1):5–12.

35. Teixeira PGR, Brown CVR, Emigh B, et al. Civilian Prehospital Tourniquet Use Is Associated with Improved Survival in Patients with Peripheral Vascular Injury. J Am Coll Surg 2018;226(5):769–76.e1.

36. Joarder M, Noureddine El, Moussaoui H, et al. Impact of time and distance on outcomes following tourniquet use in civilian and military settings: A scoping review. Injury 2023;54(5):1236–45.

37. Drew B, Bird D, Matteucci M, et al. Tourniquet Conversion: A Recommended Approach in the Prolonged Field Care Setting. J Spec Oper Med Peer Rev J SOF Med Prof 2015;15(3):81–5.

38. Welch M, Barratt J, Peters A, et al. Systematic review of prehospital haemostatic dressings. BMJ Mil Health 2020;166(3):194–200.

39. Littlejohn LF, Devlin JJ, Kircher SS, et al. Comparison of Celox-A, ChitoFlex, WoundStat, and combat gauze hemostatic agents versus standard gauze dressing in control of hemorrhage in a swine model of penetrating trauma. Acad Emerg Med Off J Soc Acad Emerg Med 2011;18(4):340–50.

40. Schauer SG, April MD, Fisher AD, et al. Junctional Tourniquet Use During Combat Operations in Afghanistan: The Prehospital Trauma Registry Experience. J Spec Oper Med Peer Rev J SOF Med Prof 2018;18(2):71–4.

41. Roberts I, Shakur H, Coats T, et al. The CRASH-2 trial: a randomised controlled trial and economic evaluation of the effects of tranexamic acid on death, vascular occlusive events and transfusion requirement in bleeding trauma patients. Health Technol Assess Winch Engl 2013;17(10):1–79.
42. Relke N, Chornenki NLJ, Sholzberg M. Tranexamic acid evidence and controversies: An illustrated review. Res Pract Thromb Haemost 2021;5(5):e12546.
43. Grassin-Delyle S, Shakur-Still H, Picetti R, et al. Pharmacokinetics of intramuscular tranexamic acid in bleeding trauma patients: a clinical trial. Br J Anaesth 2021;126(1):201–9.
44. Hoffman JR, Wolfson AB, Todd K, et al. Selective cervical spine radiography in blunt trauma: methodology of the National Emergency X-Radiography Utilization Study (NEXUS). Ann Emerg Med 1998;32(4):461–9.
45. Kwan I, Bunn F, Roberts I. Spinal immobilisation for trauma patients. Cochrane Database Syst Rev 2001;2001(2):CD002803.
46. Thiboutot F, Nicole PC, Trépanier CA, et al. Effect of manual in-line stabilization of the cervical spine in adults on the rate of difficult orotracheal intubation by direct laryngoscopy: a randomized controlled trial. Can J Anaesth J Can Anesth 2009; 56(6):412–8.
47. Mobbs RJ, Stoodley MA, Fuller J. Effect of cervical hard collar on intracranial pressure after head injury. ANZ J Surg 2002;72(6):389–91.
48. White CC, Domeier RM, Millin MG. National Association of EMS Physicians. EMS spinal precautions and the use of the long backboard - resource document to the position statement of the National Association of EMS Physicians and the American College of Surgeons Committee on Trauma. Prehosp Emerg Care 2014; 18(2):306–14.
49. Haut ER, Kalish BT, Efron DT, et al. Spine immobilization in penetrating trauma: more harm than good? J Trauma 2010;68(1):115–20, discussion 120-121.
50. Velopulos CG, Shihab HM, Lottenberg L, et al. Prehospital spine immobilization/ spinal motion restriction in penetrating trauma: A practice management guideline from the Eastern Association for the Surgery of Trauma (EAST). J Trauma Acute Care Surg 2018;84(5):736–44.
51. Bangura A, Burke CE, Enobun B, et al. Are Pelvic Binders an Effective Prehospital Intervention? Prehosp Emerg Care 2023;27(1):24–30.
52. Agri F, Bourgeat M, Becce F, et al. Association of pelvic fracture patterns, pelvic binder use and arterial angio-embolization with transfusion requirements and mortality rates; a 7-year retrospective cohort study. BMC Surg 2017;17(1):104.
53. Hsu SD, Chen CJ, Chou YC, et al. Effect of Early Pelvic Binder Use in the Emergency Management of Suspected Pelvic Trauma: A Retrospective Cohort Study. Int J Environ Res Public Health 2017;14(10):1217.
54. Cullinane DC, Schiller HJ, Zielinski MD, et al. Eastern Association for the Surgery of Trauma practice management guidelines for hemorrhage in pelvic fracture–update and systematic review. J Trauma 2011;71(6):1850–68.
55. Chi JH, Knudson MM, Vassar MJ, et al. Prehospital hypoxia affects outcome in patients with traumatic brain injury: a prospective multicenter study. J Trauma 2006;61(5):1134–41.
56. Jeremitsky E, Omert L, Dunham CM, et al. Harbingers of poor outcome the day after severe brain injury: hypothermia, hypoxia, and hypoperfusion. J Trauma 2003;54(2):312–9.
57. Muizelaar JP, Marmarou A, Ward JD, et al. Adverse effects of prolonged hyperventilation in patients with severe head injury: a randomized clinical trial. J Neurosurg 1991;75(5):731–9.

58. Garvin R, Mangat HS. Emergency Neurological Life Support: Severe Traumatic Brain Injury. Neurocrit Care 2017;27(Suppl 1):159–69.
59. Vella MA, Crandall ML, Patel MB. Acute Management of Traumatic Brain Injury. Surg Clin North Am 2017;97(5):1015–30.
60. Bulger EM, May S, Brasel KJ, et al. Out-of-hospital hypertonic resuscitation following severe traumatic brain injury: a randomized controlled trial. JAMA 2010;304(13):1455–64.
61. Caicedo Y, Gallego LM, Clavijo HJ, et al. Resuscitative endovascular balloon occlusion of the aorta in civilian pre-hospital care: a systematic review of the literature. Eur J Med Res 2022;27(1):202.
62. Wall MJ, Pepe PE, Mattox KL. Successful roadside resuscitative thoracotomy: case report and literature review. J Trauma 1994;36(1):131–4.
63. Athanasiou T, Krasopoulos G, Nambiar P, et al. Emergency thoracotomy in the pre-hospital setting: a procedure requiring clarification. Eur J Cardio-Thorac Surg Off J Eur Assoc Cardio-Thorac Surg. 2004;26(2):377–86.
64. Davies GE, Lockey DJ. Thirteen survivors of prehospital thoracotomy for penetrating trauma: a prehospital physician-performed resuscitation procedure that can yield good results. J Trauma 2011;70(5):E75–8.
65. Libby C, Skinner RB, Rawal AR. EMS Termination Of Resuscitation And Pronouncement of Death. In: StatPearls. StatPearls Publishing; 2023. Available at: http://www.ncbi.nlm.nih.gov/books/NBK541113/. Accessed May 30, 2023.
66. American College of Surgeons Committee on Trauma, American College of Emergency Physicians Pediatric Emergency Medicine Committee, National Association of Ems Physicians, et al. Withholding or termination of resuscitation in pediatric out-of-hospital traumatic cardiopulmonary arrest. Pediatrics 2014; 133(4):e1104–16.
67. Newgard CD, Fischer PE, Gestring M, et al. National guideline for the field triage of injured patients: Recommendations of the National Expert Panel on Field Triage, 2021. J Trauma Acute Care Surg 2022;93(2):e49–60.
68. Harmsen AMK, Giannakopoulos GF, Moerbeek PR, et al. The influence of prehospital time on trauma patients outcome: a systematic review. Injury 2015;46(4): 602–9.
69. Galvagno SM, Sikorski R, Hirshon JM, et al. Helicopter emergency medical services for adults with major trauma. Cochrane Database Syst Rev 2015;2015(12): CD009228.
70. Zafar SN, Haider AH, Stevens KA, et al. Increased mortality associated with EMS transport of gunshot wound victims when compared to private vehicle transport. Injury 2014;45(9):1320–6.
71. Wandling MW, Nathens AB, Shapiro MB, et al. Police transport versus ground EMS: A trauma system-level evaluation of prehospital care policies and their effect on clinical outcomes. J Trauma Acute Care Surg 2016;81(5):931–5.
72. Band RA, Pryor JP, Gaieski DF, et al. Injury-adjusted mortality of patients transported by police following penetrating trauma. Acad Emerg Med Off J Soc Acad Emerg Med 2011;18(1):32–7.
73. Wend C, Ayyagari R, Herbst L, et al. Implementation of Stop the Bleed on an Undergraduate College Campus: The Johns Hopkins Experience. J Coll Emerg Med Serv 2018;1(2). https://doi.org/10.30542/JCEMS.2018.01.02.03.

Resuscitation and Care in the Trauma Bay

Jan-Michael Van Gent, DO[a,b], Thomas W. Clements, MD, FRCSC[a,b], Bryan A. Cotton, MD, MPH[a,b,c],*

KEYWORDS

- Balanced resuscitation • Trauma • Hemorrhagic shock
- Trauma-induced coagulopathy

KEY POINTS

- Start balanced resuscitation early (pre-hospital if possible), either in the form of whole blood or 1:1:1 ratio.
- Minimize resuscitation with crystalloid to minimize patient morbidity and mortality.
- Trauma-induced coagulopathy can be largely avoided with the use of balanced resuscitation, permissive hypotension, and minimized time to hemostasis.
- Using protocolized "triggers" for massive and ultramassive transfusion will assist in minimizing delays in transfusion of products, achieving balanced ratios, and avoid trauma-induced coagulopathy.
- Once "audible" bleeding has been addressed, further blood product resuscitation and adjunct replacement should be guided by viscoelastic testing.

INTRODUCTION

Hemorrhage remains the leading cause of potentially preventable trauma death worldwide.[1,2] Since the 1980s, resuscitation strategies in the hemorrhaging patient centered around crystalloid administration.[3] The crystalloid-centric strategy yielded mortality rates approximately 50% to 80% in severely injured patients.[4] Much of the trauma community's recent success has been due to shifting away from massive crystalloid administration to early balanced blood product administration (1:1:1).[5] Additionally, mortality has further decreased into the single digits with the advances in patient transport times, prehospital care, massive transfusion (MT) protocols, permissive hypotension, and rapid progression to hemorrhage control in the operating room.[3,6–10]

[a] The Red Duke Trauma Institute, Memorial Hermann Hospital, Houston, TX, USA; [b] McGovern Medical School, University of Texas Health Science Center-Houston, Houston, TX, USA; [c] Center for Translational Injury Research, Houston, TX, USA
* Corresponding author. Department of Surgery, 6431 Fannin, MSB 4.286, Houston, TX 77030.
E-mail address: Bryan.A.Cotton@uth.tmc.edu

Surg Clin N Am 104 (2024) 279–292
https://doi.org/10.1016/j.suc.2023.09.005
0039-6109/24/© 2023 Elsevier Inc. All rights reserved.

surgical.theclinics.com

The paradigm shift toward hemostatic resuscitation (early blood products, permissive hypotension and avoidance of crystalloid) and rapid surgical hemostasis (**Fig. 1**), whether in the form of damage control or a definitive operation, has led to fewer patients with the "lethal triad," ultimately improving survivability.[11] Resuscitative adjuncts such as viscoelastic testing (VET) and tranexamic acid (TXA) have also assisted in reducing trauma-induced coagulopathy (TIC).[12]

Within the spectrum of trauma resuscitation, this article focuses on resuscitation in the trauma bay, touching on prehospital resuscitation and into the intensive care unit. The aim is to understand how historical failures have paved the way to the current approach of resuscitation and to review different resuscitation agents and techniques.

THE RESUSCITATION PENDULUM: THE HISTORY BEHIND RESUSCITATING WITH BLOOD

Resuscitation with blood has been documented since 1665, in which the first animal-to-animal transfusion was noted using dogs. Two years later, the first animal-to-human transfusion was performed. A century and a half later, in 1818, the first human-to-human blood transfusion was performed.[13] Blood transfusions were harmful and resuscitation largely centered around crystalloids, however, the ABO blood grouping system in the early 1900s was developed, altering the transfusion landscape forever.[3,13] Based on this system, the first pre-transfusion crossmatch was successfully executed in 1907.[13] This had tremendous downstream effects with the start of World War I the following decade. In 1917, Captain Ostwald Robertson (US Army) built the world's first blood bank.[14] Captain Robertson collected 22 bottles of universal whole blood (WB) and resuscitated 20 soldiers, 9 (45%) of which survived.[14] His methods of collection, storage solution, infectious disease testing, and ice storage were widely replicated, and by the final year of the war, 30,000 soldiers received transfusions.[14]

WB-based resuscitation continued to spread and evolve over the ensuing US conflicts. The US military was collecting and transporting massive amounts of WB by the end of World War II, collecting more than 13 million units during that time. This strategy was continued into the next 2 conflicts, but immeasurable product waste was noted. Over 50% of these blood products were wasted during these wars.[3] Due to the logistical constraints of storage and utilization of WB in the 1970s, resuscitation strategies were overhauled and would have a lasting effect for the next 50 years.

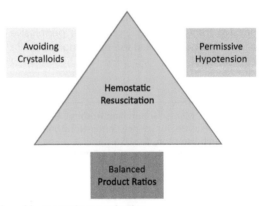

Fig. 1. The principles of hemostatic resuscitation.

ENTER THE ERA OF COMPONENT THERAPY

Efficiency and practicality of having a product that would have a smaller logistical footprint (sustainability) drove the advent of partitioning WB into red blood cells (RBCs), plasma, and platelets. WB is processed by collecting 450 to 500 mL of WB and adding 63 to 70 mL of a mixture of citrate, phosphate, and dextrose.[15] This additive solution preserves the WB and allows for storage of approximately 4 weeks, depending on the nutrient/anticoagulant solution used.[3] On the other hand, fractionating WB into each component has numerous advantages over only storing WB. By dividing WB, RBCs can be stored for 6 weeks, plasma for 1 to 7 years (depending on storage temperature), and platelets for 5 days at room temperature. Additionally, component therapy is advantageous for precision targeted treatments outside the confines of trauma. For example, patients who have non-traumatic anemia, coagulopathy/hemophilia, or thrombocytopenia require a specific product to treat illness.[13] Consequently, blood banks converted to stocking these components instead of WB.

RESUSCITATING THE BLEEDING PATIENT: CRYSTALLOID, COMPONENT THERAPY, OR WHOLE BLOOD?

Fractionated products became available at the end of the Vietnam War era, in which the US military prioritized the procurement and storage of RBCs only.[3] With that being said, resuscitation of casualties with RBCs was augmented with WB due to the benefits of being able to acquire fresh blood on the front-line. Despite literature during this period suggesting that augmenting WB resuscitation with component therapy was not necessary, once blood banking converted to fractionation as the dominant priority, the resuscitation of bleeding patients with RBCs and high volumes of crystalloid ensued.[3,16,17]

In the late 1970s and early 1980s, there was apprehension to transfuse patients in fear of transmitting (what would later be described as) hepatitis C or human immunodeficiency virus.[3] This, coupled with the ease of giving crystalloid while awaiting blood preparation, became the foundation of early resuscitation in the 1980s. Additionally, evidence from the elective and emergency general surgery arenas was extrapolated and applied to the bleeding patient in hemorrhagic shock. Patients were resuscitated with enormous amounts of crystalloid to achieve normal physiologic parameters, often using invasive monitoring methods such as pulmonary artery catheters.

With all good intentions, this paradigm shift had unintended consequences. First off, the administration of crystalloid shifts osmotic pressure, increasing capillary permeability, and ultimately, pushing the well-intended volume into the extracellular space.[18] The exorbitant amount of fluid given to achieve these physiologic goals potentiates acidosis, coagulopathy, endothelial glycocalyx dysregulation, and profound volume overload.[11,19] The volume overload alone increases morbidity with higher rates of ileus and postoperative pulmonary edema, mortality, and the incidence of abdominal compartment syndrome leading to the "open abdomen" era after damage control laparotomies.[20] Lastly, large volumes of crystalloid, in the form of lactated ringer or normal saline, can lead to a myriad of consequences including reduced cardiac output, acute respiratory distress syndrome, and multi-organ failure.[3,21] Therefore, the benefit of this resuscitation strategy for the patient was temporary at best, and largely resulted in the treatment of the surgeon and not the patient.

SALTWATER POISONING VERSUS BALANCED RESUSCITATION (1:1:1)

After the turn of the 20th century, war again pushed the needle in the treatment of hemorrhagic shock. During the Operation Iraqi Freedom and Operation Enduring

Freedom conflicts, logistics forced the pendulum back to resuscitating with products that emulate that of which is lost during hemorrhage (WB).[22] An evaluation of the Joint Theater Trauma Registry (JTTR) data produced the idea of damage-control resuscitation in which a hemostatic balanced blend of blood products would best support the coagulopathic critically injured casualty.[22] A review of the JTTR data exhibited better outcomes when a ratio of 1:1:1 (RBC, plasma, platelets) was utilized. Like previous US conflicts, fresh whole blood (FWB) was collected in theater when fractionated products were unavailable, with excellent outcomes.[22]

Balanced transfusions and avoidance of crystalloid was further urged by the civilian literature. Ho and colleagues urged "transfusing with the equivalent of whole blood" and avoiding crystalloid.[23] Holcomb and colleagues fostered this ideal and revealed that higher ratios of plasma and platelets to RBCs increased 30-day survival by nearly 20%.[24] The Pragmatic, Randomized Optimal Platelet and Plasma Ratios (PROPPR) study solidified these findings, concluding that exsanguination within 24 hours was significantly lower in the 1:1:1 (RBC, plasma, platelet) cohort compared to the 2:1:1 group. Eastern Association for the Surgery of Trauma (EAST) unified this consensus with the recommendation of balanced transfusions (1:1:1) during the early phase of resuscitation for hemorrhagic shock.[25]

THE RETURN OF WHOLE BLOOD

As stated previously, the paradigm shift away from WB to fractionated components were numerous and well-intended. The simple fact of fractionating WB into component products to then reconstitute them back into something comparable to WB is nonsensical and impractical. Resuscitating using a 1:1:1 ratio sounds excellent in theory, but realistically produces a dilute blood mixture with a low hematocrit, poor coagulation factors, and suboptimal platelet count (**Fig. 2**).[15] Additionally, the hemostatic composition of WB is more advantageous, with reaction time and maximum aplitude values (based off thromboelastography) within 15% of baseline even after 3 to 4 weeks of cold storage.[9] Moreover, the utilization of WB decreases donor exposure of transmissible infectious diseases from 3 or more donors (with fractionated products) to 1. With that being said, the benefit of longer storage times and precision treatment cannot be disputed, however, what is actually best for the patient?

Most of the known literature around the turn of the century was based off of the US military's experience displaying fresh WB saving lives in the austere environment.[9,26,27] Due to the unavailability of fractionated blood products in Somalia and later in Baghdad, "walking blood banks" were planned and implemented and were met with successful

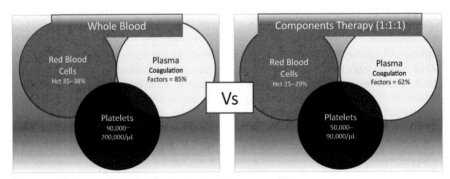

Fig. 2. Breakdown of whole blood vs 1:1:1 Component Therapy.

outcomes.[26,27] However, translating a "walking blood bank" into the civilian setting is impractical and the effectiveness of WB was challenged. Since then, multiple observational studies have shown that early WB resuscitation yields a good safely profile (no increased hemolysis, transfusion reaction, or transfusion-related events) and lower component transfusion needs.[28,29] Recent literature has shown improved 6-h, 24-h, in-hospital, and 30-day mortality with the use of early WB resuscitation.[9,30–32] With the release of this recent information, many civilian high volume trauma centers have adopted an early WB resuscitation strategy because the need for long storage times is less of a concern with quick turnover of products.

PREHOSPITAL RESUSCITATION AND TRIGGERS FOR MASSIVE TRANSFUSIONS

The logistical challenges of damage control resuscitation and large-scale blood banking are compounded in the prehospital setting. While the recognition of the dangers of crystalloid was center stage by the turn of the century, the use of blood products in the prehospital setting continued to lag. Seemingly irresistible in the prehospital setting, crystalloid solutions are inexpensive, readily available, require no specialized storage, and have an exceptionally long shelf life. As such, volume expansion with crystalloid fluid has continued to be the most common form of prehospital resuscitation.

As previously discussed, the downsides of massive crystalloid resuscitation in the inpatient setting were easily recognizable. The deleterious effects of even limited amounts of crystalloid in the prehospital setting would not be described until much later. In 2011, a review of the National Trauma Data Base associated the mere presence of prehospital IV access with increased mortality.[33] This was largely attributed to the fact that during this study period, the use of prehospital crystalloid was ubiquitous. Later studies would show increased rates of acute kidney injury, acute respiratory distress syndrome, and coagulopathy with the use of prehospital crystalloid. In 2015 the Resuscitation Outcomes Consortium would compare 2L boluses of crystalloid resuscitation with systolic blood pressure goals of 110 mm Hg head to head with 250 mL aliquots of fluid with 70 mm Hg goals, confirming the effectiveness of crystalloid avoidance and permissive hypotension in the prehospital setting.[34] More recently, Deeb and colleagues have demonstrated a mortality nadir between 250 and 1250 mL of prehospital crystalloid.[35] Ironically, this benefit of restraint is predicted by the wise observations of Moore and Shires as early as 1967, whose editorial urged "moderation" in resuscitation with crystalloid, yet would require another half century to be accepted by the trauma community as a whole.[36]

As with most trauma innovations, experience in modern war-time theaters has led to a massive overhaul of prehospital resuscitation in cutting edge civilian trauma centers. By 2012, blood product transfusion and damage control resuscitation principles began to be instituted as a *prehospital* intervention in military trauma systems. O'Reilly and colleagues[37] showed in their retrospective study of matched casualties of the conflict in Afghanistan, that prehospital WB was associated with a 58% decrease in mortality rates compared to prehospital crystalloid resuscitation. The landmark Pre-Hospital Air Medical Plasma trial would later compare prehospital plasma to standard crystalloid based resuscitation in the civilian setting.[38] This trial confirmed that plasma resuscitation was superior to crystalloid in regards to 30-day mortality rates.

Both prehospital data, and extrapolation of in-hospital resuscitation programs, had led to the application of hemostatic, balanced resuscitation practices in the prehospital setting.[39,40] Today, the most modern trauma systems have not only moved beyond crystalloid, but have introduced prehospital WB resuscitation as the cutting edge of trauma care.

As the resuscitation pendulum has swung back toward WB, the benefits of early application of this near-perfectly balanced resuscitation medium have continued to manifest. "Walking blood blanks" in the military have provided excellent opportunities to study WB in combat settings. Once again, military surgeons lead the charge with the use of WB demonstrating improved mortality in severely injured casualties.[41] Prehospital WB in the civilian setting has been shown to be associated with improved thromboelastographic profiles, decreased 24-h transfusion requirements, and mortality.[42–44] In patients receiving ultra-MTs (>20U in 24 hours), mortality differences are even more pronounced than patients receiving prehospital WB.[45]

PREDICTION MODELS

The timely administration of blood products to hemorrhaging patients is lifesaving. In efforts for early identification of hemorrhaging patients and algorithmic approaches to resuscitation, prediction models have been developed to predict patients with blood product requirements. The ideal prediction model is concise, rapidly applicable, and requires minimal logistical support, while providing excellent sensitivity and acceptable specificity for prediction of transfusion requirement. While a number of prediction models exist, the applicability of these can be severely limited by the absence of early laboratory or diagnostic imaging capabilities.

Assessment of Blood Consumption Score

The Assessment of Blood Consumption (ABC) score was published in 2009 in an effort to provide a standardized assessment of patients who require MT.[46] The ABC score consists of 4 paraments, each of which is assigned a value of 1 point. Systolic blood pressure less than or equal to 90 mm Hg, heart rate more than or equal to 120 bpm, penetrating mechanism, and a positive Focused Assessment with Sonography for Trauma (FAST) examination are equally weighted to generate an integer score out of 4. Using a score cutoff of more than or equal to 2, the ABC score predicts the need for MT with 75% sensitivity and 86% specificity. This score generates a rapid, easy to calculate, and memoizable score, and still has appropriate sensitivity and specificity to be of clinical use. While its use in the prehospital setting is limited by the requirement of an ultrasound, this capability has expanded into a large number of air-ambulance services, giving it superior applicability in the prehospital setting. Additionally, given that the most commonly used score cutoff is 2, many patients can be identified as high risk for MT without the use of an ultrasound, using vitals and mechanism alone.

Trauma Associated Severe Hemorrhage

The European derived Trauma Associated Severe Hemorrhage (TASH) score predicts the need for MT using biochemical, imaging, and clinical parameters.[47] A score out of 28 is generated using systolic blood pressure, heart rate, hemoglobin level, base excess, sex, FAST result, and the presence of clinically unstable pelvis or femur fractures. The score is then placed into the TASH formula ($P = 1/[1\exp(4.90.3 * TASH)]$) to generate a probability of requiring MT. The TASH score provides a robust, continuous prediction of MT requirement. It also allows each individual user to set their own threshold for sensitivity of MT. The downsides of requirements for laboratory investigations in addition to ultrasound add another level of difficulty in applying this score in the clinical setting. Decisions regarding the activation of MT protocols are often made prior to these data-points being available.

Shock Index

The shock index is a simple calculation made by dividing the heart rate in bpm by the systolic blood pressure in mm Hg. A cutoff of more than or equal to 1 has been used to predict the need for MT with 67.7% sensitivity and 81.3% specificity.[48] The advantages of shock index its simplicity and ease of use, allowing for ultrarapid application in all clinical settings. In a head-to-head comparison with the ABC score, SI was shown to be a stronger predictor of MT requirement, with an area under receiver operating characterictic curve of 0.83, compared to 0.74 for the ABC score, but had significantly weaker specificity in the same head-to-head comparison.

In addition to the aforementioned scores, many other systems have been used to predict the need for blood transfusion including clinical gestalt, Schreiber, and McLaughlin scores.[49,50] Resuscitation intensities (units transfused in the first 30 minutes of arrival) and critical administration thresholds ($\geq$3units per hour at any point in the first 24 hours) have been used to both predict and study MT requirements and outcomes with success.[51] While each score has its strengths and challenges, the developments of algorithmic triggers for MT are helpful adjuncts in the development of both hospital and prehospital transfusion protocols. These allow for more rapid and effective hemostatic resuscitation in hemorrhaging patients, and thus improve outcomes.

TRAUMA BAY RESUSCITATION

The robust logistical capability of large trauma centers facilitates the transition to rapid balanced resuscitation. The ability to have blood products immediately on hand to be rapidly administered to the hemorrhaging patient improves outcome and saves lives (**Fig. 3**). The tenants of crystalloid avoidance, permissive hypotension, and balanced resuscitation remain paramount in the early stages of any trauma situation. These practices become facilitated at a systemic level by instituting algorithmic triggers for activation of massive hemorrhage protocols. The clinical gestalt of trauma practitioners has been shown to be an inconsistent indicator of need for, and activation of, MT in trauma patients.[52] As such, the need for standardized clinical prediction scores remains high. While triggers vary by center, the American College of Surgeons Trauma Quality Improvement Guidelines recommend activation of MT protocols in

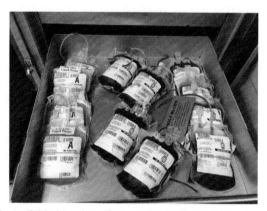

Fig. 3. Immediately available blood products in trauma bay refrigerator while awaiting delivery of massive transfusion protocol (MTP) products (4 each of plasma, whole blood, and RBCs).

patients with; an ABC score more than or equal to 2, persistent hemodynamic instability, active bleeding requiring operation or angioembolization, and requirement for blood transfusion in the trauma bay.[53]

While the revolutionary effect of 1:1:1 transfusion in trauma resuscitation demonstrated by the PROPPR study cannot be understated, the understanding of optimal balanced resuscitation continues to evolve.[5] WB has continued to demonstrate its role as the most ideal resuscitation medium available. Large military and civilian studies have shown that the use of WB as an early pillar of resuscitation leads to improved mortality, coagulopathy, and improvement in arrival shock index, as well as decreased need for overall transfusion.[9,42,43,45,54,55] Additionally, the cadence with which WB is initiated has been recognized as an important determinant of patient outcomes. Recently published data in the civilian setting have demonstrated a 2% increase in mortality for every minute delay in the administration of WB.[56]

The experience with prehospital WB also signals the benefit of early replacement of all blood components, with an increased focus on coagulopathy, as opposed to oxygen carrying capacity alone. In settings without access to WB programs, 1:1:1 ratios are still advocated as the resuscitation of choice. The PROPPR study demonstrated that 1:1:1 is superior to unbalanced resuscitation in regards to death due to hemorrhage.[5] As the presenting pathology of trauma patients is most often hemorrhage, a focus on the early replacement of coagulation factors, as opposed to RBCs or simple volume expansion, or has led to promising improvements in the care of the severely injured.

In summary, adequate trauma bay resuscitation starts from the systemic level with readily available blood products which are easily and rapidly accessible by trauma team members. MT protocols should rely on easy-to-use algorithms that utilize evidence-based clinical scoring systems. Resuscitation should be thoughtfully carried out with a focus on the treatment of coagulopathy while also replacing lost blood volume. Utilizing balanced resuscitation and WB, where available, improves the outcomes of hemorrhaging patients. The tenants of hemostatic resuscitation, avoidance of crystalloid, and permissive hypotension are applicable in all phases of a trauma patient's care, and are vital to ensure optimal probability of survival.

TRANSITIONING TO GOAL-DIRECTED RESUSCITATION

After hemostatic resuscitation in the trauma bay or the operating room (which is based off "what they have lost"), TIC typically persists for the next several hours.[57] The coagulopathy that ensues after balanced resuscitation is thought to be dependent on injury mechanism/patterns and phenotypical inflammatory response differences.[57] Despite the benefits of empiric balanced resuscitation with WB or fixed ratio products in the early phase of resuscitating the hemorrhaging patient, this strategy does not provide precision-based resuscitation to treat TIC which is often required in the hours following big resuscitation efforts.

As the resuscitation progresses, more data-points become available. These data-points allow for a more nuanced and individualized approach to each individual patient. While simple blood counts and coagulation parameters have been used for nearly a century, the paradigm-shifting application of thromboelastographic-based resuscitation began to be applied by the late 1990s.[58] The research application of viscoelastic testing (VET) subsequently exploded in the trauma field, with the clinical application of this new technology entering soon after. VET rapidly generates a patient's coagulation profile based on the mechanical resistance of the clot over time.[12] This allows the trauma specialist to identify specific components of the clotting cascade which are deranged and precisely replace these factors accordingly. This application of "personalized medicine" to trauma has led to significant improvements in hemostatic resuscitation, as well as end-points for goal-directed resuscitation.

VET-guided management has shown multiple different benefits compared to empiric-driven or gestalt-driven resuscitation. Compared to 1:1:1 therapy given empirically, VET-based resuscitation has been shown in retrospective settings to confer significant survival differences.[59] Compared to resuscitation based on conventional coagulation assays, the prospective randomized trial by Gonzalez and colleagues showed improved survival with less transfusion requirements in VET-guided resuscitation.[60] Many trauma centers have transitioned to goal-directed resuscitation accordingly. However, some prospective data have challenged the use of VET-based resuscitation, showing no difference in survival or secondary outcomes between VET and conventional coagulation assays.[61] The differences between these prospective studies can be attributed to differences in MT activation (trigger for enrollment in trials), injury severity, and time to presentation between the 2 populations, making the question of applicability center specific.

The uptake of VET-based resuscitation has been exceptionally slow despite the demonstrated benefits.[57] Despite slow adoption, VET-based resuscitation continues to demonstrate improved outcomes with less resource consumption and allows for the application of "personalized medicine" for the trauma sphere, making it a valuable addition to high-volume trauma centers.

Therapeutic Adjuncts

As the resuscitation paradigm shifted from volume expansion to correction of coagulopathy, other adjuncts to correct coagulopathy were investigated. The corticosteroid randomization after significant head injury-2 (CRASH-2) and CRASH-3 trials led to an increase in the use of TXA in hopes of improving mortality of patients with early empiric treatment of trauma-induced hyperfibrinolysis.[62,63] The US military, and many civilian centers for that matter, have adopted empiric administration of TXA,[64] while other centers use VET to guide the treatment of hyperfibrinolysis. If used, the patient populations where TXA has been shown to provide benefit are limited. Both CRASH-2 and Study of Tranexamic Acid During Air and Ground Medical PreHospital Transport trials showed its benefit lies in those with arrival systolic blood pressures less than 70 to 75 mm Hg. Moreover, the use of TXA should be limited to the first 3 hours since injury, with increased mortality/harm when administered after that time. Finally, increasing evidence and experience has transitioned away from the original 1g bolus and 1 g infusion over 8 hours to a single immediate bolus of 2 to 3g of TXA. This assists in saturating the receptors systemically of uPA, kallikrein, and tPA.

The Early high-dose cryoprecipitate in adult patients with major trauma haemorrhage requiring major haemorrhage protocol activation (CRYOSTAT), early fibrinogen in trauma (E-FiT), and fibrinogen in the initial resuscitation of severe trauma (FiiRST) trials have all investigated the used of cryoprecipitate in the early resuscitation of trauma patients, showing improved fibrinogen levels, but without mortality differences.[65–67] The CRYOSTAT-2 trial has yet to report at the time of this publication, but is meant to shed further light on the use of cryoprecipitate. While many centers have adopted these protocols, many institutions have avoided the implementation of empiric resuscitation practices; the argument against these studies being that the era of prehospital WB, early VET testing, and short prehospital times may obviate the need for these empiric measures.[57]

SUMMARY

The paradigm shift to hemostatic resuscitation with balanced ratios or WB has vastly improved outcomes in patients presenting in hemorrhagic shock. Executing this strategy has reduced mortality rates from 50% to 80% to now 10% to 20% in the last 20 years. With the avoidance of crystalloid, using products that match the makeup of WB, and utilizing permissive hypotension, many of the causes of morbidity which occurred in the past have been reduced. Throughout the continuum of trauma resuscitation, the mantra is simple, replace lost blood with blood.

CLINICS CARE POINTS

- The resuscitation of severely injured patients should begin in the prehospital setting en route to the nearest trauma center.
- Early identification of patients at risk for massive transfusion by either the ABC score or Shock Index is critical to stay ahead in resuscitation, as every minute delay in delivering MT coolers is associated with a 5% increase in mortality.
- Early identification of coagulation abnormalities within minutes of arrival via ROTEM or TEG is key to truncating and preventing the development of coagulopathy.
- Early transfusion of whole blood can reduce patient morbidity, mortality, decreases donor exposure, and reduces nursing logistics during transfusions.
- Adjuncts to resuscitation should be guided by laboratory testing and carefully developed, institution-specific guidelines. These include empiric calcium replacement, tranexamic acid (or other anti-fibrinolytics), and fibrinogen supplementation.

FUNDING

This work was supported by funding from the John B Holmes Endowed Chair in Clinical Sciences.

REFERENCES

1. Eastridge BJ, Holcomb JB, Shackelford S. Outcomes of traumatic hemorrhagic shock and the epidemiology of preventable death from injury. Transfusion 2019;59(S2):1423–8.
2. Cothren CC, Moore EE, Hedegaard HB, et al. Epidemiology of urban trauma deaths: A comprehensive reassessment 10 years later. World J Surg 2007; 31(7):1507–11.
3. Cantle PM, Cotton BA. Balanced Resuscitation in Trauma Management. Surg Clin North Am 2017;97(5):999–1014.
4. Cinat ME, Wallace WC, Nastanski F, et al. Improved survival following massive transfusion in patients who have undergone trauma. Arch Surg 1999;134(9):964–70.
5. Holcomb JB, Tilley BC, Baraniuk S, et al. Transfusion of plasma, platelets, and red blood cells in a 1:1:1 vs a 1:1:2 ratio and mortality in patients with severe trauma: The PROPPR randomized clinical trial. JAMA, J Am Med Assoc 2015;313(5): 471–82.
6. Sauaia A, Moore FA, Moore EE, et al. Epidemiology of Trauma Deaths. J Trauma Inj Infect Crit Care 1995;38(2):185–93.
7. Acosta J a, Yang JC, Winchell RJ, et al. Lethal injuries and time to death in a level I trauma center. J Am Coll Surg 1998;186(5):528–33.

8. Zink KA, Sambasivan CN, Holcomb JB, et al. A high ratio of plasma and platelets to packed red blood cells in the first 6 hours of massive transfusion improves outcomes in a large multicenter study. Am J Surg 2009;197(5):565–70.

9. Brill JB, Tang B, Hatton G, et al. Impact of Incorporating Whole Blood into Hemorrhagic Shock Resuscitation: Analysis of 1,377 Consecutive Trauma Patients Receiving Emergency-Release Uncrossmatched Blood Products. J Am Coll Surg 2022;234(4):408–18.

10. Duchesne JC, Kimonis K, Marr AB, et al. Damage control resuscitation in combination with damage control laparotomy: A survival advantage. J Trauma Inj Infect Crit Care 2010;69(1):46–52.

11. Kasotakis G, Sideris A, Yang Y, et al. Aggressive early crystalloid resuscitation adversely affects outcomes in adult blunt trauma patients: An analysis of the Glue Grant database. J Trauma Acute Care Surg 2013;74(5):1215–22.

12. Taylor JRI, Cotton BA. Coagulation Issues and the trauma patient. In: Cameron J, Cameron A, editors. Current surgical therapy. 13th edition. Philadelphia: Elsevier; 2020. p. 146–54.

13. Cap AP, Beckett A, Benov A, et al. Whole blood transfusion. Mil Med 2018;183(1): 44–51.

14. Stansbury LG, Hess JR. The 100th anniversary of the first blood bank. Transfusion 2017;57(11):2562–3.

15. Hess JR. Resuscitation of trauma-induced coagulopathy. Hematol Am Soc Hematol Educ Progr 2013;2013(1):664–7.

16. Hess JR, Thomas MJG. Blood use in war and disaster: Lessons from the past century. Transfusion 2003;43(11):1622–33.

17. Counts RB, Haisch C, Simon TL, et al. Hemostasis in massively transfused trauma patients. Ann Surg 1979;190(1):91–9.

18. Shires T, Williams J, Brown F. Acute change in extracellular fluids associated with major surgical procedures. Ann Surg 1961;154(5):803–10.

19. Anand T, Reyes AA, Sjoquist MC, et al. Resuscitating the Endothelial Glycocalyx in Trauma and Hemorrhagic Shock. Ann Surg Open 2023;4(3):e298.

20. Kirkpatrick AW, Roberts DJ, De Waele J, et al. Intra-abdominal hypertension and the abdominal compartment syndrome: Updated consensus definitions and clinical practice guidelines from the World Society of the Abdominal Compartment Syndrome. Intensive Care Med 2013;39(7):1190–206.

21. Holcomb JB, Jenkins D, Rhee P, et al. Damage control resuscitation: Directly addressing the early coagulopathy of trauma. J Trauma Inj Infect Crit Care 2007; 62(2):307–10.

22. Pidcoke HF, Aden JK, Mora AG, et al. Ten-year analysis of transfusion in Operation Iraqi Freedom and Operation Enduring Freedom: Increased plasma and platelet use correlates with improved survival. J Trauma Acute Care Surg 2012; 73(6 SUPPL. 5):445–52.

23. Ho AMH, Karmakar MK, Dion PW. Are we giving enough coagulation factors during major trauma resuscitation? Am J Surg 2005;190(3):479–84.

24. Holcomb JB, Wade CE, Michalek JE, et al. Increased plasma and platelet to red blood cell ratios improves outcome in 466 massively transfused civilian trauma patients. Ann Surg 2008;248(3):447–56.

25. Cannon JW, Khan MA, Raja AS, et al. Damage control resuscitation in patients with severe traumatic hemorrhage: A practice management guideline from the Eastern Association for the Surgery of Trauma. J Trauma Acute Care Surg 2017;82(3):605–17.

26. Repine TB, Perkins JG, Kauvar DS, et al. The use of fresh whole blood in massive transfusion. J Trauma Inj Infect Crit Care 2006;60(6 SUPPL). https://doi.org/10.1097/01.ta.0000219013.64168.b2.

27. Mabry RL, Holcomb JB, Baker AM, et al. United States army rangers in Somalia: An analysis of combat casualties on an urban battlefield. J Trauma Inj Infect Crit Care 2000;49(3):515–29.

28. Dishong D, Cap AP, Holcomb JB, et al. The rebirth of the cool: a narrative review of the clinical outcomes of cold stored low titer group O whole blood recipients compared to conventional component recipients in trauma. Hematol (United Kingdom) 2021;26(1):601–11.

29. Crowe E, DeSantis SM, Bonnette A, et al. Whole blood transfusion versus component therapy in trauma resuscitation: a systematic review and meta-analysis. J Am Coll Emerg Physicians Open 2020;1(4):633–41.

30. Gurney JM, Staudt AM, del Junco DJ, et al. Whole blood at the tip of the spear: A retrospective cohort analysis of warm fresh whole blood resuscitation versus component therapy in severely injured combat casualties. Surg (United States) 2022;171(2):518–25.

31. Hanna K, Bible L, Chehab M, et al. Nationwide analysis of whole blood hemostatic resuscitation in civilian trauma. J Trauma Acute Care Surg 2020;89(2):329–35.

32. Shea SM, Staudt AM, Thomas KA, et al. The use of low-titer group O whole blood is independently associated with improved survival compared to component therapy in adults with severe traumatic hemorrhage. Transfusion 2020;60(S3):S2–9.

33. Haut ER, Kalish BT, Cotton BA, et al. Prehospital intravenous fluid administration is associated with higher mortality in trauma patients: A national trauma data bank analysis. Ann Surg 2011;253(2):371–8.

34. Schreiber MA, Meier EN, Tisherman SA, et al. A controlled resuscitation strategy is feasible and safe in hypotensive trauma patients: Results of a prospective randomized pilot trial. J Trauma Acute Care Surg 2015;78:687–97. Lippincott Williams and Wilkins.

35. Deeb AP, Guyette FX, Daley BJ, et al. Time to early resuscitative intervention association with mortality in trauma patients at risk for hemorrhage. J Trauma Acute Care Surg 2023;94(4):504–12.

36. Moore F, Shires G. Moderation. Ann Surg 1967;166(2):300–1.

37. O'Reilly DJ, Morrison JJ, Jansen JO, et al. Prehospital blood transfusion in the en route management of severe combat trauma: A matched cohort study. J Trauma Acute Care Surg 2014;77(3 SUPPL. 2). https://doi.org/10.1097/TA.0000000000000328.

38. Sperry JL, Guyette FX, Brown JB, et al. Prehospital Plasma during Air Medical Transport in Trauma Patients at Risk for Hemorrhagic Shock. N Engl J Med 2018;379(4):315–26.

39. Kim BD, Zielinski MD, Jenkins DH, et al. The effects of prehospital plasma on patients with injury: A prehospital plasma resuscitation. J Trauma Acute Care Surg 2012;73.

40. Brown JB, Sperry JL, Fombona A, et al. Pre-trauma center red blood cell transfusion is associated with improved early outcomes in air medical trauma patients. J Am Coll Surg 2015;220(5):797–808.

41. Spinella PC, Perkins JG, Grathwohl KW, et al. Warm fresh whole blood is independently associated with improved survival for patients with combat-related traumatic injuries. J Trauma Inj Infect Crit Care 2009;66(SUPPL. 4). https://doi.org/10.1097/TA.0b013e31819d85fb.

42. Braverman MA, Smith A, Pokorny D, et al. Prehospital whole blood reduces early mortality in patients with hemorrhagic shock. Transfusion 2021;61(S1):S15–21.

43. Clements T, McCoy C, Assen S, et al. The prehospital use of younger age whole blood is associated with an improved arrival coagulation profile. J Trauma Acute Care Surg 2021;90:607–14. Lippincott Williams and Wilkins.

44. Guyette FX, Zenati M, Triulzi DJ, et al. Prehospital low titer group O whole blood is feasible and safe: Results of a prospective randomized pilot trial. J Trauma Acute Care Surg 2022;92(5):839–47.

45. Clements TW, Van Gent J-M, Lubkin DE, et al. The Reports of my Death are Greatly Exaggerated: An Evaluation of Futility Cut-Points in Massive Transfusion. J Trauma Acute Care Surg 2023. https://doi.org/10.1097/TA.0000000000003980.

46. Nunez TC, Voskresensky IV, Dossett LA, et al. Early prediction of massive transfusion in trauma: Simple as ABC (Assessment of Blood Consumption)? J Trauma Inj Infect Crit Care 2009;66(2):346–52.

47. Yücel N, Lefering R, Maegele M, et al. Trauma Associated Severe Hemorrhage (TASH)-score: Probability of mass transfusion as surrogate for life threatening hemorrhage after multiple trauma. J Trauma Inj Infect Crit Care 2006;60(6):1228–36.

48. Schroll R, Swift D, Tatum D, et al. Accuracy of shock index versus ABC score to predict need for massive transfusion in trauma patients. Injury 2018;49(1):15–9.

49. Schreiber MA, Perkins J, Kiraly L, et al. Early Predictors of Massive Transfusion in Combat Casualties. J Am Coll Surg 2007;205(4):541–5.

50. McLaughlin DF, Niles SE, Salinas J, et al. A predictive model for massive transfusion in combat casualty patients. J Trauma 2008;64(2 Suppl). https://doi.org/10.1097/ta.0b013e318160a566.

51. Meyer DE, Cotton BA, Fox EE, et al. A comparison of resuscitation intensity and critical administration threshold in predicting early mortality among bleeding patients: A multicenter validation in 680 major transfusion patients. J Trauma Acute Care Surg 2018;85:691–6. Lippincott Williams and Wilkins.

52. Pommerening MJ, Goodman MD, Holcomb JB, et al. Clinical gestalt and the prediction of massive transfusion after trauma. Injury 2015;46:807–13. Elsevier Ltd.

53. American College of Surgeons Committee on Trauma. Massive Transfusion in Trauma Guidelines. Available at: https://www.facs.org/media/zcjdtrd1/transfusion_guildelines.pdf.

54. Cotton BA, Podbielski J, Camp E, et al. A randomized controlled pilot trial of modified whole blood versus component therapy in severely injured patients requiring large volume transfusions. Ann Surg 2013;258:527–32.

55. Pivalizza EG, Stephens CT, Sridhar S, et al. Whole blood for resuscitation in adult civilian trauma in 2017: A narrative review. Anesth Analg 2018;127(1):157–62.

56. Hosseinpour H, Magnotti LJ, Bhogadi SK, et al. Time to Whole Blood Transfusion in Hemorrhaging Civilian Trauma Patients: There Is Always Room for Improvement. J Am Coll Surg 2023;237(1):24–34.

57. Walsh M, Moore E, Moore H, et al. Whole blood, fixed ratio, or goal-directed blood component therapy for the initial resuscitation of severely hemorrhaging trauma patients: A narrative review. J Clin Med 2021;10(2):1–17.

58. Kaufmann CR, Dwyer KM, Crews JD, et al. Usefulness of thrombelastography in assessment of trauma patient coagulation. J Trauma 1997;42(4):716–20, discussion 720-2.

59. Johansson PI. Goal-directed hemostatic resuscitation for massively bleeding patients: The Copenhagen concept. Transfus Apher Sci 2010;43(3):401–5.

60. Gonzalez E, Moore EE, Moore HB, et al. Goal-directed hemostatic resuscitation of trauma-induced coagulopathy a pragmatic randomized clinical trial comparing a

viscoelastic assay to conventional coagulation assays. Ann Surg 2016;263(6): 1051–9.

61. Baksaas-Aasen K, Gall LS, Stensballe J, et al. Viscoelastic haemostatic assay augmented protocols for major trauma haemorrhage (ITACTIC): a randomized, controlled trial. Intensive Care Med 2021;47(1):49–59.

62. Shakur H, Roberts I, Bautista R, et al, CRASH-2 trial collaborators. Effects of tranexamic acid on death, vascular occlusive events, and blood transfusion in trauma patients with significant haemorrhage (CRASH-2): a randomised, placebo-controlled trial. Lancet 2010;376(9734):23–32.

63. Roberts I, Shakur-Still H, Aeron-Thomas A, et al. Effects of tranexamic acid on death, disability, vascular occlusive events and other morbidities in patients with acute traumatic brain injury (CRASH-3): A randomised, placebo-controlled trial. Lancet 2019;394(10210):1713–23.

64. Joint Trauma System. Damage Control Resuscitation Clinical Practice Guideline. Available at: https://jts.health.mil/index.cfm/PI_CPGs/cpgs#:~:text=Damage Control Resuscitation%2C 12 Jul 2019.

65. Curry N, Rourke C, Davenport R, et al. Early cryoprecipitate for major haemorrhage in trauma: A randomised controlled feasibility trial. Br J Anaesth 2015; 115(1):76–83.

66. Curry N, Foley C, Wong H, et al. Early fibrinogen concentrate therapy for major haemorrhage in trauma (E-FIT 1): Results from a UK multi-centre, randomised, double blind, placebo-controlled pilot trial. Crit Care 2018;22(1). https://doi.org/10.1186/s13054-018-2086-x.

67. Nascimento B, Callum J, Tien H, et al. Fibrinogen in the initial resuscitation of severe trauma (FiiRST): a randomized feasibility trial. Br J Anaesth 2016;117(6): 775–82.

Trauma Bay Evaluation and Resuscitative Decision-Making

William Robert Leeper, MD, MEd, FRCSC[a,b,*],
Nicholas James, MD, MSc[c,d]

KEYWORDS

- Trauma resuscitation • Hemorrhagic shock • Team dynamics
- Operative preparation • Crisis resource management

KEY POINTS

- Trauma resuscitation is a team sport. Success in the trauma bay, like success in the field of play, often comes down to a simple matter of contact.
- Maintaining contact with the patient, staying connected to your team, and providing hands-on, focused, deliberate care is what will save patients' lives.
- Understanding both the common pitfalls of patient physiology and our own cognitive and emotional states is the key to high performance in trauma resuscitation.

INTRODUCTION

There is perhaps no more satisfying or more daunting resuscitative opportunity than that which presents itself in the trauma resuscitation bay. The arrival of a critically injured patient, occasionally at the brink of death, demands high performance in cognitive, psychomotor, and affective domains from all team members involved if a life is to be saved. Although the performance of each individual is important, it is often the interactions within the team and how that team assembles, aligns itself, and ultimately falls into position to perform that will have the greatest impact on patient outcome. This article focuses on the individual skills from each domain (cognitive,

[a] Department of Surgery, Western University, Victoria Campus, London Health Sciences Center, Room E2-215, 800 Commissioners Road East, London, Ontario N6A 5W9, Canada; [b] Trauma Program at London Health Sciences Center, Division of Critical Care, Department of Surgery, Schulich School of Medicine and Dentistry, Western University, London, Ontario, Canada; [c] London Health Sciences Center, Victoria Campus, Room E2-214, 800 Commissioners Road East, London, Ontario N6A 5W9, Canada; [d] Trauma Program at London Health Sciences Center, Schulich School of Medicine and Dentistry, Western University, London, Ontario, Canada
* Corresponding author. Department of Surgery, Western University, Victoria Campus, London Health Sciences Center, Room E2-215, 800 Commissioners Road East, London, Ontario N6A 5W9, Canada.
E-mail address: rob.leeper@lhsc.on.ca

Surg Clin N Am 104 (2024) 293–309
https://doi.org/10.1016/j.suc.2024.01.002
0039-6109/24/© 2024 Elsevier Inc. All rights reserved.

psychomotor, and affective) that are required for each phase of trauma bay evaluation (initial survey, specific interventions, resuscitative maneuvers) and attempts to synthesize how best the knowledge, skill, and attitudes of the clinicians can be put to use in a coordinated team approach to resolving crisis.

INITIAL EVALUATION

Trauma physicians, the world over, are blessed to have a single, dominant system of communication and mental modeling for trauma resuscitation. The American College of Surgeons' (ACS) Committee on Trauma has been producing, refining, and distributing the Advanced Trauma Life Support (ATLS) course for greater than 40 years.[1] The ATLS course is now in its 11th edition and is taught in more than 150 countries and across all populated continents. More than anything, the ATLS course provides trauma providers with a single common "play book" from which to work. All clinicians caring for injured patients do so within the framework of the *ATLS primary survey*: focusing on *Airway, Breathing, Circulation, Disability, and Exposure/Environment*.[2] The authors of this article approach injured patients with that same strategy; however, in the construction of this article, the authors expand on mental models not specifically covered in the ATLS course. The purpose here is to provide a slightly more authentic and perhaps boiled down version of "how we think about it" and "how we do it" in the setting of a trauma resuscitation.

Pre-arrival Considerations

When trauma teams are provided with the luxury of a 5-, 10-, or even 15-minute warning about the impending arrival of an injured patient or patients, it is critical that those minutes be spent in thoughtful and deliberate preparation. Although each trauma bay and trauma team is unique, some general and universal principles apply.

- *Material preparation*—based on the available patient data, choose which material items to specifically open and prepare for use. Emergency access O-positive blood may be beneficial to load on the rapid infusion device, surgical chest tube trays may be wise to open and prep, and airway equipment may thoughtfully be "ready checked" and brought to the head of the bed.
- *Cognitive preparation*—take this time to work through the forming and norming phases of team assembly.[3] Introduce team members to one another. Carefully negotiate roles but remain flexible for dynamic role assignment if/when things evolve in ways that were not anticipated. Position yourself and your team members wisely. The *foot of the bed* is the position that the lead author finds themself in routinely when assuming a command-and-control posture for resuscitative activities.
- *Broaden system wide situational awareness*—now is a key time to inform the operating room of the possibility of incoming casualties. Making critical surgical teams aware, in advance, of their expected roles (orthopedics, neurosurgery, and so forth) may pay dividends. The lead author would emphasize the importance of attending-to-attending communication with other surgical services whenever possible. The blood bank, intensive care unit, and radiology department are three other organizational units who may benefit from direct pre-arrival communication. Unquestionably, the reader of this article can think of several more units within their hospital system who may benefit from early notification.

Handover of Care

Literature from every domain of medicine points to the importance of and the hazards of transitions of care.[4–10] Handovers are as dangerous if not more dangerous than fatigue. Errors are known to occur with a high frequency and high severity whenever patient data are handed over between care teams and especially when total responsibility of care is shifted from one provider group to another.[11–14]

All of these concepts can be seen in sharp relief when one examines handover of a trauma patient between the prehospital care providers and the in-hospital trauma team receiving the patient. Elements which make this phase of care both critical and challenging include: High emotional state and stakes, a high task burden, and a high cognitive burden for prehospital providers.

In aviation, the concept of a Sterile Cockpit refers to the tight prohibition of nonessential communication and activity whenever aircraft are in critical phases.[12] Handover in the trauma bay is a definitive moment for medical teams to practice "Sterile Cockpit" behavior.[15,16] If this is not a part of an established culture, it is worthwhile for those with a leadership voice to address this directly once prehospital personal have begun their approach. A simple script for trauma team leaders to use may go something like:

Eyes up team, patient arriving now. Let's have quiet for handover, non-critical communication is on hold. Let's get the patient moved over, on monitor, and situated before we get report. Once that's done, we will all listen in for handover.

Sharing this mental model with prehospital providers on their entry to the trauma bay is key. Assuring that there is no truly emergent threat that needs to be immediately addressed (active arterial bleeding, pending or ongoing cardiac arrest, and so forth) is a key first communication. Following this, establishing a plan to make a quiet and sterile transition to the trauma bay stretcher and then to receive a full verbal handover thereafter should be carried out. Pitfalls in this phase include multiple voices making information sharing difficult and unhelpful expressions of concern or pending needs.

Primary Survey and Adjuncts

Once the patient has successfully accomplished the transition of care to the in-hospital trauma team, the next pressing concern is to deliberately carry out the ATLS primary survey.[2]

It is the preference of the authors to assign one member of the trauma team to physically move from area to area on the patient, performing or reviewing the basic maneuvers within the primary survey and calling out the results with eye contact and vocal communication targeted at the trauma bay charge nurse or recorder. This primary survey provider (PSP) while communicating with the charge RN is still making their thoughts clear and audible to all members of the trauma team, allowing others to cross monitor the data being shared about the primary survey. This promotes a shared mental model and allows other individuals to thoughtfully add to the discussion as needed. Specifics of the authors' preferred survey are as follows.

- *Airway*: PSP should call out patient airway status (speaking in short sentences, intubated, stridulous, and so forth) and provide a specific comment about cervical spine precautions and whether a collar is in place and/or is required. A brief synthesis may be appropriate here, as well, such as "airway is not protected due to depressed level of consciousness and Dr. X and RT Y are currently making preparations for intubation while I move on in our survey."
- *Breathing*: PSP should lay hands on the chest of the patient and auscultate, as appropriate. PSP should perform or else witness the performance of the thoracic portion of the extended focused assessment with sonography for trauma (eFAST)

examination to confirm bilateral lung slide and the absence of hemothoracies.[17,18] Specific data regarding patient vital signs, such as oxygen saturation, respiratory rate, and end-tidal CO_2, should be stated aloud by the PSP to the charge RN.

- *Circulation*: PSP should manually palpate the abdomen for tenderness and rigidity, should manually assess the pelvis and femurs for stability and signs of fracture, and should perform "wet checks" by passing gloved hands over extremities and through patient's hair and clothing to check for external hemorrhage. The PSP should perform or witness the performance of the remaining mediastinal, pleural, and abdominal components of the eFAST examination.[17,18] Specific data regarding patient vital signs, such as heart rate and blood pressure, as well as a comprehensive summary of all venous access points currently present should be stated aloud by the PSP to the charge RN. A brief synthesis may be appropriate here, such as "hemorrhagic shock seems clinically evident. Dr. X has placed in intra-osseus line and Nurse W is priming the rapid infuser with uncrossed matched blood. Dr. C is making material preparations for a right subclavian central line. A massive hemorrhage protocol is being ordered by Nurse M and TXA 1g has been given through the IO."
- *Disability*: PSP should passively observe pupillary status and rapidly test each eye for ipsilateral and consensual response to light. An estimated pupillary size and comment on reactivity should be given to the charge nurse. Following this, a cursory examination sufficient to calculate the Glasgow Coma Scale (GCS) score should be performed.[19,20] This should entail verbal challenges/orders and, if required, physical stimuli such as a sternal rub and nail bed pressure in order to elicit response. The PSP should call out the responses to each maneuver and then, ideally, state what they believe the GCS value to be for each of eye, motor, and verbal systems in order to achieve a degree of group consensus on a final total score.
- *Exposure/Environment*: PSP should help direct the actions of ED technicians and nurses as all clothing and pre-hospital dressings are removed from the patient and all skin surfaces are briefly exposed for examination. It is the lead author's preference to borrow slightly from the ATLS secondary survey, at this point, and perform a log roll in order to both examine the patient's back and to perform a rectal temperature and rectal examination, as appropriate. Once the patient has been fully exposed and assessed, data from this phase should be shared with the charge nurse verbally and the PSP should then direct ED technicians and nurses to rapidly apply or adjust all appropriate dressings, splints, and so forth and cover the patient with a forced air heating blanket to decrease the risk of hypothermia.

Adjuncts to the primary survey, as described in the ATLS terminology, are a small but important number of point-of-care tests and bedside interventions that may provide critical ancillary information to supplement and bolster decision-making which arises from the primary survey.

- The *drawing of blood* for laboratory assessment, including blood gases, standard chemistry and hematology, plus thromboelastography should occur at the earliest possible moment in patient assessment, likely before the completion of the primary survey.
- The insertion of *nasogastric and urinary catheters* can prove critical in the appropriate context (massive hematuria from renal injury, high aspiration risk pre-intubation, and so forth) but also result in patient discomfort and distress that can distract and delay resuscitation. Similarly, an *electrocardiogram* may demonstrate an ST segment elevation MI as the cause of a patient presenting

after a single vehicle collision, but more often than not it will show only sinus tachycardia. For these reasons, the author deploys these particular adjuncts selectively and at a time point in resuscitation where they are least disruptive.

- *Chest x-Ray, Pelvic x-Ray, and the eFAST* are the three components of the adjuncts to the primary survey which deserve a status all their own. As the three most critical and most universally useful tools, the lead author performs these adjuncts hyper early in the care of the most critically injured patients, moving eFAST components directly into the primary survey and treating them as a natural extension of physical examination of the chest and abdomen.

Life-Threatening Syndromes of the Primary Survey

In performing the ATLS primary survey and its adjuncts, as outlined above, providers will identify those patients with immediate and life-threatening syndromes. The goal of the primary survey is NOT to specifically localize or completely characterize these conditions, but rather to broadly identify which, of the often multiple, syndromes exist/coexist and to initiate directed therapies well before details are completely established. In other words, trauma surgeons do not need to know precisely what is wrong as long as they know what to do.

Life-threatening syndromes that arise in the primary survey should be broadly classified into two groups: hemorrhagic etiology and non-hemorrhagic etiology.

Non-hemorrhagic etiology

Although other syndromes certainly exist, the list of common, life-threatening, and immediately treatable syndromes which kill by means OTHER than completely depleting the body's circulating blood volume is as follows.

- Airway Obstruction
  - Mechanical obstruction (fracture, soft tissue injury, foreign body, and so forth)
  - Airway hemorrhage and massive traumatic hemoptysis leading to blood asphyxia
- Obstructive Physiologic States
  - Cardiac tamponade
  - Tension pneumothorax
- Hypoxemic Syndromes
  - Massive blunt pulmonary injury (flail chest, blast injury, and so forth.)
  - Pulmonary fat emboli
- Increased Intra-cranial Pressure Syndromes
  - Evacuate-able space occupying intracranial hemorrhage (epidural, subdural, or intraparenchymal spaces)
  - Severe diffuse or localized traumatic brain edema

This list is not exhaustive, and one could argue, for example, to include distributive shock states such as neurogenic syndromes resulting from high cervical spinal cord injury in this list. Whichever mechanisms one wishes to add or subtract from the list of non-hemorrhagic syndromes of early trauma death, the fact remains that each of these conditions has its own unique set of considerations, risk factors, and relatively specific solutions to consider. The bulk of the remainder of this article is dedicated to a region-by-region breakdown of such syndromes and concise advice on their individualized management. Although individual hemorrhagic syndromes also have their own bespoke considerations, they broadly follow such identical and physiologically simple principles that it is possible, and in fact advisable, to consider them as a whole.

Hemorrhagic etiology

Hemorrhage is the enemy. As surgeons providing care to injured patients, our principal mission should be the resuscitation from, and treatment of, life-threatening hemorrhage.[21] Although patients bleed from various parts of their bodies and wasted blood may collect in a variety of locations, the principles of managing hemorrhage are simple, universal, and crucial to practice assiduously and regularly in order to maximize the numbers of injured patients whose lives can be saved. What follows is a simple and universal algorithm, or module, on how the authors approach massive hemorrhage in all its forms.

Step 1: make the diagnosis. Although greater specificity is always appreciated, it is not required. Knowing precisely where a patient is bleeding from is not required to initiate measures of resuscitation. Using information from the ATLS primary survey,[2] in combination with evidence-based clinical tools such as the ABC score,[22] providers should have a very good sense about whether a patient is suffering from massive hemorrhage. If an injured patient is in shock, even if the diagnosis of hemorrhage has not been definitively made, the authors recommend treating the patient as if they are bleeding until better data become available.

Step 2: institute best available immediate hemorrhage control. Deploy all appropriate methods at your disposal to address diagnosed or suspected causes of bleeding.

- Direct pressure to bleeding wounds
  - One well-placed finger works far better than a wad of loose gauze
  - Foley catheters inserted into deeper lacerations to provide hemostasis to less accessible venous injuries[23–25]
- Tourniquet any bleeding extremity
  - Document time of tourniquet placement
  - Maximize tension on the primary fixation apparatus first, THEN tighten windlass and secure
  - If bleeding persists, consider a second, more proximal tourniquet
- Pelvic binder empirically for all blunt trauma
- Administer TXA with first IV access

Step 3: obtain resuscitative vascular access. Intraosseous access is a universal and simple first access point for patients in extremis and allows volume replacement to begin immediately.[26,27] If possible, peripheral IV sites may also be used in the earliest phases of hemorrhagic shock resuscitation. However, the ultimate access point for any patient requiring massive resuscitation should be a large caliber central venous cannula.[28,29] Efforts to obtain this access point should begin immediately and should be occurring simultaneously with the primary survey. The specific type and features of the central venous cannula are largely inconsequential provided that it has a generous lumen (8 or 9 Fr), is approved by the local radiology department for power contrast injection, and ideally functions as an introducer sheath for the later insertion of a multi-lumen catheter. The specific location of the central venous cannula bears consideration only if there is high suspicious of an injury to the SVC or IVC, which would potentially impair venous return and delivery of blood products to the right heart from a supradiaphragmatic or subdiaphragmatic location. In this situation alone, it is reasonable to specify a preferred location for the initial site of resuscitative access (internal jugular or subclavian vs femoral vein).

Step 4: initiate massive hemorrhage protocol in a crew-based model. Emergency release blood products and the institutional massive hemorrhage protocol should be accessed immediately. For patients with massive hemorrhage, all blood products must be delivered warm via a high-capacity rapid transfusion device.[30] This is of the utmost importance due to both the necessity of avoiding hypothermia but, with a perhaps more nuanced understanding, owing to the importance of human psychology and organizational behavior that is required for task completion under duress.

The concept of a "Crew Served Weapon" was initially defined during the study of modern warfare up to, and including, the Second World War. After action analysis revealed that individual soldiers who were killed in action were overwhelmingly likely to have never fired their personal service weapons. Much like single nursing or medical professional hanging a unit of blood via a single peripheral IV, the lack of secondary observation and social pressure to perform the task at hand led to unintentional distraction. Other tasks may appear more urgent, and the unit of blood or the M1 rifle is simply ignored. As a result of the lack of continuous attention, the blood all too often remains in the bag, just as the ammunition all too often remained in the magazine.

Conversely, when more than one individual is assigned to complete a task, it is exceptionally unlikely that this task will go unattended. Borrowing again from the military example, when soldiers who are tasked to operate a belt-fed automatic machine gun, typically from a nest or fixed/reinforced position, the weapon is nearly universally fired to the point of exhaustion before the position is taken. The military refers to these types of firearms as "Crew Served Weapons" and they are well known to be among the most effective and most deadly tools for infantry combat. In the practice of hemorrhagic shock resuscitation, we find a very apt analogy with the Rapid Infusion Device. This is a medical "Crew Served Weapon" which requires the attention of two or more providers to prime the device, check and re-check blood products, and then continually feed fresh product and unload spent rounds of packed red cells and fresh frozen plasma. When such a device is paired with a large caliber central venous cannula and run by a crew of service providers (nurses, physicians, respiratory therapists, and so forth), it is exceptionally likely to function and function rapidly with little interruption in the flow of blood product until either hemorrhage control is achieved or the patient succumbs to physiologic exhaustion.

Step 5: transition the patient to definitive hemorrhage control. Once resuscitation has begun in earnest, bringing the patient to definitive hemorrhage control is the next immediate step. Facilitating emergency access to the operating room or interventional radiology suite should be a major focus of a mid-to-senior-level provider. Assigning such a provider, with knowledge and familiarity with the system, to perform this communication and facilitation as their sole responsibility is an appropriate resource allocation in this phase. Making preparations to continue the resuscitation during patient transport and to transition to a new resuscitative area (OR, IR, and so forth) should also be done at this time.

REGION-SPECIFIC ASSESSMENT AND INTERVENTION

What follows, now in the latter half of this article, is a region-by-region breakdown of our approach to care in the trauma bay. These considerations and interventions may fit best within the primary survey or the secondary survey, or they may exist somewhat outside those two constructs. Ultimately, the authors wish to provide some guidance and clarity on the important activities to be carried out in the trauma bay for each anatomic region, as providers may find this breakdown more digestible and selectively readable than an exhaustive, start to finish, linear description of trauma bay care.

Airway Considerations

All trauma airways are potentially difficult airways.[31] Physiologic challenges, such as hypovolemia, commonly lead to hypotension or even arrest during the act of airway acquisition and it is certainly the authors' position that physiologic restoration via hemorrhage control and blood resuscitation should take precedence over airway management whenever possible. The lead author routinely delays definitive airway management until shocked patients are prepped and draped in the operating room, where possible.

It is beyond the scope of this article to examine the myriad of algorithms and flow charts that are published on airway management options.[32] Given the routinely physiologically and anatomically challenging nature of trauma airway acquisition,[31,33] it is often simplest to prepare for the worst and hope for the best. In this way, the authors would recommend a so-called "Double Setup" approach to most trauma airways. The principles of this approach are outlined below.

- *Two providers simultaneously make material and cognitive preparation for airway acquisition:* one at the head of the bed preparing for an attempt at orotracheal intubation and the other at the patient's right side preparing for an attempt at a front-of-the-neck surgical airway.
- *The most experienced physicians are chosen for these roles.* High-functioning senior trainees may be appropriate. A great disservice is done to both the patient and the learner if junior or less experienced trainees are allowed to attempt an airway of this caliber.
- *Maximum preoxygenation, ideally without bag mask ventilation, is completed and rapid sequence induction (RSI) is performed* with predetermined doses of neuromuscular blocking agents plus some combination of analgesics, amnestics, and lidocaine.
- *First-pass attempts are made by the orotracheal intubator,* using their preferred techniques. Typically, up to three attempts will be allowed, and the variation of techniques between failed attempts is encouraged (change from video laryngoscopy to direct, change from rigid stylet to flexible, change from bougie to ETT direct, and so forth)
- *After three failed attempts, the second provider proceeds with a surgical airway,* using their preferred technique. Typically, an open cricothyrotomy is preferred and can be accomplished with relative ease in the vast majority of trauma patients using only a scalpel, the index finger, and a 6 mm or so outer diameter tracheostomy tube. The addition of a bougie, a cricoid hook, retractors, an assistant, suction, and a curved hemostat are considered a luxury but not a necessity for this procedure.
- *Emergency surgical airways are like chest tubes, done in the neck.* Surgeons will not see well but should be able to feel their way through landmarks within the neck to achieve airway cannulation. There will be blood, and this should be ignored until end-tidal CO_2 is obtained. At that time, several heavy polypropylene sutures encompassing skin on either side of the generous incision will near universally achieve hemorrhage control.

Neck and Junctional Considerations

Traditional teaching on hemorrhage from the neck relied on the division of this body region into three zones.

1. Zone 1: cervicothoracic junctional wounds from the thoracic inlet to the cricoid cartilage

2. Zone 2: operative neck wound from the cricoid cartilage to the angle of the mandible
3. Zone 3: cervicocranial junctional wound from the angle of the mandible to the skull base

The authors still prefer to think of wounds in these three categories as it helps direct one's situational awareness (SA) to the fact that for instance, Zone 1 injuries will often require chest surgery (sternotomy, thoracotomy), Zone 3 injuries will often be best managed by endovascular means (interventional radiologic stenting or embolization), and Zone 2 injuries are most likely to be conventionally operative. Other authors have, of late, espoused a "no zone" approach to penetrating neck trauma.[34,35] Ultimately, for the purpose of this article, the authors will try to simply describe a "no nonsense" approach to neck injuries.

Step 1: Decide Whether You Have Big Trouble or Little Problems: in the first 45 seconds of assessment in the trauma bay, providers should be able to account for any hard sign (airway loss or violation, massive blood loss or hematoma, and so forth) and detect the presence of "Big Trouble" or its absence.

Step 2: Deal With Big Trouble: if airway violation or loss is detected, it must be addressed immediately. See "Double Setup" from the preceding paragraphs. Where possible, the direct intubation via a cervical wound that widely lacerates the airway is acceptable. In addition, if severe anatomic derangement has occurred, it may be possible and advisable to move directly to the operating room for an awake surgical airway. If massive hemorrhage is ongoing, a single well-aimed finger is often the single best approach for control. In junctional locations, a 20 mL Foley catheter balloon inflated and fixed in place can be very helpful.[23-25] The authors have seen complete disruption of the jugular vein controlled successfully with this strategy, for example. Tight intracavitary packing of the nasal and oral cavities may be required, and rapid transition to an operating room or interventional radiology suite should be immediately planned whenever "Big Trouble" is identified in the neck.

Step 3: Take a Consistent Approach to Little Problems in Neck Trauma: all comers with violations of the platysma muscle should receive CT arteriograms of the head and neck. Any concern for aerodigestive injury should prompt the addition of a CT swallow protocol. For any area of concern, such as large or difficult tissue flaps to close (from long or disfiguring knife wounds) or for any lingering concern about aerodigestive injury, surgeons should maintain a very low threshold to simply bring the patient to the operating room. All concerns can be put rapidly to rest with a combination of pan-endoscopy (bronchoscopy/laryngoscopy/esophagoscopy) and surgical repair of soft tissues of the neck ± exploration and repair of lacerated deep neck structures and nerve(s). There is no better way to get a specialist colleague in to look at a neck wound, at night, than to book the case yourself and invite them to join.

Thoracic Considerations

Trauma bay thoracic considerations generally fall into three categories.

1. Ventilation and oxygenation concerns
2. Pleural space concerns
3. The need for resuscitative thoracotomy (RT)

In the case of thoracic injuries that lead to respiratory embarrassment or failure of oxygenation, these are almost universally addressed by invasive mechanical ventilation. In scenarios such as flail chest with underlying severe pulmonary contusion, the only error is to wait too long to initiate invasive ventilation. Advanced methods of pain control (regional, neuraxial, infusional) and indications for rib fixation should be considered outside the trauma bay setting. A few unique, but important oxygenation considerations do bear mentioning in this paragraph. These include the treatment of traumatic bronchopleural fistulas (BPFs) and the bridging to recovery of traumatic total pulmonary failure from issues such as fat emboli or massive hemoptysis leading to blood asphyxia.

A. Traumatic BPFs occur when large airways, such as the mainstem bronchi are disrupted by blunt or penetrating trauma. In this scenario, large proportions of each tidal volume administered (25%–50% or more) by the ventilator will be lost into the pleural space, chest tube(s), and subcutaneous tissues. This can also, rarely, be seen with multifocal severe peripheral injury to the entire lung or to a pulmonary lobe, whereby innumerable small air leaks lead to the same accumulative phenomenon. In these cases, one-lung ventilation is the preferred approach. Bronchoscopic guidance will be required, and instrumentation should generally be focused on the left mainstem as it is the longer and more forgiving mainstem to work with. If the injury is to the left lung, then we recommend placing a bronchial blocker in the left main stem and ventilating via an endotracheal tube placed above the carina. If the injury is to the right lung, we recommend selective left mainstem intubation of the left main bronchus with subsequent single-lung ventilation through this tube. If the injury is to the carina itself or is a destructive injury to the distal trachea that has somehow survived to the trauma bay, then we recommend reading further regarding bridging for total pulmonary failure.

B. Rarely, but tragically, injured patients will present with potentially reversible causes of total pulmonary failure. Overwhelming venous fat emboli and resultant ARDS are a possible early cause of this.[36,37] Severe pulmonary or airway laceration leading to massive hemoptysis and blood asphyxia is another. In situations such as these, the authors have found good success with the use of veno-venous extracorporeal membrane oxygenation (VV-ECMO).[38,39] Although specifics of this are well beyond the scope of this article, the authors have routinely applied this technology without the use of adjunctive heparin in the earliest phases of trauma care and seen several cases of intact survival from otherwise lethal pulmonary syndromes. The major error, with respect to the bridging of pulmonary failure patients with VV-ECMO, is to wait too long to initiate this therapy.

In respect to pleural space diseases in the trauma bay, it is perhaps enough to say that when in doubt, placing bilateral tube thoracostomies is something that the authors have rarely, if ever, regretted. The cognitive unloading that comes from having ruled out pleural-based contributions to shock, and the positive data that is obtained when large volumes of blood or enteric contents emanate from a chest tube is tremendously helpful in advancing the care of the patient down an appropriate pathway.

Finally, in respect to the performance of an emergency department RT, there is a great deal which has been written and a great deal more which has been said on this topic.[40–43] Although the performance of RT is both exciting and potentially effective, it should always remain a technique of last resort. When indicated, the lead author prefers to use a unilateral left, anterolateral approach for patients with wounds located exclusively below the diaphragm. In this case, aortic control is the principal objective and open cardiac massage the secondary benefit. In contrast, for patients with injuries above the diaphragm, the lead author routinely and exclusively performs a bilateral, clamshell thoracotomy in order to gain rapid and complete exposure to the thoracic cavity so that proper surgical repair of lacerated vital organs can be done with the utmost rapidity. It is anatomically undeniable that clamshell thoracotomy provides the ultimate and commanding exposure for thoracic injuries,[44] and although many authors argue that they have the surgical skill to perform most required repairs through a unilateral thoracotomy,[45,46] this has not been the experience of the lead author. Optimizing exposure is key to identifying and repairing life-threatening thoracic injuries.

Abdominal Considerations

Given the training background of many trauma surgeons, the abdomen is a region which is very comfortable to most trauma attendings. It is, therefore, relatively second nature to divide abdominal findings into those hard signs that direct early surgical exploration (peritonitis, shock with positive abdominal eFAST, evisceration) from those in which advanced CT imaging is preferred as a next step. A few unique scenarios bear mentioning.

A. Penetrating anterior abdominal wall injuries — while many trauma society guidelines do not include CT imaging for this injury, the lead author freely admits that they use CT imaging routinely in this setting in hemodynamically stable patients. As an adjunct to serial physical examination, the author finds the data from CT often expedites care in a variety of ways. These patients do not require CT, but it provides a useful roadmap.
B. Penetrating flank wound: Although it is often a challenge with respect to patient compliance, rectal contrast is a beneficial adjunct in identifying retroperitoneal injuries to the right and left colon for these patients.
C. Penetrating left-sided thoracoabdominal stab wounds: The use of diagnostic laparoscopy for these patients has proven critical time and again. In the instance of negative imaging, it is the authors' preference to wait until the following morning to perform the laparoscopy, as this gives time for subtle colonic and/or gastric injuries to declare themselves with peritonitis and facilitates a switch to laparotomy for exploration. If peritonitis has not developed during serial examination, then laparoscopy the following morning allows a typically very simple laparoscopic repair of any diaphragmatic injuries and facilitates rapid discharge of the patient thereafter.

Pelvic Considerations

Experienced trauma surgeons should maintain a healthy respect for the lethal potential of bony pelvic disruptions and the resultant hemorrhage. In general, these injuries are best managed in trauma bay by the simple application of a pelvic binder placed accurately and tightly across the greater trochanters.[47,48] Beyond this, the authors can only recommend the earliest possible communication with orthopedic surgery, interventional radiologic, and surgical colleagues for these challenging cases. Although data have been increasingly negative for the use of resuscitative endovascular balloon occlusion of the aorta (REBOA) as an approach for all noncompressible truncal hemorrhage,[49–52] the authors have found their most success with Zone 3 (aortic bifurcation) REBOA in the setting of exsanguinating pelvic hemorrhage. For this reason, the authors still retain a high degree of fluency with REBOA technology and have systems in place to ensure material readiness of the most effective and easiest to use systems available for REBOA application.

Extremity and Integumentary Considerations

Perhaps the most often ignored or forgotten systems in early trauma care is the extremity and integumentary system. Blood loss from open fractures of the upper and lower extremities can be extreme. On more than one occasion, the principal source of near-fatal hemorrhage has been a posterior scalp wound.[53,54] For these reasons, it is worthwhile paying specific attention to how a trauma surgeon can and should approach extremity and integumentary injury.

Step 1: Apply tourniquets first, ask questions very shortly thereafter—the application of effective tourniquets is critical for extremity hemorrhage. As taught in the ACS Stop the Bleed course, to be effective, tourniquets must be placed above the zone of injury, must be maximally tightened in order to occlude arterial inflow, and should be carefully monitored in terms of duration of use. Immediate interventions/investigations should ensue after tourniquet application with a search for other sources of blood loss as well as a plan being put in place to address the wound below the tourniquet.

Step 2: Avoid fixation error on mangled extremities—once a tourniquet is in place, it is important to move on and complete a thorough primary and secondary survey of all other areas of the injured patient. All too often, the mangled extremity may capture the attention and create both cognitive and task overload if the trauma team allow themselves to direct all their efforts and attention to that limb.

Step 3: Use specific and general hemostatic techniques—in certain body regions, such as the scalp, commercially available devices known as Raney clips can be very effective in controlling hemorrhage.[55] Interestingly, although they are often touted as a preferred technique, the authors find skin staples/clips to be one of the least effective means of controlling scalp hemorrhage. In general, however, all areas of the integumentary and extremities tend to respond well to basic approaches at hemorrhage control including:

- Packing with appropriate hemostatic gauze
- Direct finger pressure
- Splinting and reduction of fractures to obtain bony realignment
- Hemostatic suturing with deep, absorbable figure-of-8 stitches to bleeding sites and large, wide, polypropylene sutures to bring together skin

Neurologic Considerations

Simple spinal precautions and the application of accepted cervical spine imaging guidelines are all that is typically required to address traumatic spinal cord injuries or the risk thereof in the trauma bay.[56,57] The use of corticosteroids for acute spinal cord injury goes against best evidence and should be discouraged.[58–60]

With respect to the avoidance of secondary brain injury in the setting of confirmed or suspected intracranial injury, the authors consider the following general approach.

- Avoid hypotension and hypoxia at all costs. Target systolic blood pressures above 100 mm Hg, in contrast to standard practice of permissive hypotension for bleeding patients. Use vasopressors early and liberally to achieve these goals, if required.
- Minimize ICP elevation during airway management with additional dosing of analgesic medications and the use of lidocaine as an adjunctive medication in a neuroprotective RSI.
- Treat empirically for ICP with all available measures when clinical grounds exist which suggest raised ICP. Transient hyperventilation (CO_2 target 30–35), heavy sedation, neuromuscular blockade, head of bed elevation, loosening of cervical collar, and osmotic therapy (hypertonic saline 3%, 250 cc bolus) are all appropriate maneuvers in the earliest phases in the trauma bay.
- Advocate for early neuroimaging and early neurosurgical evacuation if findings are positive.

CRISIS RESOURCE MANAGEMENT

As a final topic for a chapter on trauma bay resuscitative management, crisis resource management (CRM) is a far more important skill than its place in the article would suggest. Although it is impossible to summarize much, if any, of the content of CRM in these short paragraphs, we must at least acknowledge its importance. In fact, it is these authors' belief that CRM is the single most important skill that providers in trauma can possess. The 11th edition of ATLS now devotes an entire module to CRM and the body of literature looking at trauma bay performance is increasingly pointing to the centrality of the cognitive and affective domains of CRM as being the center piece of high-quality trauma care.[61–63]

A few very brief points can be emphasized about high-quality CRM as it relates to trauma bay performance:

Situational Awareness is of paramount importance. The ability to understand where a patient has been and to recognize where that patient and the care team are now allows providers to predict accurately where the crisis is going next and to be able to prepare and act to address the next need before it arises. It is not enough that the crisis leader has SA. In fact, group and cultural SA is the key to success. As much as possible, crisis teams should check in with one another to assure that a Shared Mental Model is maintained throughout a crisis.[64,65]

Communication and Leadership styles vary among providers and among team and hospital settings. The universal guiding principles that can be identified are that compassionate communication which honors the importance of group input is critical. Although hierarchies should never be truly flat in crisis management, those with a larger share of power and therefore pressure do well to share the burden of decision-making and the affective elements therein with the larger group.

Debriefings done both "hot," immediately after crisis and "cold" as a special rounds or case review can often lead to high-quality learning for the crisis team. Identifying latent safety threats within the patient care environment allows meaningful quality improvement cycles to occur.[66,67] It is equally likely to identify and promote high-quality and adaptive behaviors within a trauma team so that those can be focused on and amplified in future events.

CLINICS CARE POINTS

- Identification of the etiology of shock in the trauma bay is important, but decision-making and rapid resuscitative action BEFORE precise diagnoses have been made is the true art of initial trauma care.

- Bleeding is the universal enemy of the trauma patient. Prompt repletion of circulating blood volume with balanced product, and careful monitoring of coagulopathy is the cornerstone of trauma resuscitation.

- Non-hemorrhagic causes of shock (tamponade, tension pneumothorax, neurogenic shock, and so forth) have unique presentations and treatments.

- Non-shock-related issues in the initial trauma evaluation, such as severe brain injury, airway loss, respiratory failure, and many others, will compete for attention and cognitive focus during trauma resuscitation. Delegation of tasks and the use of other providers to cognitively and materially unload the crisis leader should be encouraged in complex patient scenarios.

- Prompt transition from initial evaluation and resuscitation to damage control surgery is critical. Specific focus on communication, including assigning a senior member of the team to EXCLUSIVELY manage telecommunications with operating room teams and consulting surgical services, is highly recommended.

- Crisis resource management skills are as important if not more important than surgical skills in the initial care of trauma patients. Focusing on high-quality communication, team situational awareness, shared mental modeling, and a culture of regular after action debriefing will improve initial trauma care perhaps more than any other intervention.

DISCLOSURE

The authors have no conflicts to disclose.

REFERENCES

1. Radvinsky DS, Yoon RS, Schmitt PJ, et al. Evolution and development of the Advanced Trauma Life Support (ATLS) protocol: a historical perspective. Orthopedics 2012;35(4):305–11.
2. Galvagno SM Jr, Nahmias JT, Young DA. Advanced Trauma Life Support® Update 2019: Management and Applications for Adults and Special Populations. Anesthesiol Clin 2019;37(1):13–32.
3. Tuckman BW. Developmental sequence in small groups. Psychol Bull 1965;63: 384–99.
4. Desmedt M, Ulenaers D, Grosemans J, et al. Clinical handover and handoff in healthcare: a systematic review of systematic reviews. Int J Qual Health Care 2021;33(1):mzaa170.
5. Leonard M, Graham S, Bonacum D. The human factor: the critical importance of effective teamwork and communication in providing safe care. Qual Saf Health Care 2004;13(Suppl 1):i85–90.
6. Nasiri E, Lotfi M, Mahdavinoor SMM, et al. The impact of a structured handover checklist for intraoperative staff shift changes on effective communication, OR team satisfaction, and patient safety: a pilot study. Patient Saf Surg 2021; 15(1):25.
7. Carter AJ, Davis KA, Evans LV, et al. Information loss in emergency medical services handover of trauma patients. Prehosp Emerg Care 2009;13(3):280–5.
8. Cohen MD, Hilligoss PB. The published literature on handoffs in hospitals: deficiencies identified in an extensive review. Qual Saf Health Care 2010;19(6): 493–7.
9. Hunt GE, Marsden R, O'Connor N. Clinical handover in acute psychiatric and community mental health settings. J Psychiatr Ment Health Nurs 2012;19(4): 310–8.
10. Siddiqui N, Arzola C, Iqbal M, et al. Deficits in information transfer between anaesthesiologist and postanaesthesia care unit staff: an analysis of patient handover. Eur J Anaesthesiol 2012;29(9):438–45.
11. Janagama SR, Strehlow M, Gimkala A, et al. Critical Communication: A Cross-sectional Study of Signout at the Prehospital and Hospital Interface. Cureus 2020;12(2):e7114.
12. Wheeler DS, Sheets AM, Ryckman FC. Improving transitions of care between the operating room and intensive care unit. Transl Pediatr 2018;7(4):299–307.
13. Smith CJ, Britigan DH, Lyden E, et al. Interunit handoffs from emergency department to inpatient care: A cross-sectional survey of physicians at a university medical center. J Hosp Med 2015;10(11):711–7.
14. Horwitz LI, Moin T, Krumholz HM, et al. Consequences of inadequate sign-out for patient care. Arch Intern Med 2008;168(16):1755–60.

15. Kapur N, Parand A, Soukup T, et al. Aviation and healthcare: a comparative review with implications for patient safety. JRSM Open 2015;7(1). 2054270415616548.

16. Hardie JA, Oeppen RS, Shaw G, et al. You Have Control: aviation communication application for safety-critical times in surgery. Br J Oral Maxillofac Surg 2020; 58(9):1073–7.

17. Kirkpatrick AW, Sirois M, Laupland KB, et al. Hand-held thoracic sonography for detecting post-traumatic pneumothoraces: the Extended Focused Assessment with Sonography for Trauma (EFAST). J Trauma 2004;57(2):288–95.

18. Abdulrahman Y, Musthafa S, Hakim SY, et al. Utility of extended FAST in blunt chest trauma: is it the time to be used in the ATLS algorithm? World J Surg 2015;39(1):172–8.

19. Teasdale G, Maas A, Lecky F, et al. The Glasgow Coma Scale at 40 years: standing the test of time [published correction appears in Lancet Neurol. 2014 Sep;13(9):863]. Lancet Neurol 2014;13(8):844–54.

20. Teasdale G, Jennett B. Assessment of coma and impaired consciousness. A practical scale. Lancet 1974;2(7872):81–4.

21. Kauvar DS, Lefering R, Wade CE. Impact of hemorrhage on trauma outcome: an overview of epidemiology, clinical presentations, and therapeutic considerations. J Trauma 2006;60(6 Suppl):S3–11.

22. Nunez TC, Voskresensky IV, Dossett LA, et al. Early prediction of massive transfusion in trauma: simple as ABC (assessment of blood consumption)? J Trauma 2009;66(2):346–52.

23. Kong V, Ko J, Cheung C, et al. Foley Catheter Balloon Tamponade for Actively Bleeding Wounds Following Penetrating Neck Injury is an Effective Technique for Controlling Non-Compressible Junctional External Haemorrhage. World J Surg 2022;46(5):1067–75.

24. Scriba M, McPherson D, Edu S, et al. An Update on Foley Catheter Balloon Tamponade for Penetrating Neck Injuries. World J Surg 2020;44(8):2647–55.

25. Gilroy D, Lakhoo M, Charalambides D, et al. Control of life-threatening haemorrhage from the neck: a new indication for balloon tamponade. Injury 1992; 23(8):557–9.

26. Wang D, Deng L, Zhang R, et al. Efficacy of intraosseous access for trauma resuscitation: a systematic review and meta-analysis. World J Emerg Surg 2023;18(1):17.

27. Tyler JA, Perkins Z, De'Ath HD. Intraosseous access in the resuscitation of trauma patients: a literature review. Eur J Trauma Emerg Surg 2021;47(1):47–55.

28. Berman DJ, Schiavi A, Frank SM, et al. Factors that influence flow through intravascular catheters: the clinical relevance of Poiseuille's law. Transfusion 2020; 60(7):1410–7.

29. Milne A, Teng JJ, Vargas A, et al. Performance assessment of intravenous catheters for massive transfusion: A pragmatic in vitro study. Transfusion 2021;61(6): 1721–8.

30. Dunham CM, Belzberg H, Lyles R, et al. The rapid infusion system: a superior method for the resuscitation of hypovolemic trauma patients. Resuscitation 1991;21(2–3):207–27.

31. Kovacs G, Sowers N. Airway Management in Trauma. Emerg Med Clin North Am 2018;36(1):61–84.

32. Brown CVR, Inaba K, Shatz DV, et al. Western Trauma Association critical decisions in trauma: airway management in adult trauma patients. Trauma Surg Acute Care Open 2020;5(1):e000539.

33. Estime SR, Kuza CM. Trauma Airway Management: Induction Agents, Rapid Versus Slower Sequence Intubations, and Special Considerations. Anesthesiol Clin 2019;37(1):33–50.

34. Ko JW, Gong SC, Kim MJ, et al. The efficacy of the "no zone" approach for the assessment of traumatic neck injury: a case-control study. Ann Surg Treat Res 2020;99(6):352–61.

35. Ibraheem K, Khan M, Rhee P, et al. "No zone" approach in penetrating neck trauma reduces unnecessary computed tomography angiography and negative explorations. J Surg Res 2018;221:113–20.

36. Taviloglu K, Yanar H. Fat embolism syndrome. Surg Today 2007;37(1):5–8.

37. Tsai SHL, Chen CH, Tischler EH, et al. Fat Embolism Syndrome and in-Hospital Mortality Rates According to Patient Age: A Large Nationwide Retrospective Study. Clin Epidemiol 2022;14:985–96.

38. Wang C, Zhang L, Qin T, et al. Extracorporeal membrane oxygenation in trauma patients: a systematic review. World J Emerg Surg 2020;15(1):51.

39. Fan E, Gattinoni L, Combes A, et al. Venovenous extracorporeal membrane oxygenation for acute respiratory failure : A clinical review from an international group of experts. Intensive Care Med 2016;42(5):712–24.

40. Atkins K, Schneider A, Gallaher J, et al. Who benefits from resuscitative thoracotomies following penetrating trauma: The patient or the learner? Injury 2023; 54(11):111033.

41. Liu A, Nguyen J, Ehrlich H, et al. Emergency Resuscitative Thoracotomy for Civilian Thoracic Trauma in the Field and Emergency Department Settings: A Systematic Review and Meta-Analysis. J Surg Res 2022;273:44–55.

42. Aseni P, Rizzetto F, Grande AM, et al. Emergency Department Resuscitative Thoracotomy: Indications, surgical procedure and outcome. A narrative review. Am J Surg 2021;221(5):1082–92.

43. Panossian VS, Nederpelt CJ, El Hechi MW, et al. Emergency Resuscitative Thoracotomy: A Nationwide Analysis of Outcomes and Predictors of Futility. J Surg Res 2020;255:486–94.

44. Simms ER, Flaris AN, Franchino X, et al. Bilateral anterior thoracotomy (clamshell incision) is the ideal emergency thoracotomy incision: an anatomic study. World J Surg 2013;37(6):1277–85.

45. Vassiliu P, Yilmaz T, Degiannis E. On the ideal emergency thoracotomy incision. World J Surg 2014;38(4):1001–2.

46. Morgan BS, Garner JP. Emergency thoracotomy–the indications, contraindications and evidence. J R Army Med Corps 2009;155(2):87–93.

47. Biffl WL. Control of pelvic fracture-related hemorrhage. Surg Open Sci 2022; 8:23–6.

48. Hsu SD, Chen CJ, Chou YC, et al. Correction: Hsu et al. Effect of Early Pelvic Binder Use in the Emergency Management of Suspected Pelvic Trauma: A Retrospective Cohort Study. Int. J. Environ. Res. Public Health 2017, 14, 1217. Int J Environ Res Public Health 2022;19(11):6654.

49. Jansen JO, Hudson J, Cochran C, et al. Emergency Department Resuscitative Endovascular Balloon Occlusion of the Aorta in Trauma Patients With Exsanguinating Hemorrhage: The UK-REBOA Randomized Clinical Trial. JAMA 2023; 330(19):1862–71.

50. Joseph B, Zeeshan M, Sakran JV, et al. Nationwide Analysis of Resuscitative Endovascular Balloon Occlusion of the Aorta in Civilian Trauma. JAMA Surg 2019; 154(6):500–8.

51. Morrison JJ, Galgon RE, Jansen JO, et al. A systematic review of the use of resuscitative endovascular balloon occlusion of the aorta in the management of hemorrhagic shock. J Trauma Acute Care Surg 2016;80(2):324–34 [published correction appears in J Trauma Acute Care Surg. 2016 Mar;80(3):554. Morrison, Jonathan James [corrected to Morrison, Jonathan J]; Jansen, Jan Olaf [corrected to Jansen, Jan O]; Rasmussen, Todd Erik [corrected to Rasmussen, Todd E]].

52. Norii T, Crandall C, Terasaka Y. Survival of severe blunt trauma patients treated with resuscitative endovascular balloon occlusion of the aorta compared with propensity score-adjusted untreated patients. J Trauma Acute Care Surg 2015; 78(4):721–8.

53. Basyuni S, Panayi A, Sharma V, et al. A missed scalp laceration causing avoidable sequelae. Int J Surg Case Rep 2016;23:61–4.

54. Turnage B, Maull KI. Scalp laceration: an obvious 'occult' cause of shock. South Med J 2000;93(3):265–6.

55. Sykes LN Jr, Cowgill F. Management of hemorrhage from severe scalp lacerations with Raney clips. Ann Emerg Med 1989;18(9):995–6.

56. Zileli M, Osorio-Fonseca E, Konovalov N, et al. Early Management of Cervical Spine Trauma: WFNS Spine Committee Recommendations. Neurospine 2020; 17(4):710–22.

57. Stiell IG, Wells GA, Vandemheen KL, et al. The Canadian C-spine rule for radiography in alert and stable trauma patients. JAMA 2001;286(15):1841–8.

58. Sultan I, Lamba N, Liew A, et al. The safety and efficacy of steroid treatment for acute spinal cord injury: A Systematic Review and meta-analysis. Heliyon 2020; 6(2):e03414.

59. Liu Z, Yang Y, He L, et al. High-dose methylprednisolone for acute traumatic spinal cord injury: A meta-analysis. Neurology 2019;93(9):e841–50.

60. Evaniew N, Belley-Côté EP, Fallah N, et al. Methylprednisolone for the Treatment of Patients with Acute Spinal Cord Injuries: A Systematic Review and Meta-Analysis. J Neurotrauma 2016;33(5):468–81.

61. Huffman EM, Anton NE, Athanasiadis DI, et al. Multidisciplinary simulation-based trauma team training with an emphasis on crisis resource management improves residents' non-technical skills. Surgery 2021;170(4):1083–6.

62. Gillman LM, Brindley PG, Blaivas M, et al. Trauma team dynamics. J Crit Care 2016;32:218–21.

63. Ziesmann MT, Widder S, Park J, et al. S.T.A.R.T.T.: development of a national, multidisciplinary trauma crisis resource management curriculum-results from the pilot course. J Trauma Acute Care Surg 2013;75(5):753–8.

64. Johnsen BH, Westli HK, Espevik R, et al. High-performing trauma teams: frequency of behavioral markers of a shared mental model displayed by team leaders and quality of medical performance. Scand J Trauma Resusc Emerg Med 2017;25(1):109.

65. Westli HK, Johnsen BH, Eid J, et al. Teamwork skills, shared mental models, and performance in simulated trauma teams: an independent group design. Scand J Trauma Resusc Emerg Med 2010;18:47.

66. Petrosoniak A, Fan M, Hicks CM, et al. Trauma Resuscitation Using in situ Simulation Team Training (TRUST) study: latent safety threat evaluation using framework analysis and video review. BMJ Qual Saf 2021;30(9):739–46.

67. Shah S, McGowan M, Petrosoniak A. Latent safety threat identification during in situ simulation debriefing: a qualitative analysis. BMJ Simul Technol Enhanc Learn 2020;7(4):194–8.

The Role of Resuscitative Endovascular Balloon Occlusion of the Aorta

Megan Brenner, MD, MS

KEYWORDS

- Hemorrhage • Resuscitative endovascular balloon occlusion of the aorta
- Resuscitative thoracotomy • Endovascular technology

KEY POINTS

- Resuscitative endovascular balloon occlusion of the aorta (REBOA) is utilized in clinical practice by acute care surgeons for temporization of hemorrhage.
- The balloon is used to occlude the aorta at Zone 1 (descending thoracic aorta) for intra-abdominal hemorrhage and all etiologies of cardiac arrest, and at Zone 3 (distal abdominal aorta) for pelvic, junctional, and extremity hemorrhage.
- Clinical data suggest that REBOA is at least as effective as or more effective than emergency department thoracotomy in select patients.
- Clinical data suggest that REBOA increases survival in hypotensive patients compared with no REBOA when used in select centers with significant REBOA experience.

INTRODUCTION

Hemorrhagic shock stands as the predominant cause of death on the battlefield and the second most common cause among civilian trauma patients. The management of hemorrhagic bleeding becomes particularly challenging in cases of truncal injury, where manual pressure application proves ineffective.[1] Traditionally, noncompressible torso hemorrhage below the diaphragm necessitated a resuscitative thoracotomy (RT) with aortic cross-clamping, a highly morbid procedure aimed at preserving perfusion to coronary and cerebral vessels. However, as an alternative for temporarily addressing hemorrhage in such cases, resuscitative endovascular balloon occlusion of the aorta (REBOA) has emerged.[2,3]

REBOA involves the insertion of an endovascular balloon catheter into the aorta through a sheath in the common femoral artery. The balloon is then inflated to occlude the aorta.[4] The use of endoluminal aortic occlusion dates to 1954 when Hughes first applied the technique during the Korean War.[5] Although the initial cases

UCLA Department of Surgery, UCLA David Geffen School of Medicine, 10833 Le Conte Avenue #72, Los Angeles, CA 90024, USA
E-mail address: mbrenner@mednet.ucla.edu

Surg Clin N Am 104 (2024) 311–323
https://doi.org/10.1016/j.suc.2024.01.003
0039-6109/24/© 2024 Elsevier Inc. All rights reserved.
surgical.theclinics.com

resulted in fatalities, this seminal report marked the beginning of intravascular balloon occlusion, initially limited to treating ruptured abdominal aortic aneurysms. Documentation of its application for trauma patients dates to the 1980s in select centers, where interventionalists, not always readily available, utilized larger-profile devices.[6,7]

Advancements in endovascular technology spurred interest in using balloon occlusion for hemorrhage below the diaphragm. Over the past decade, trauma surgeons have been performing REBOA with standardized training platforms, improved technology, and clinical guidelines.[8] Surprisingly, contemporary use of REBOA has not been widely adopted in scenarios such as bleeding during pelvic surgery,[9] hepatobiliary surgery,[10] postpartum hemorrhage,[11,12] gastrointestinal bleeding,[13] and vascular disease-related hemorrhage.[14–16]

The development of a bedside aortic occlusion device arose from the need for a portable and easily deployable solution to address noncompressible hemorrhage in combat settings, where hemorrhagic shock leads to the highest mortality.[1] Civilian and military collaboration has refined the REBOA technique and increased surgical training, prompting guidelines and paradigm shifts in clinical practice.[8]

REBOA has proven to be equivalent or superior to RT in various injury patterns,[17] including traumatic brain injury (TBI),[18] and in select populations as a superior technique for hemorrhage control in hypotensive patients.[19] As a temporizing measure to reduce life-threatening hemorrhage, REBOA offers the potential to provide resuscitative support until definitive care is administered. This additional time may allow for crucial discussions regarding goals of care and obtaining additional imaging, influencing subsequent medical decisions, or permitting organ donation.[20]

According to a 2019 survey of 158 trauma medical directors in the United States, nearly half of the respondents stated that their institutions used REBOA for managing pelvic fractures.[21] Currently, American College of Surgeons (ACS) Level I trauma hospitals in the United States have acquired the 7Fr catheter, as have Level II centers.[22] The Aortic Occlusion for Resuscitation in Trauma and Acute Care Surgery registry, which enrolls patients from 58 hospitals, with 90% being ACS Level I trauma centers,[23] reflects widespread utilization. However, usage patterns vary even within institutions, with some faculty incorporating REBOA into their practice, while others do not. Barriers to implementation range from a lack of Level 1 evidence to a reluctance to adopt new procedures and technology.[24]

THE PROCEDURE

The conventional application of aortic balloon occlusion by vascular surgeons for intra-abdominal hemorrhage involves needle cannulation of the common femoral artery, insertion of a steerable wire under fluoroscopy, and subsequent upsizing and placement of a compliant balloon. Initially, the Coda balloon (Cook Medical) was used in trauma patients for several years before the advent of wire-free balloon catheters, eliminating the need for fluoroscopy. Portable digital radiographs have addressed concerns about inadvertent wire and device misplacement, making them readily available in trauma bays. The impracticality of closure devices in the crowded and hurried atmosphere of the trauma bay led to open surgical repair of arteriotomy due to the large sheath size.

Today's REBOA catheters are wire-free, compatible with 7Fr or 4Fr sheaths, feature an atraumatic tip and compliant balloon marked with proximal and distal radiopaque markers for radiograph visualization. These compact devices prove ideal for emergent aortic balloon occlusion when hemodynamic collapse is imminent or has occurred.

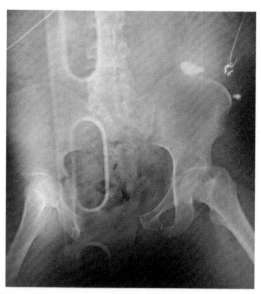

Fig. 1. Portable pelvis radiograph demonstrating severe pelvic fracture with potential for life-threatening hemorrhage. In these patients, consideration for early placement of a sheath in the common femoral artery is recommended for measurement of systemic arterial pressure. If REBOA is needed, insertion of the device is facilitated by the sheath already in place.

Following the primary survey, chest or pelvis x-ray imaging (**Fig. 1**), and focused abdominal sonography for trauma, consideration of balloon occlusion is warranted upon detecting life-threatening hemorrhage below the diaphragm. REBOA is notably faster than emergency department thoracotomy (EDT)[25] when rapid percutaneous cannulation is achieved.

Some trauma centers now place small-bore common femoral arterial lines in all hypotensive patients upon arrival. This facilitates quicker REBOA placement, aligning with at least one clinical algorithm.[26] REBOA should be contemplated for patients with abdominal or pelvic bleeding who transiently respond or do not respond to traditional resuscitation methods. It can be performed in hypotensive patients before arrest, serving as an attractive alternative to EDT.

Balloon occlusion should be performed at the appropriate level (Zone 1 or 3; **Fig. 2**) for stabilization before definitive therapy. Zone 1, from the takeoff of the left subclavian artery to the diaphragm,[4] addresses bleeding below the diaphragm, with limited occlusion times due to compromised blood flow to the viscera, kidneys, and lower extremities. Zone 3, from the renal arteries to the aortic bifurcation, targets pelvic or groin junctional bleeding. Image-guided device placement in the resuscitation area using portable digital x-ray is recommended. External landmarks are utilized for approximate distances, ensuring proper device placement before inflation.

Confirmation of full aortic occlusion involves systolic blood pressure improvement on inflation, measured by upper extremity cuff or radial arterial line, or noting the disappearance of the contralateral femoral pulse. Inflation with a 1:4 contrast and saline ratio aids radiographic visualization. Tactile feedback for inflation may be misleading due to the exceptional compliance of smaller devices, emphasizing the need for thoughtful inflation to prevent overinflation and subsequent complications.[27]

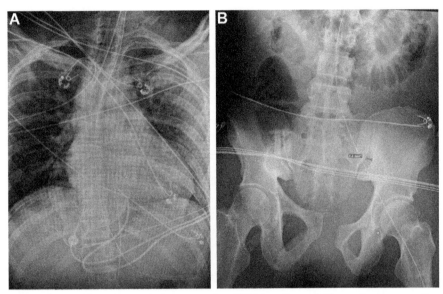

Fig. 2. (*A*) Portable radiograph demonstrating REBOA at Zone 1. The radiopaque markers delineate the compliant balloon. (*B*) Portable radiograph demonstrating the COBRA-OS catheter in the aorta from a sheath in the left common femoral artery.

Sheath placement can be open or percutaneous, with or without ultrasound guidance. Percutaneous cannulation is increasing with experience,[28] but challenges arise in patients without a palpable pulse during cardiac arrest, necessitating an open surgical cutdown if percutaneous methods fail.[25] After balloon occlusion, prompt transportation to the operating room or other care location is crucial for definitive therapy and minimizing ischemia.

Deflating the balloon requires communication with anesthesia colleagues, with slow deflation to mitigate ischemia and reperfusion impact. Specific antidotes to ischemia reperfusion injury are under active investigation.[29,30] Closure devices are technically challenging and require experience to use responsibly[31] thus are not recommended for sheaths of 7Fr or smaller. Postsheath removal, distal neurovascular checks are performed hourly, with ultrasound evaluation of the puncture site within 24 to 48 hours to rule out potential complications.[32]

Successful technical REBOA placement is not necessarily correlated with the physician's skillset, suggesting accessibility to surgeons and nonsurgeons alike.[26,33,34] Training programs are essential, and a consensus guideline recommends that REBOA practitioners be physicians or directly supervised by those completing standardized training programs,[8] ensuring a standardized and safe approach.

RESUSCITATIVE ENDOVASCULAR BALLOON OCCLUSION OF THE AORTA FOR BLUNT INJURY

In patients with blunt abdominal and pelvic injuries presenting without a pulse (in cardiac arrest), REBOA has demonstrated success as a temporizing hemostatic measure. This intervention can be applied without interrupting cardiopulmonary resuscitation, serving as a valuable adjunct to high-quality chest compressions.[35] It is important to note, however, that REBOA does not address cardiac causes of arrest, such as cardiac tamponade, tension hemothorax, or pneumothorax. These potential causes of arrest should be ruled out through diagnostic imaging before deploying the REBOA device.[36]

A clinical algorithm has been developed for patients in arrest to assist in identifying those who could benefit from REBOA.[37] In addition, REBOA has been used in managing blunt abdominal and pelvic injuries in patients with hypotension unresponsive to resuscitative measures.[38] In these cases, the primary goals of resuscitation are to restore and maintain intravascular volume, correct metabolic derangements, and promptly identify and treat hemorrhage.[20,39,40] It may be advisable to exercise caution in using REBOA in settings where these goals are not clearly achievable.[36]

Determining whether there is an intrathoracic contraindication to REBOA in patients with blunt injury poses a challenge. Blunt thoracic aortic injury, although rare, carries a high mortality rate and remains the second most common cause of death among all nonpenetrating traumatic injuries.[41] The mechanism of injury is typically rapid deceleration, resulting in the shearing of the ligamentum arteriosum and traumatic rupture of the aorta.[42] If the primary survey and imaging suggest an intrathoracic location as the source of primary hemorrhage, REBOA use should be avoided. Placing an endovascular balloon distal to a severe thoracic aortic injury may worsen the injury or lead to further decompensation with aortic rupture.[43]

In patients with TBI, REBOA can play a crucial role in hemorrhage control, potentially preventing the deterioration of primary TBI or the development of secondary TBI. One multi-institutional trial has demonstrated the superiority of REBOA over RT in patients with TBI.[17] In some cases, REBOA can serve as a tool to facilitate organ perfusion while awaiting harvest and donation.

RESUSCITATIVE ENDOVASCULAR BALLOON OCCLUSION OF THE AORTA FOR PENETRATING INJURY

Patients presenting with penetrating torso hemorrhage below the diaphragm may be considered candidates for REBOA.[44] In contrast to the more invasive traditional RT, which serves both diagnostic and therapeutic purposes, REBOA provides a less morbid incision for temporizing hemorrhage.[45] Of note, in specific populations, REBOA has demonstrated superiority to RT in terms of overall survival across multiple studies; metrics such as in-hospital survival, survival to discharge, Glasgow Coma Scale score at discharge, and the duration of stays in the intensive care unit and hospital have all been found to be superior for REBOA patients compared with those undergoing RT.[17,39,46]

It is important to exercise caution and adhere to the same considerations regarding the etiology of cardiac arrest or refractory hypotension. If conditions such as massive hemothorax, pneumothorax, or cardiac tamponade are suspected to be the cause of a pulseless or hypotensive state, REBOA placement is not advisable.[36] In addition, penetrating thoracic aortic injury above the diaphragm is considered a relative contraindication. Some specialized centers, with substantial experience in penetrating trauma and REBOA, have successfully utilized REBOA for resuscitation in cases of penetrating thoracic and great vessel trauma.[47] Moreover, these centers have demonstrated a survival benefit in comparison to patients who do not undergo REBOA.[48]

The utilization of REBOA in penetrating trauma is on the rise in the United States, with ongoing efforts to further investigate its effectiveness in this domain.[44] In an initial case series from 2 high-volume REBOA centers, all patients with penetrating injuries who underwent REBOA survived.[49,50] Additional studies have shown that cohorts with penetrating injuries exhibit improved survival outcomes with REBOA compared with traditional RT.[18]

RESUSCITATIVE ENDOVASCULAR BALLOON OCCLUSION OF THE AORTA FOR NONTRAUMATIC HEMORRHAGE

In addition to its applications in trauma, REBOA has been utilized for many years by interventionalists in cases of nontraumatic hemorrhage.[11] The increased adoption and growing expertise of trauma surgeons in using REBOA have expanded the technique's application in various settings dealing with life-threatening hemorrhage.[51] Conventional surgical approaches to stem blood loss in patients with pelvic bleeding involve aortic cross-clamping at the infrarenal level and preperitoneal pelvic packing. Comparative studies between REBOA and preperitoneal packing for pelvic fractures have shown that REBOA yields improved outcomes.[52] Other methods for achieving hemostasis, such as temporary open bilateral common iliac artery ligation, have been found to be less effective than REBOA.[53] It is crucial to recognize that REBOA serves as a temporary measure and a bridge to other hemorrhage control methods.

Nontraumatic hemorrhage encompasses a diverse range of causes and may involve both medical management and conservative treatment, potentially leading to transient periods of stability before necessitating surgical intervention. Moreover, nontraumatic bleeding is often characterized by smaller volume, slower bleeding, and more confined spaces compared with trauma-related bleeding. The open strategies used to control nontraumatic bleeding vary due to the different causes and acuity levels. In certain studies, REBOA has been applied in patients with nontraumatic hemorrhage both before the first incision of exploratory laparotomy and to achieve proximal control in intraoperative hemorrhage among unstable patients.[51] The use of REBOA in postpartum hemorrhage caused by placental disorders is part of a multidisciplinary approach in select centers treating pelvic hemorrhage. Data indicate that prophylactic REBOA use, when compared with patients not receiving REBOA, is associated with reduced blood product transfusions, lower rates of ileus, and shorter hospital stays.[54] A recent meta-analysis also reported a significantly lower risk of lower extremity access complications in patients undergoing REBOA for nontraumatic hemorrhage.[55]

DURATION OF AORTIC OCCLUSION

Securing definitive hemorrhage control with expediency is paramount once aortic occlusion has been achieved. The life-threatening consequences of ischemia below the occlusion level necessitate swift intervention. Recent recommendations from expert consensus guidelines advise limiting full aortic occlusion to less than 30 minutes in Zone 1 and less than 60 minutes in Zone 3.[8] Consequently, undertaking full aortic occlusion should only be considered when the patient is in close proximity to a location where definitive hemostasis can be promptly administered. Although future technologies and partial or intermittent REBOA techniques may potentially alleviate the physiologic burden of ischemia, their significant benefit compared with full occlusion has not been conclusively demonstrated in clinical studies and is discussed further in the subsequent section.[56]

COMPLICATIONS

Systemic complications associated with REBOA arise as consequences of aortic occlusion. Reperfusion following prolonged aortic occlusion may lead to multiple organ failure, encompassing conditions like acute respiratory distress syndrome, acute kidney injury necessitating hemodialysis, and limb ischemia.[43] Rare complications include aortic rupture during balloon overinflation and aortic dissection as a consequence of wire manipulation.[45] Data indicate that these complications occur less frequently in centers with more experience in REBOA placement.[8] Standardized training platforms have been established to instruct trauma surgeons in the safe performance of the technique.[26]

Recognized access complications of REBOA encompass distal embolism resulting in acute limb ischemia, reperfusion injury, and potential lower limb amputation.[45] Studies from the National Trauma Database reveal that mortality and limb loss in REBOA patients cannot be solely attributed to REBOA.[57,58] In a recent meta-analysis, Foley and colleagues reported a significantly increased amputation rate in patients experiencing access-related complications after REBOA placement.[55] Other documented access complications include common femoral artery pseudoaneurysms, intimal flaps, and vessel transection.[59]

In the initial adoption of REBOA by trauma surgeons, only large introducer sheaths (>11Fr) were available for placing balloon catheters. Several studies have demonstrated higher rates of distal embolism with these larger access sheaths compared with smaller ones (7Fr),[60] which have since become widely adopted in US trauma centers. Moreover, while larger access sheaths necessitate open vessel cutdown and repair after removal, hemostasis can be achieved at smaller sheath access sites through manual compression alone.[55]

The incidence of serious ischemic complications underscores the necessity for expertise in REBOA device placement and the presence of vascular surgical expertise to address adverse events if they occur. Detecting subtle perfusion changes, troubleshooting device placement and removal, and managing complications such as device mitigation are not typically covered in most trauma surgery training programs. Therefore, experts in sheath management and those experienced in treating access complications and ischemic events must be available to minimize morbidity and mortality associated with device use.

Managing access complications is further complicated by the critical severity of illness in this patient population. In many cases involving extensive traumatic injury and concern for hemorrhagic shock, traditional strategies for embolic sequelae, such as systemic heparinization, are not suitable. Successful management requires a critical evaluation of the risk and benefit to the patient, considering their overall medical stability alongside subspecialty expert support. Overall, the implementation of REBOA necessitates a multidisciplinary approach before clinical adoption.[61]

TECHNOLOGY

Partial and intermittent REBOA, abbreviated as pREBOA and iREBOA, respectively, represent newer techniques designed to prolong the therapeutic effectiveness of REBOA while simultaneously addressing nontruncal hemorrhage. In the pREBOA technique, an aortic balloon catheter is partially inflated, allowing some distal perfusion while still reducing ongoing hemorrhage. Some animal models indicate that pREBOA is associated with less rebound hypertension and lower serum lactate levels.[62] However, studies in humans do not suggest increased survival in patients with prolonged occlusion who received pREBOA compared with traditional REBOA.[63] It is important to note that the existing body of literature on the use of pREBOA in human subjects is limited and primarily consists of case studies.[64]

Similarly, iREBOA involves cyclical balloon inflation and deflation to allow transient distal flow between aortic occlusions. Like pREBOA, iREBOA has not demonstrated a survival benefit in animal models.[65] In a solid organ injury model, iREBOA was associated with decreased survival compared with standard REBOA.[66] Partial REBOA devices are currently undergoing clinical trials at select centers.[63] These devices, which require a 7Fr introducer sheath, possess the capability to program and transduce blood pressure above and below the balloon occlusion using 2 separate systemic monitoring units.[66] A recently US Food and Drug Administration-approved balloon catheter, compatible with a 4Fr introducer sheath, is now available for clinical use, and suitable for both pREBOA and iREBOA.[67] Future research will focus on these devices and others, aiming to determine their most effective applications in specific populations.

FUTURE DIRECTIONS

REBOA stands out as a promising technique for managing noncompressible truncal hemorrhage in both traumatic and nontraumatic patients. Its resurgence in recent years has triggered heightened research efforts and the development of evolving technology, including pREBOA and iREBOA, aimed at mitigating its known potential complications. As the utilization of REBOA expands and more high-quality data become available, future research will focus on crafting devices designed for an improved safety profile. Additionally, efforts will be directed toward identifying the specific patient populations that can derive the greatest benefits from these tools.

CLINICS CARE POINTS

- REBOA is used as a tool to temporize intra-abdominal and pelvic hemorrhage
- REBOA is used for patients in arrest and those in shock
- REBOA is a skill that is used as an adjunct to resuscitation in trauma and non-trauma patients
- Data suggests REBOA is at least as beneficial, and at times more beneficial for patient outcomes compared to resuscitative thoracotomy and patients hypotensive from hemorrhagic shock
- Complications from REBOA are systemic and access-related
- REBOA should be used in a multi-disciplinary system with experience, efficient time to hemorrhage control, and the ability to monitor and treat complications

---

DISCLOSURE

Dr Brenner is a chapter co-author and receives royalties from UptoDate Inc. She was previously a Clinical Advisory Board Member with Prytime Medical Inc. and received stock options, this relationship ended in 05/2022.

Declaration of AI and AI-assisted technologies in the writing process: During the preparation of this work the author used ChatAI in order to revise an existing chapter written by the same author. After using this tool/service, the author reviewed and edited the content as needed and takes full responsibility for the content of the publication.

REFERENCES

1. Malik A, Rehman FU, Shah KU, et al. Hemostatic strategies for uncontrolled bleeding: A comprehensive update. J Biomed Mater Res B Appl Biomater 2021;109(10):1465–77.
2. Cralley AL, Vigneshwar N, Moore EE, et al. Zone 1 Endovascular Balloon Occlusion of the Aorta vs Resuscitative Thoracotomy for Patient Resuscitation After

Severe Hemorrhagic Shock. JAMA Surg 2022. https://doi.org/10.1001/jamasurg.2022.6393.

3. Castellini G, Gianola S, Biffi A, et al. Resuscitative endovascular balloon occlusion of the aorta (REBOA) in patients with major trauma and uncontrolled haemorrhagic shock: a systematic review with meta-analysis. World J Emerg Surg 2021; 16(1):41.

4. Stannard A, Eliason JL, Rasmussen TE. Resuscitative endovascular balloon occlusion of the aorta (REBOA) as an adjunct for hemorrhagic shock. J Trauma 2011;71(6):1869–72.

5. Hughes C. Use of intra-aortic balloon catheter tamponade for controlling intra-abdominal hemorrhage in man. Surgery 1954;36(1):65–8.

6. Low RB, Longmore W, Rubinstein R, et al. Preliminary report on the use of the Percluder occluding aortic balloon in human beings. Ann Emerg Med 1986;15(12):1466–9.

7. Gupta BK, Khaneja SC, Flores L, et al. The role of intra-aortic balloon occlusion in penetrating abdominal trauma. J Trauma 1989;29(6):861–5.

8. Bulger EM, Perina DG, Qasim Z, et al. Clinical use of resuscitative endovascular balloon occlusion of the aorta (REBOA) in civilian trauma systems in the USA, 2019: a joint statement from the American College of Surgeons Committee on Trauma, the American College of Emergency Physicians, the National Association of Emergency Medical Services Physicians and the National Association of Emergency Medical Technicians. Trauma Surg Acute Care Open 2019;4(1):e000376.

9. Tang X, Guo W, Yang R, et al. Use of aortic balloon occlusion to decrease blood loss during sacral tumor resection. J Bone Joint Surg Am 2010;92(8):1747–53.

10. Matsuoka S, Uchiyama K, Shima H, et al. Temporary percutaneous aortic balloon occlusion to enhance fluid resuscitation prior to definitive embolization of post-traumatic liver hemorrhage. Cardiovasc Intervent Radiol 2001;24(4):274–6.

11. Paull JD, Smith J, Williams L, et al. Balloon occlusion of the abdominal aorta during caesarean hysterectomy for placenta percreta. Anaesth Intensive Care 1995; 23(6):731–4.

12. Sovik E, Stokkeland P, Storm BS, et al. The use of aortic occlusion balloon catheter without fluoroscopy for life-threatening post-partum haemorrhage. Acta Anaesthesiol Scand 2012;56(3):388–93.

13. Sano H, Tsurukiri J, Hoshiai A, et al. Resuscitative endovascular balloon occlusion of the aorta for uncontrollable nonvariceal upper gastrointestinal bleeding. World J Emerg Surg 2016;11:20.

14. Greenberg RK, Srivastava SD, Ouriel K, et al. An endoluminal method of hemorrhage control and repair of ruptured abdominal aortic aneurysms. J Endovasc Ther 2000;7(1):1–7.

15. Malina M, Veith F, Ivancev K, et al. Balloon occlusion of the aorta during endovascular repair of ruptured abdominal aortic aneurysm. J Endovasc Ther 2005;12(5):556–9.

16. Assar AN, Zarins CK. Endovascular proximal control of ruptured abdominal aortic aneurysms: the internal aortic clamp. J Cardiovasc Surg 2009;50(3):381–5.

17. Brenner M, Zakhary B, Coimbra R, et al. Resuscitative endovascular balloon occlusion of the aorta (REBOA) may be superior to resuscitative thoracotomy (RT) in patients with traumatic brain injury (TBI). Trauma Surg Acute Care Open 2022; 7(1):e000715.

18. Brenner M, Zakhary B, Coimbra R, et al. Balloon Rises Above: REBOA at Zone 1 May Be Superior to Resuscitative Thoracotomy. J Am Coll Surg 2023. https://doi.org/10.1097/XCS.0000000000000925.

19. Harfouche MN, Madurska MJ, Elansary N, et al. Resuscitative endovascular balloon occlusion of the aorta associated with improved survival in hemorrhagic shock. PLoS One 2022;17(3):e0265778.

20. Berlin A. Goals of Care and End of Life in the ICU. Surg Clin North Am 2017;97(6): 1275–90.

21. Jarvis S, Kelly M, Mains C, et al. A descriptive survey on the use of resuscitative endovascular balloon occlusion of the aorta (REBOA) for pelvic fractures at US level I trauma centers. Patient Saf Surg 2019;13:43.

22. ER-REBOA PLUS CATHETER Instructions For Use. Updated 28 February 2020, 2023. Available at: https://prytimemedical.com/wp-content/uploads/2020/12/PN-06-7005-Rev-A_ER-REBOA-PLUS-Catheter-IFU-WEB.pdf. Accessed April 4, 2023.

23. Aortic Occlusion for Resuscitation in Trauma and Acute Care Surgery. NIH US National Library of Medicine. Updated 3 March 2022, 2023. Available at: https://clinicaltrials.gov/ct2/show/NCT05263765. Accessed 4 April 2023.

24. Sutherland M, Shepherd A, Kinslow K, et al. REBOA Use, Practices, Characteristics, and Implementations Across Various US Trauma Centers. Am Surg 2022; 88(6):1097–103.

25. Romagnoli A, Teeter W, Pasley J, et al. Time to aortic occlusion: It's all about access. J Trauma Acute Care Surg 2017;83(6):1161–4.

26. Brenner M, Hoehn M, Pasley J, et al. Basic endovascular skills for trauma course: bridging the gap between endovascular techniques and the acute care surgeon. J Trauma Acute Care Surg 2014;77(2):286–91.

27. Meyer DE, Mont MT, Harvin JA, et al. Catheter distances and balloon inflation volumes for the ER-REBOA catheter: A prospective analysis. Am J Surg 2020; 219(1):140–4.

28. Bukur M, Gorman E, DiMaggio C, et al. Temporal Changes in REBOA Utilization Practices are Associated With Increased Survival: an Analysis of the AORTA Registry. Shock 2021;55(1):24–32.

29. Franko JJ, Vu MM, Parsons ME, et al. Adenosine, lidocaine, and magnesium for attenuating ischemia reperfusion injury from resuscitative endovascular balloon occlusion of the aorta in a porcine model. J Trauma Acute Care Surg 2022; 92(4):631–9.

30. Simon MA, Tibbits EM, Hoareau GL, et al. Lower extremity cooling reduces ischemia-reperfusion injury following Zone 3 REBOA in a porcine hemorrhage model. J Trauma Acute Care Surg 2018;85(3):512–8.

31. Saleem TBD. Vascular access closure devices. StatPearls Publishing; 2022. Available at: https://www.ncbi.nlm.nih.gov/books/NBK470233/. Accessed 31 March 2023.

32. Reva VA, Perevedentcev AV, Pochtarnik AA, et al. Ultrasound-guided versus blind vascular access followed by REBOA on board of a medical helicopter in a hemorrhagic ovine model. Injury 2021;52(2):175–81.

33. Hilbert-Carius P, McGreevy D, Abu-Zidan FM, et al, group ABRr. Successfully REBOA performance: does medical specialty matter? International data from the ABOTrauma Registry. World J Emerg Surg 2020;15(1):62.

34. Engberg M, Mikkelsen S, Horer T, et al. Learning insertion of a Resuscitative Endovascular Balloon Occlusion of the Aorta (REBOA) catheter: Is clinical

experience necessary? A prospective trial. Injury 2023. https://doi.org/10.1016/j.injury.2023.02.048.

35. Wasicek PJ, Yang S, Teeter WA, et al. Traumatic cardiac arrest and resuscitative endovascular balloon occlusion of the aorta (REBOA): a preliminary analysis utilizing high fidelity invasive blood pressure recording and videography. Eur J Trauma Emerg Surg 2019;45(6):1097–105.

36. Mill V, Wellme E, Montan C. Trauma patients eligible for resuscitative endovascular balloon occlusion of the aorta (REBOA), a retrospective cohort study. Eur J Trauma Emerg Surg 2021;47(6):1773–8.

37. Brenner M, Moore L, Dubose J, et al. Resuscitative Endovascular Balloon Occlusion of the Aorta (REBOA) for Use in Temporizing Intra-Abdominal and Pelvic Hemorrhage: Physiologic Sequelae and Considerations. Shock 2020;54(5):615–22.

38. Ordonez CA, Parra MW, Caicedo Y, et al. REBOA as a New Damage Control Component in Hemodynamically Unstable Noncompressible Torso Hemorrhage Patients. Colomb Méd 2020;51(4):e4064506.

39. Ogura T, Lefor AT, Nakano M, et al. Nonoperative management of hemodynamically unstable abdominal trauma patients with angioembolization and resuscitative endovascular balloon occlusion of the aorta. J Trauma Acute Care Surg 2015;78(1):132–5.

40. Ordonez CA, Herrera-Escobar JP, Parra MW, et al. A severe traumatic juxtahepatic blunt venous injury. J Trauma Acute Care Surg 2016;80(4):674–6.

41. Mouawad NJ, Paulisin J, Hofmeister S, et al. Blunt thoracic aortic injury - concepts and management. J Cardiothorac Surg 2020;15(1):62.

42. Niranjan N, Samarasinghe P, Di Mascio D, et al. Blunt thoracic aortic injury resulting in free rupture into the pleural space and cardiac arrest, managed successfully with endovascular stenting. BMJ Case Rep 2022;15(3). https://doi.org/10.1136/bcr-2021-248211.

43. Davidson AJ, Russo RM, Reva VA, et al. The pitfalls of resuscitative endovascular balloon occlusion of the aorta: Risk factors and mitigation strategies. J Trauma Acute Care Surg 2018;84(1):192–202.

44. Schellenberg M, Owattanapanich N, DuBose JJ, et al. Resuscitative Endovascular Balloon Occlusion of the Aorta in Penetrating Trauma. J Am Coll Surg 2022;234(5):872–80.

45. Ribeiro Junior MAF, Feng CYD, Nguyen ATM, et al. The complications associated with Resuscitative Endovascular Balloon Occlusion of the Aorta (REBOA). World J Emerg Surg 2018;13:20.

46. Brenner M, Inaba K, Aiolfi A, et al. Resuscitative Endovascular Balloon Occlusion of the Aorta and Resuscitative Thoracotomy in Select Patients with Hemorrhagic Shock: Early Results from the American Association for the Surgery of Trauma's Aortic Occlusion in Resuscitation for Trauma and Acute Care Surgery Registry. J Am Coll Surg 2018;226(5):730–40.

47. Parra MW, Ordonez CA, Pino LF, et al. Damage control surgery for thoracic outlet vascular injuries: the new resuscitative median sternotomy plus REBOA. Colomb Méd 2021;52(2):e4054611.

48. Ordonez CA, Rodriguez F, Parra M, et al. Resuscitative endovascular balloon of the aorta is feasible in penetrating chest trauma with major hemorrhage: Proposal of a new institutional deployment algorithm. J Trauma Acute Care Surg 2020;89(2):311–9.

49. Garcia AF, Manzano-Nunez R, Orlas CP, et al. Association of resuscitative endo-vascular balloon occlusion of the aorta (REBOA) and mortality in penetrating trauma patients. Eur J Trauma Emerg Surg 2021;47(6):1779–85.

50. Brenner M, Moore L, Teeter W, et al. Exclusive clinical experience with a lower profile device for resuscitative endovascular balloon occlusion of the aorta (RE-BOA). Am J Surg 2019;217(6):1126–9.

51. Hoehn MR, Hansraj NZ, Pasley AM, et al. Resuscitative endovascular balloon oc-clusion of the aorta for non-traumatic intra-abdominal hemorrhage. Eur J Trauma Emerg Surg 2019;45(4):713–8.

52. Asmar S, Bible L, Chehab M, et al. Resuscitative Endovascular Balloon Occlusion of the Aorta vs Pre-Peritoneal Packing in Patients with Pelvic Fracture. J Am Coll Surg 2021;232(1):17–26 e2.

53. Riazanova OV, Reva VA, Fox KA, et al. Open versus endovascular REBOA control of blood loss during cesarean delivery in the placenta accreta spectrum: A single-center retrospective case control study. Eur J Obstet Gynecol Reprod Biol 2021;258:23–8.

54. Ioffe YJM, Burruss S, Yao R, et al. When the balloon goes up, blood transfusion goes down: a pilot study of REBOA in placenta accreta spectrum disorders. Trauma Surg Acute Care Open 2021;6(1):e000750.

55. Foley MP, Walsh SR, Doolan N, et al. Systematic Review and Meta-Analysis of Lower Extremity Vascular Complications after Arterial Access for Resuscitative Endovascular Balloon Occlusion of the Aorta (REBOA): An Inevitable Concern? Eur J Vasc Endovasc Surg 2023. https://doi.org/10.1016/j.ejvs.2023.02.

56. Levin SR, Farber A, Burke PA, et al. The majority of major amputations after resus-citative endovascular balloon occlusion of the aorta are associated with pread-mission trauma. J Vasc Surg 2021;74(2):467–76.e4.

57. Linderman GC, Lin W, Becher RD, et al. Increased mortality with resuscitative en-dovascular balloon occlusion of the aorta only mitigated by strong unmeasured confounding: An expanded analysis using the National Trauma Data Bank. J Trauma Acute Care Surg 2021;91(5):790–7.

58. Laverty RB, Treffalls RN, McEntire SE, et al. Life over limb: Arterial access-related limb ischemic complications in 48-hour REBOA survivors. J Trauma Acute Care Surg 2022;92(4):723–8.

59. Matsumura Y, Matsumoto J, Kondo H, et al. Fewer REBOA complications with smaller devices and partial occlusion: evidence from a multicentre registry in Japan. Emerg Med 2017;34(12):793–9.

60. Zakaluzny SA, Beldowicz BC, Salcedo ES, et al. Guidelines for a system-wide multidisciplinary approach to institutional resuscitative endovascular balloon oc-clusion of the aorta implementation. J Trauma Acute Care Surg 2019;86(2):337–43.

61. Russo RM, Neff LP, Lamb CM, et al. Partial Resuscitative Endovascular Balloon Occlusion of the Aorta in Swine Model of Hemorrhagic Shock. J Am Coll Surg 2016;223(2):359–68.

62. Madurska MJ, McLenithan A, Scalea TM, et al. A feasibility study of partial RE-BOA data in a high-volume trauma center. Eur J Trauma Emerg Surg 2022;48(1):299–305.

63. Russo RM, White JM, Baer DG. Partial Resuscitative Endovascular Balloon Oc-clusion of the Aorta: A Systematic Review of the Preclinical and Clinical Literature. J Surg Res 2021;262:101–14.

64. Johnson MA, Hoareau GL, Beyer CA, et al. Not ready for prime time: Intermittent versus partial resuscitative endovascular balloon occlusion of the aorta for

prolonged hemorrhage control in a highly lethal porcine injury model. J Trauma Acute Care Surg 2020;88(2):298–304.

65. Kuckelman J, Derickson M, Barron M, et al. Efficacy of intermittent versus standard resuscitative endovascular balloon occlusion of the aorta in a lethal solid organ injury model. J Trauma Acute Care Surg 2019;87(1):9–17.

66. Kemp MT, Wakam GK, Williams AM, et al. A novel partial resuscitative endovascular balloon aortic occlusion device that can be deployed in zone 1 for more than 2 hours with minimal provider titration. J Trauma Acute Care Surg 2021; 90(3):426–33.

67. Power A, Parekh A, Scallan O, et al. Size matters: first-in-human study of a novel 4 French REBOA device. Trauma Surg Acute Care Open 2021;6(1):e000617.

Management of Head Trauma

Deborah Stein, MD, MPH*, Meaghan Broderick, MD

KEYWORDS

- Traumatic brain injury • Head trauma • Critical care • Coma

KEY POINTS

- Rapid and accurate neurologic examination is essential in the initial evaluation of patients with head trauma.
- Prevention of secondary brain injury (ie, hypoxia and hypotension) is the mainstay of managing patients with traumatic brain injury (TBI).
- Management of intracranial hypertension (ICH) in patients with TBI should follow a tiered approach and incorporate all 3 components of ICH: blood, brain, and cerebrospinal fluid.
- TBI represents a wide-ranging spectrum of conditions, which can have long-lasting physical, social, and economic consequences for patients and their families.

INTRODUCTION AND EPIDEMIOLOGY

Traumatic brain injury (TBI) poses a significant global health challenge with profound implications for individuals, families, and health-care systems. This article aims to provide a comprehensive overview of TBI, covering key aspects such as epidemiology, evaluation and diagnosis, management strategies, prognosis, concussion, and ongoing research. By synthesizing current knowledge and exploring emerging research areas, this review seeks to enhance our understanding and improve clinical practices in the field of TBI.

TBI is defined as a head injury caused by a bump, blow, or jolt to the head or a penetrating injury that disrupts normal brain function and is commonly caused by falls and motor vehicle collisions (MVCs), which account for most cases.[1] Falls represent 51% of TBI cases, making it the primary mechanism, whereas MVCs contribute to 24% of cases. Other mechanisms include motorcycle or bicycle collisions, pedestrian accidents, and assault. Remarkably, 25% of all injury-related deaths involve or are directly caused by TBI, resulting in TBI being the leading cause of death following injury. One-third of TBI-related deaths are the result of suicide, with many of these being caused by firearms.[1,2]

Department of Surgery, R Adams Cowley Shock Trauma Center, 22 South Greene Street, Baltimore, MD 21201, USA
* Corresponding author.
E-mail address: dstein@som.umaryland.edu

Surg Clin N Am 104 (2024) 325–341
https://doi.org/10.1016/j.suc.2023.09.006
surgical.theclinics.com

Age and sex play significant roles in the distribution and impact of TBI. Accidental falls are a leading cause of death in older adults, who are also more likely to require hospitalization. Conversely, MVCs are the primary cause of death among teenagers and young adults. Regarding sex distribution, men are twice as likely to be hospitalized for a TBI as women and have 3 times higher mortality rates. These disparities underscore the specific influence of TBI on the male population.[1,2]

Nonfatal TBIs impose a substantial economic burden on the United States, totaling US$40.6 billion annually. This financial impact encompasses direct medical expenses and the loss of income for patients and their caregivers.[3,4] Additionally, survivors of severe TBI suffer from many long-lasting consequences. Survivors of moderate-to-severe TBI are 50 times more likely to die from seizures, 9 times more likely to die from any infection, and 6 times more likely to die from pneumonia when compared with the general population. Of patients employed before their injury, 55% cannot return to work. Almost one-third of patients who survive a moderate or severe TBI use illicit drugs or abuse alcohol.[5] Recognizing the long-standing consequences of TBI is crucial for policymakers and health-care systems to prioritize prevention, early intervention, and comprehensive care.

EVALUATION AND DIAGNOSIS
Initial Evaluation

The initial examination of a traumatically injured patient begins with the primary survey looking for immediate threats to life. After evaluating the patient's airway, breathing and circulation, disability, or the patient's neurologic status must be rapidly assessed. The key components of the disability examination include the Glasgow Coma Scale (GCS) score, the pupil examination (assessing for size, symmetry, and reactivity), and the motor and sensory examination, evaluating for deficits in all 4 extremities. It is ideal to perform this examination before administering medications that may interfere with the ability to get a reliable examination, such as sedatives or paralytics. The GCS (**Table 1**) is the sum of motor, verbal, and eye subscores and is used to stratify TBIs by severity, with mild TBI ranging from 13 to 15, moderate TBI ranging from 9 to 12, and severe TBI ranging from 3 to 8.[6,7] The Full Outline of Unresponsiveness (FOUR) score is a newer grading system that provides a more detailed evaluation of comatose patients and considers 4 components: eye response, motor response, brainstem reflexes, and patterns of respiration. The FOUR score is advantageous in that it can detect locked-in syndrome and a vegetative state. A patient's FOUR score is inversely related to poor outcomes and in-hospital mortality.[8]

Table 1
Glasgow Coma Scale

	Motor	Verbal	Eyes
6	Follows commands		
5	Localizes	Orientation	
4	Normal flexion	Confused conversation	Spontaneous
3	Abnormal flexion	Inappropriate speech	Verbal stimuli
2	Extensor posturing	Incomprehensible speech	Painful stimuli
1	None	None	None

Data from Teasdale G, Jennett B. Assessment of coma and impaired consciousness. The Lancet. 1974;304(7872):81-84. https://doi.org/10.1016/S0140-6736(7491639-0)

With the maturation of trauma and acute care surgery as a specialty, efforts have been made to determine which patients with TBI can be safely managed by trauma surgeons alone and which patients require neurosurgical consultation. The birain injury guidelines (BIG) criteria (**Table 2**) are prospectively validated guidelines guiding acute care surgeon management of TBI to minimize unneeded hospitalization, repeat head CT, and neurosurgical consultation. It is important to note that a patient must meet all BIG 1 or BIG 2 criteria to be included in those categories. The presence of one or more BIG 3 criteria automatically upgrades the patient to the BIG 3 category and treatment plan.[9]

Imaging

Imaging plays a crucial role in evaluating and managing TBI. The decision to perform an initial imaging study depends on specific criteria. For mild TBI, the Canadian Head CT rule is widely accepted. This rule applies to patients with a GCS of 13 to 15 and excludes patients taking blood thinners or who have had a postinjury seizure. High-risk factors, including failure to reach a GCS score of 15 within 2 hours of injury, suspected open skull fracture, basal skull fracture, recurrent vomiting (>2 episodes), or age older than 65 years, indicate the need for a CT scan. Approximately 32% of patients with these high-risk factors have positive CT findings. Medium-risk factors, including amnesia before impact exceeding 30 minutes or a dangerous mechanism of injury, provide a sensitivity of 98.4% and a specificity of 49.6% for predicting clinically significant brain injury.[10] The American College of Radiology Appropriateness Criteria recommends noncontrasted head CT for all patients with penetrating head trauma and those with moderate (GCS 9–12) or severe (GCS 3–8) blunt TBI.[11]

Table 2
Brain Injury Guidelines

Variables	BIG 1	BIG 2	BIG 3
	Brain Injury Guidelines		
LOC	Yes/No	Yes/No	Yes/No
Neurologic examination	Normal	Normal	Abnormal
Intoxication	No	No/Yes	No/Yes
CAMP (Coumadin, ASA, Motrin, Plavix)	No	No	No
Skull fracture	No	Nondisplaced	Displaced
SDH	≤4 mm	5–7 mm	≥8 mm
EDH	≤4 mm	5–7 mm	≥8 mm
IPH	≤4 mm, 1 location	3–7 mm, 2 locations	≥8 mm, multiple locations
SAH	Trace	Localized	Scattered
IVH	No	No	Yes
Therapeutic plan			
Hospitalization	No, 6 h observation	Yes	Yes
Repeat head CT	No	No	Yes
Neurosurgical consultation	No	No	Yes

Data from Joseph B, Friese RS, Sadoun M, et al. The BIG (brain injury guidelines) project: Defining the management of traumatic brain injury by acute care surgeons. J Trauma Acute Care Surg. 2014;76(4):965-969. https://doi.org/10.1097/TA.0000000000000161

Multiple scoring systems have been developed to prognosticate based on findings on head CT. Two of the most well-known systems are the Marshall and Rotterdam classifications. These scores consider the presence or absence of basal cisterns and midline shift. Additionally, the Rotterdam classification incorporates epidural, intraventricular, and subarachnoid hemorrhages (SAHs), whereas the Marshall classification includes surgical evacuation of the lesion and volumetric assessment of the hemorrhage. These scores have been found to correlate with outcomes in patients with severe TBI, with higher scores portending a worse prognosis.[12]

The role of repeat imaging depends on initial CT findings and changes in mental status. Routine repeat imaging is not recommended for mild TBI because it does not alter management. Instead, the clinical examination should guide decision-making, with repeat head imaging obtained only when there are changes in the patient's clinical status. For moderate TBI with negative initial imaging, repeat imaging should be performed if there are changes in the clinical examination. Routine repeat head CT is recommended for severe TBI, although the optimal timing for such imaging remains unclear. A study by Brown and colleagues reported that routine repeat head CT led to surgical interventions in 2 patients with a GCS score of 8 or lower.[13,14]

MRI is not recommended because the initial imaging modality for TBI. However, it may be helpful in cases with persistent neurologic deficits that CT findings cannot explain. MRI is more sensitive than CT in detecting small intracranial lesions, including shearing injuries such as diffuse axonal injury (DAI) and may also provide valuable prognostic information.[11]

Types of Brain Injury

Epidural hematomas (EDHs) are collections of blood that accumulate between the dura and the inner table of the skull. They often occur associated with skull fractures and arterial injury, most commonly the middle meningeal artery. These lesions typically present as a hyperdense biconvex or lens-shaped mass adjacent to the skull, bounded by suture lines (**Fig. 1**). Classic symptoms of EDH include loss of consciousness followed by a lucid interval. However, without intervention, the lucid interval progresses to a neurologic decline characterized by contralateral hemiparesis, ipsilateral pupillary dilation, and altered mental status. The mortality rate associated with EDHs ranges from 5% to 12%.[15]

However, subdural hematomas (SDHs) are located between the dura and arachnoid mater, resulting from tearing of the bridging veins in the subdural space. Unlike EDHs, SDHs do not conform to suture lines and typically presents as crescent-shaped collections that may layer along the falx or the tentorium (**Fig. 2**). Notably, SDHs are more prevalent in older adults due to cerebral atrophy. In SDH, the underlying brain parenchyma is often injured along with the blood vessels because the shear forces that cause tearing of the venous structures are also applied across the brain parenchyma, leading to worse outcomes than in EDHs of similar size. Mortality rates are higher in older adults and patients receiving preinjury anticoagulation therapy.[15]

SAH originates from tears in small blood vessels within the subarachnoid space between the arachnoid and pia mater. On CT scans, SAH is characterized by diffuse hyperdensities within the gyri. Traumatic SAH tends to be around the cerebral convexity (**Fig. 3**), whereas aneurysmal SAH is more commonly observed within the basal cistern. Although vasospasm of cerebral vessels is a common complication of SAH, it is more frequently observed in cases of nontraumatic aneurysmal SAHs rather than in traumatic SAHs.[15]

Intraparenchymal hemorrhage refers to collections of blood that can occur anywhere within the brain parenchyma (**Fig. 4**). Close monitoring of patients with intraparenchymal

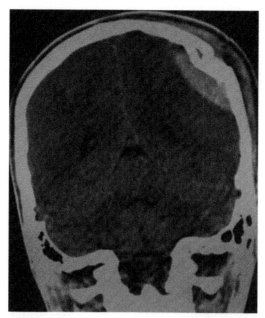

Fig. 1. Epidural hematoma.

hemorrhage is vital due to the potential for rapid expansion of these lesions, leading to swift clinical deterioration. Additionally, perilesional edema can cause significant mass effect, further exacerbating the patient's mental status. Details regarding operative indications for intracranial lesions are discussed in the subsequent management section.[15]

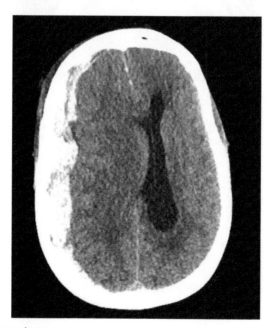

Fig. 2. Subdural hematoma.

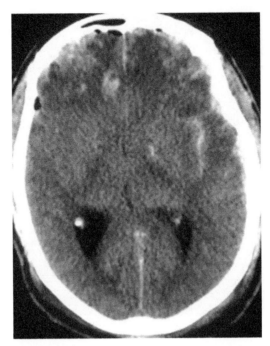

Fig. 3. Subarachnoid hemorrhage.

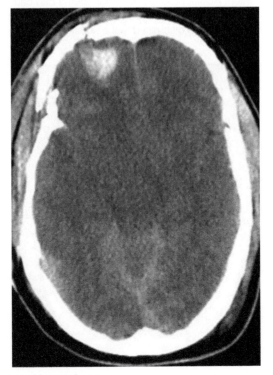

Fig. 4. Intraparenchymal hemorrhage.

DAI is a blunt TBI caused by acceleration-deceleration mechanisms that lead to shearing forces that damage the white matter in the brain. These forces cause damage to the axons at the interface between the gray and white matter. Although the exact incidence of DAI is unknown, approximately 10% of people hospitalized with TBI have some degree of DAI, and about 25% of people with DAI will die. DAI is graded on a scale of 1 to 3 using the Adams DAI classification.

- Grade 1: mild; microscopic changes in the cortex, corpus callosum, and brain stem
- Grade 2: moderate; gross lesions in the corpus callosum
- Grade 3: severe; findings of grade 2, plus additional lesions in the brainstem

DAI is a clinical diagnosis, often considered when a patient remains with a GCS less than 8 for more than 6 hours. It can be suggested on CT with microhemorrhages in the white matter but MRI is the imaging modality most used to make the diagnosis. DAI is associated with a poor prognosis.[16]

These injuries can occur in isolation but also in combination due to a single traumatic event.

Biomarkers

Biomarkers are currently under investigation to aid in diagnosing and prognosis of TBI due to its heterogeneous nature. An ideal biomarker should possess specific characteristics. First, it should be released into accessible body fluids in response to head trauma. Additionally, the biomarker must demonstrate a significant increase in patients with TBI compared with healthy controls. It should also correlate quantitatively and qualitatively with injury severity, aligning with other diagnostic tools such as CT, MRI, and the GCS. The most commonly discussed biomarkers are summarized in **Table 3**.[17,18]

MANAGEMENT

Prevention of secondary injury is crucial in managing patients with TBIs. Secondary injuries encompass insults after the initial traumatic event, including hypoxemia, ischemia, seizures, fever, and hypoglycemia.[15] Studies have shown that a single episode of hypotension or hypoxemia independently predicts worse outcomes following TBI.[19,20] Therefore, prehospital and emergency department providers should aim to maintain oxygenation, which may involve intubation if necessary, and to maintain normotension, defined by the Brain Trauma Foundation as systolic blood pressure greater than 110 mm Hg in adults.[15,21]

Tranexamic acid (TXA) has been investigated as a potential treatment of TBI, and there is no consensus in the literature. In a multicenter, international, randomized controlled trial, patients with moderate or severe TBI (GCS 3–12) or positive imaging without evidence of extracranial hemorrhage were randomized to receive either placebo or TXA if they reached treatment within 3 hours of injury. The group receiving TXA demonstrated lower head-injury-related mortality without an increase in thromboembolic events.[22] A multicenter, prospective trial in Europe demonstrated higher rates of 30-day mortality in patients with isolated TBI who received TXA than those who did not.[23] Finally, a randomized controlled trial comparing prehospital TXA administration with placebo administration demonstrated no difference in the proportion of patients having favorable neurologic outcomes at 6 months between the medication and placebo groups. Further studies are required to determine which, if any, subset of patients with TBI will derive the most benefit from TXA administration.[24]

Table 3
Biomarkers in traumatic brain injury

Biomarker	Location	Information
Neuron-specific enolase	Neuron cytoplasm	• Peaks within 12 h of injury • Persistent elevation associated with poor outcomes • Also found in RBCs, can have elevation of levels with hemolysis
Ubiquitin C-terminal hydrolase-L1	Neuron cytoplasm	• Levels increase in blood and CSF within 6–24 h • Levels correlate w/injury severity and outcomes
Glial fibrillary acidic protein (GFAP)	Astroglial cells	• Levels increase related to trauma or other insults • Positive correlation between GFAP levels and injury severity
S100-B	Astroglial cells	• Released in response to brain trauma or ischemia • Can predict postconcussive syndrome • Also released from cardiac and skeletal muscle, as well as adipose tissue
Neurofilament proteins	Neuron axon	• Specific to neurons and axons • May have predictive value for long-term effects of TBI
Myelin basic protein	Neuron axon	• Released in response to axonal damage • Delayed release: 1–3 d postinjury • Association between levels and mortality risk
Tau protein	Neuron axon	• CSF levels are more diagnostic and prognostic than serum levels • Unclear correlation between levels and CT lesions or postconcussive syndrome

Data from Ghaith HS, Nawar AA, Gabra MD, et al. A Literature Review of Traumatic Brain Injury Biomarkers. Mol Neurobiol. 2022;59(7):4141-4158. https://doi.org/10.1007/s12035-022-02822-6 and Dadas A, Washington J, Diaz-Arrastia R, Janigro D. Biomarkers in traumatic brain injury (TBI): a review. Neuropsychiatr Dis Treat. 2018;Volume 14:2989-3000. https://doi.org/10.2147/NDT.S125620

Hyperventilation has historically been used to reduce intracranial pressure (ICP) by lowering cerebral blood flow and the risk of cerebral hyperemia.[25–27] However, recent data indicate cerebral ischemia is more common than cerebral hyperemia. Consequently, prolonged hyperventilation aiming for a $Paco_2$ of 25 mm Hg or lower is no longer recommended without signs of herniation.[28–32] Hyperventilation can still be used temporarily as a rescue strategy to decrease ICP in cases of impending herniation or active herniation.[32]

Monitoring plays a vital role in managing TBIs, particularly ICP and cerebral perfusion pressure (CPP). According to the Monroe-Kellie doctrine, the intracranial volume occupied by the brain, cerebrospinal fluid (CSF), and intravascular blood is fixed. Any increase in one component or addition of a new component, that is, extravascular blood, results in compensatory decreases in the other components to maintain a constant ICP. Elevated pressure can lead to local tissue compression, shifting of intracranial structures, herniation, and neurologic dysfunction. Transtentorial herniation, the most severe consequence, compresses the brainstem, causing tissue damage, arterial occlusion, cerebral infarction, and potentially death.[15] Normal ICP levels for adults and older children range from 10 to 15 mm Hg, and sustained levels greater than 20 mm Hg are associated with worse outcomes and increased mortality.[33] The Brain

Trauma Foundation recommends treatment of ICP levels equal to or greater than 22 mm Hg.[32]

Determining which patients require ICP monitoring is essential. The Brain Trauma Foundation recommends that salvageable patients with a GCS score between 3 and 8 and a positive CT scan indicating hematoma, contusion, swelling, herniation, or compressed basal cisterns should receive ICP monitoring. There is also a suggestion that patients with a GCS score between 3 and 8, a normal CT scan, and 2 or more of the following criteria should also undergo ICP monitoring[19].

- Age older than 40 years
- Unilateral or bilateral motor posturing
- Systolic blood pressure less than 90 mm Hg

These recommendations have been called into question due to conflicting literature on the benefit of ICP monitoring. Chesnut and colleagues demonstrated no benefit to care incorporating ICP monitoring compared with care focused on imaging and clinical examination alone.[34] However, 2 additional multicenter trials have demonstrated mortality benefit in patients with severe TBI that undergo ICP monitoring.[35,36] CPP is another critical parameter to monitor in severe TBI cases. CPP is calculated by subtracting ICP from mean arterial pressure. Guideline-based management strategies recommend CPP monitoring for all patients with severe TBI, with a goal CPP of 60 mm Hg to 70 mm Hg.[19]

Ongoing investigations explore advanced monitoring techniques to improve TBI outcomes. The multicenter BOOST-3 trial aims to determine whether adding brain tissue oxygenation monitoring to traditional ICP monitoring can prevent secondary injury and improve outcomes. This trial will provide valuable insights into the potential benefits of advanced monitoring techniques in TBI management.[37]

Managing ICP in TBI involves multiple strategies, targeting each intracranial component: blood, brain, and CSF. Sedation and analgesia are crucial to address pain, agitation, and stress, which can increase ICP and metabolic demand. Balancing the benefits with potential side effects such as hypotension, alteration in the neurologic examination, and rebound hypertension on medication discontinuation is important, favoring shorter acting agents that allow for frequent neurologic assessments and using continuous infusions over bolus dosing. Fentanyl, midazolam, and propofol are commonly used medications.[15]

Maintaining normothermia through targeted temperature management is another aspect of TBI management. Hyperthermia can harm the injured brain for various reasons, including increased excitatory amino acids, oxygen free radicals, enzyme inhibition, blood–brain barrier breakdown, and ischemia. The goal is to maintain normothermia between 36°C and 37°C because fever in the early postinjury period is associated with worse outcomes. Although hypothermia lacks significant benefits and may cause harm, temperature management within the desired range is vital.[38]

In cases of refractory elevated ICP, barbiturate coma may be considered. Barbiturates control ICP by reducing movement, coughing, fighting against endotracheal tube placement, decreasing cerebral metabolism, and augmenting cerebral vascular tone.[39,40] Barbiturate coma should be reserved as a treatment option when other measures fail, and the focus should remain on maintaining hemodynamic stability through adequate fluid resuscitation and the availability of vasopressors.[32]

Hyperosmolar therapy is critical to managing ICP in patients with TBI. The mainstays of hyperosmolar therapy are mannitol and hypertonic saline. Empiric hyperosmolar therapy should only be administered without measurement of ICP in cases of herniation or neurologic deterioration when extracranial causes have been ruled out.[32] Mannitol creates an osmotic gradient that draws fluid out of brain parenchyma, thereby reducing ICP. However, monitoring the patient's fluid status is a necessity because mannitol can cause hypotension due to fluid shifts. Additionally, mannitol can lead to acute tubular necrosis in patients with chronic kidney disease or when combined with other nephrotoxic agents. Raising serum osmolality greater than 320 mOsm/L should be avoided.[15] Hypertonic saline, such as mannitol, creates a pressure gradient across the blood–brain barrier and draws fluid out of the brain parenchyma. It also serves as a resuscitative fluid due to its volume-expanding properties. The target sodium level commonly ranges from 145 to 160 mEq/L. Serum sodium levels must be monitored serially, especially when sodium is elevated rapidly because patients with chronic hyponatremia are at risk for central pontine myelinolysis.[15]

The final nonsurgical option for managing intracranial hypertension is CSF drainage. This is often done with an external ventricular drain (EVD), which serves the dual purpose of monitoring ICP and allowing for CSF drainage. The placement of an EVD zeroed at the midbrain with continuous CSF drainage is more effective at lowering ICP than intermittent drainage.[32] This approach is based on the Monroe-Kellie doctrine as described above.

In patients with intracranial hemorrhage, operative evacuation plays a vital role in specific types of lesions. The decision to perform evacuation depends on the volume of the hemorrhage, the degree of midline shift, the patient's mental status, and the ICP. EDHs greater than 30 mL in volume require operative evacuation, regardless of the patient's GCS. EDHs smaller than 30 mL may be managed nonoperatively if all of the following conditions are met: hematoma thickness less than 15 mm, midline shift less than 5 mm, GCS greater than 8, and absence of focal deficit. Regarding SDH, all patients with hematomas greater than 10 mm thick or with greater than 5 mm of midline shift should undergo evacuation, irrespective of GCS. Additional indications for evacuation of SDH include the following:

- GCS less than 9;
- Decrease in GCS by 2 or more points between the time of injury and hospital admission;
- Asymmetric or fixed and dilated pupils; and
- ICP greater than 20 mm Hg.

The last type of injury that may require operative intervention is intraparenchymal hemorrhage. All IPH greater than 50 mL in volume should be treated operatively. Additionally, patients with progressive neurologic decline attributable to the IPH, signs of mass effect on CT scan, and patients with intracranial hypertension refractory to medical management would benefit from evacuation. Finally, patients with GCS 6 to 8 with frontal or temporal contusions greater than 20 mL in volume who also have 5 mm or greater of midline shift or compression of the cisterns are candidates for surgical management.

Decompressive craniectomy (DC) is another operative approach to managing refractory intracranial hypertension. The DECRA (Decompressive Craniectomy in Diffuse Traumatic Brain Injury) study, a randomized controlled trial, compared DC with medical management in severe diffuse TBI cases. The study revealed that the DC group required fewer interventions for elevated ICP, had less time spent with elevated ICP, and experienced shorter lengths of hospital stay. However, the DC group had a higher risk of unfavorable outcomes, and DC did not improve mortality risk at 6 months compared with medical therapy. The protocol applied in this study was atypical, as was the surgical procedure. Additionally, there were issues with randomization. Another randomized controlled trial, RESCUEicp (Randomised Evaluation of Surgery with Craniectomy for Uncontrollable Elevation of Intracranial Pressure), assessed DC versus medical management in patients with refractory intracranial hypertension following TBI using a more typical definition of refractory intracranial hypertension. The study found that DC was associated with lower mortality rates but higher rates of poor neurologic outcomes as measured by the Glasgow Outcome Scale Extended in survivors. However, there was no significant difference in rates of moderate disability or good recovery between the DC and medical management groups.

Management of intracranial hypertension should follow a tiered approach, starting with the least invasive measures and progressing to more invasive or risky maneuvers. First-tier therapies include adequate analgesia and sedation, maintenance of normocarbia, administration of hyperosmolar agents, and CSF drainage when an EVD is in place. Should these measures be inadequate to control ICP, mild permissive hypocapnia with $Paco_2$ of 32 to 35 mm Hg, neuromuscular blockade, and elevation of CPP with fluids, vasopressors, or inotropes are the next steps. The final tier of therapy involves the most invasive measures, including DC, barbiturate coma, and active cooling to 35°C to 36°C.[41]

Posttraumatic seizures (PTS) can be classified into 3 categories: early seizures (occurring within 7 days), late seizures (occurring after 7 days), and posttraumatic epilepsy (characterized by persistent seizures beyond 7 days).[42] Several risk factors have been identified for early PTS, including a GCS score of 10 or lower, immediate seizures, posttraumatic amnesia lasting 30 minutes or longer, skull fractures, penetrating head injury, and various types of intracranial hemorrhage or contusion. Risk factors for posttraumatic epilepsy include severe TBI with early seizures before discharge, acute intracranial hemorrhage or cortical contusion, prolonged posttraumatic amnesia, age older than 65 years, and a history of depression.[43]

Phenytoin is effective as prophylaxis against early PTS, as supported by studies.[32] As newer antiepileptics emerge, they have become increasingly popular for seizure prophylaxis in patients with TBI. A 2013 study comparing phenytoin and levetiracetam found no significant difference in seizure rates, adverse drug reactions, complications, or mortality between phenytoin and levetiracetam. It is important to note that only a small percentage of patients in this study met the criteria for severe TBI.[44] Levetiracetam may offer potential advantages over phenytoin, such as not requiring therapeutic drug monitoring. The choice of medication for seizure prophylaxis should be based on individual patient factors, medication availability, and cost considerations.[45]

Paroxysmal sympathetic hyperactivity (PSH) is a syndrome observed in a subgroup of individuals who have experienced severe acquired brain injury. It is characterized by simultaneous, paroxysmal transient increases in sympathetic (elevated heart rate, blood pressure, respiratory rate, temperature, sweating) and motor (posturing) activity. The diagnosis can be made at any point during TBI, and the duration of symptoms can vary. The reported prevalence of PSH among TBI patients ranges from 6% to 33% in different studies. Although no precise data suggests that PSH is associated with worse outcomes, anecdotal evidence suggests that it may have a negative impact. The exact underlying pathophysiology of PSH is unknown. However, the prevailing theory suggests a loss of descending inhibition and altered perception of stimuli, leading to an exaggerated sympathetic and motor response.[46,47]

The treatment goals for PSH are to minimize triggers of paroxysms, reduce excessive sympathetic outflow, and address the effects of PSH on other organ systems. Multiple medications from different classes are often required. The main classes of medications used for PSH include opioids, benzodiazepines, nonselective β-blockers, α2 agonists, and GABA agonists. Each medication class has its proposed mechanism of action, specific symptoms it targets, and relevant side effects. Treatment of PSH should be individualized, and the choice of medication depends on the patient's clinical presentation and response to therapy.[46,47]

An increasing number of patients presenting to the trauma bay are taking anticoagulants or antiplatelet agents, which can complicate TBI. A meta-analysis comparing patients who take antiplatelet agents with those who do not showed no difference in mortality, neurosurgical intervention, or length of stay between the 2 groups. This meta-analysis did not analyze the effects of individual antiplatelet agents and focused on patients being treated with antiplatelets as a single group.[48] This is significant because data examining specific antiplatelets suggest that aspirin does not portend worse outcomes but that clopidogrel increases the risk of progression of lesions or need for neurosurgical intervention.[49,50] A multicenter trial also demonstrated an increased mortality risk in patients taking oral anticoagulants and sustaining a TBI.[51] Given this information, it is essential to identify and correct coagulopathy in patients with TBI, regardless of the cause.

ADJUNCTS

Given the significant morbidity and mortality associated with TBI, various adjuncts have been proposed to supplement current treatment strategies. Steroids have garnered interest in TBI but their use, specifically methylprednisolone, has been associated with an increased risk of death or disability within the first 2 weeks after injury, as demonstrated in a randomized controlled trial.[52] This risk persists at 6 months,[53] leading the Brain Trauma Foundation to recommend against their use in TBI.[32]

Beta-blockers have also been considered adjuncts in severe TBI management. The Eastern Association for the Surgery of Trauma Practice Management Guidelines conditionally recommends inpatient beta-blocker usage for patients with severe TBI. However, further research is needed to determine the optimal timing, duration, medication selection, dose, and titration of beta-blockers concerning heart rate or blood pressure.[54] Recent prospective randomized controlled trials have shown potential benefits of initiating 20 mg propranolol twice daily at 24 hours postinjury in hemodynamically stable patients, resulting in improved in-hospital mortality and long-term functional outcomes as measured by the GOSC-E at 6 months postinjury.[55]

Amantadine and modafinil have been investigated for their potential to improve cognitive impairment in patients with TBI. Amantadine has demonstrated the ability to accelerate recovery based on the Disability Rating Scale but does not provide a benefit in terms of recovery endpoint at 6 months.[56] Modafinil, a medication commonly used for narcolepsy, has been evaluated for TBI-related chronic cognitive impairment. However, a Cochrane review found insufficient evidence to support its use in improving chronic cognitive impairment. No significant global improvement was observed with modafinil compared with placebo.[57] The mechanism of action of these medications remains unclear.

Explorations into nonpharmacologic treatments of TBI are also underway. Additionally, a phase 3 clinical trial is currently evaluating the use of hyperbaric oxygen therapy in TBI.[58]

MILD TRAUMATIC BRAIN INJURY/CONCUSSION

Mild traumatic brain injury (mTBI), or concussion, comprises 75% of all TBIs and imposes an annual cost of US$17 billion in the United States.[59] According to the Centers for Disease Control and Prevention, an mTBI is a head injury caused by blunt trauma or forces of acceleration or deceleration. To diagnose mTBI, patients must exhibit one or more of the following conditions due to the head trauma.

- Transient confusion, disorientation, or impaired consciousness;
- Amnesia around the time of injury;
- Observed signs of other neurologic dysfunction, such as seizures in adults or irritability, lethargy, or vomiting in infants or young children; and
- Observed or self-reported loss of consciousness lasting 30 minutes or lesser.

Although symptoms such as headache, dizziness, irritability, fatigue, or poor concentration may be present in adults or older children, they are not sufficient for an mTBI diagnosis in the absence of loss or alteration of consciousness.[60] Other common symptoms include nausea/vomiting, vertigo, balance or coordination issues, anxiety, or depression. CT scans are typically normal, although MRI may show structural abnormality in approximately 25% of cases.[15]

Two clinically important syndromes can profoundly influence patients who have suffered from mTBI. Second impact syndrome is a dangerous condition that occurs when a patient sustains a second concussion while recovering from a previous one. This concussion further damages an already compromised brain, leading to rapid neurologic deterioration, herniation, and potentially fatal consequences.[15] The second entity is postconcussive syndrome, characterized by symptoms persisting beyond 3 months after injury. Risk factors for developing postconcussive syndrome include being female, experiencing multiple TBIs, older age, a history of psychiatric disorders, and chronic pain syndrome.[59] Even patients who do not meet the criteria for these syndromes may still experience deficits that limit their ability to return to work or resume their normal activities.[60] Consequently, a gradual return to function is recommended for individuals with mTBI to facilitate their recovery.[61]

PROGNOSIS

Prognostication for patients who have sustained a TBI remains challenging for clinicians. There are a variety of factors that portend a poor prognosis, including bilaterally dilated pupils, absent pupillary light, oculocephalic or oculovestibular reflexes, Injury Severity Score greater than 40, age greater than 60 years or less than 2, hypotension, hypoxemia, persistently elevated ICP, ICP elevation within first 24 hours, presence of apolipoprotein E4 allele, GCS 8 or lesser, and abnormal imaging.[62–64] Despite knowledge regarding these prognostic indicators, the ability of a clinician to predict outcomes in a patient with a TBI is "still often unduly optimistic, unnecessarily pessimistic, or inappropriately ambiguous."[64] Current research, especially in biomarkers and imaging modalities, aims to improve our ability to accurately predict outcomes in this patient population.[62–64]

CURRENT RESEARCH

Ongoing research in TBI has been focused on expanding our understanding of the underlying mechanisms and developing novel interventions for improved patient outcomes. One prominent area of active investigation involves the role of neuroinflammation in TBI pathogenesis. Researchers are exploring the complex interplay between immune cells, glial cells, and neuronal responses after injury, aiming to identify key molecular targets that could be manipulated to reduce neuroinflammatory processes and mitigate secondary brain damage. Furthermore, advancements in neuroimaging techniques have allowed for more precise characterization of TBI-related structural and functional alterations in the brain. Integration of advanced imaging modalities with biomarker analysis holds promise for enhancing diagnostic accuracy, prognostication, and treatment monitoring in patients with TBI. Additionally, there is increasing emphasis on personalized medicine approaches, with studies investigating the genetic and epigenetic factors influencing TBI susceptibility, severity, and recovery trajectories. By unraveling the complex mechanisms and individual variability associated with TBI, ongoing research endeavors aim to pave the way for targeted therapies and interventions tailored to the unique needs of patients with TBI.

CLINICS CARE POINTS

- The Brain Injury Guidelines are a validated set of criteria that indicate when a patient with a TBI can be safely managed by the acute care surgeon, and when specialty neurosurgical consultation is recommended.

- Prevention of secondary insults is crucial when managing TBI. Patients should be maintained within normal physiologic parameters: normoxia, normothermia, and normotension.

- A tiered approach to managing intracranial hypertension should incorporate modalities that affect intracranial blood volume, cerebral edema, and CSF volume.

- Steroids should not be used in the treatment of TBI because these have been shown to worsen outcomes.

- Patients taking anticoagulants or antiplatelet agents with intracranial hemorrhage should have their coagulopathy reversed promptly to avoid worsened bleeding.

DISCLOSURES

Deborah Stein and Meaghan Broderick has no disclosures to report.

REFERENCES

1. SURVEILLANCE REPORT. Published online 2018.
2. Peterson AB, Thomas KE. Incidence of Nonfatal Traumatic Brain Injury–Related Hospitalizations — United States, 2018. MMWR Morb Mortal Wkly Rep 2021; 70(48):1664–8.
3. Miller GF, DePadilla L, Xu L. Costs of nonfatal traumatic brain injury in the United States, 2016. Med Care 2021;59(5):451–5.
4. Asmamaw Y, Yitayal M, Debie A, et al. The costs of traumatic head injury and associated factors at University of Gondar Specialized Referral Hospital, Northwest Ethiopia. BMC Publ Health 2019;19(1):1399.
5. Potential Effects of a Moderate or Severe TBI | Concussion | Traumatic Brain Injury | CDC Injury Center. Published April 10, 2023 Available at: https://www.cdc.gov/traumaticbraininjury/moderate-severe/potential-effects.html. Accessed June 10, 2023.
6. Teasdale G, Jennett B. Assessment of coma and impaired consciousness. Lancet 1974;304(7872):81–4.
7. Advanced trauma life support: student course manual. Tenth edition. American College of Surgeons; 2018.
8. Wijdicks EFM, Bamlet WR, Maramattom BV, et al. Validation of a new coma scale: The FOUR score. Ann Neurol 2005;58(4):585–93.
9. Joseph B, Friese RS, Sadoun M, et al. The BIG (brain injury guidelines) project: Defining the management of traumatic brain injury by acute care surgeons. J Trauma Acute Care Surg 2014;76(4):965–9.
10. Stiell IG, Wells GA, Vandemheen K, et al. The Canadian CT Head Rule for patients with minor head injury. Lancet Lond Engl 2001;357(9266):1391–6.

11. Shih RY, Burns J, Ajam AA, et al. ACR Appropriateness Criteria® Head Trauma: 2021 Update. J Am Coll Radiol 2021;18(5):S13–36.
12. Elkbuli A, Shaikh S, McKenney K, et al. Utility of the Marshall & Rotterdam Classification Scores in Predicting Outcomes in Trauma Patients. J Surg Res 2021; 264:194–8.
13. Rosen CB, Luy DD, Deane MR, et al. Routine repeat head CT may not be necessary for patients with mild TBI. Trauma Surg Acute Care Open 2018;3(1):e000129.
14. Brown CVR, Zada G, Salim A, et al. Indications for routine repeat head computed tomography (CT) stratified by severity of traumatic brain injury. J Trauma Inj Infect Crit Care 2007;62(6):1339–45.
15. Yang L, Opalak CF, Valadka AB. Brain. In: Feliciano DV, Mattox KL, Moore EE, editors. Trauma. Ninth edition. McGraw-Hill; 2021. p. 457–78.
16. Mesfin FB, Gupta N, Hays Shapshak A, Taylor RS. Diffuse Axonal Injury. In: StatPearls. StatPearls Publishing; 2023 http://www.ncbi.nlm.nih.gov/books/NBK44 8102/. Accessed June 10, 2023.
17. Ghaith HS, Nawar AA, Gabra MD, et al. A literature review of traumatic brain injury biomarkers. Mol Neurobiol 2022;59(7):4141–58.
18. Dadas A, Washington J, Diaz-Arrastia R, et al. Biomarkers in traumatic brain injury (TBI): a review. Neuropsychiatric Dis Treat 2018;14:2989–3000.
19. McHugh GS, Engel DC, Butcher I, et al. Prognostic value of secondary insults in traumatic brain injury: results from the IMPACT study. J Neurotrauma 2007;24(2): 287–93.
20. Chesnut RM, Marshall LF, Klauber MR, et al. The role of secondary brain injury in determining outcome from severe head injury. J Trauma 1993;34(2):216–22.
21. Lulla A, Lumba-Brown A, Totten AM, et al. Pre-hospital guidelines for the management of traumatic brain injury – 3rd Edition. Prehosp Emerg Care 2023;1–32.
22. Effects of tranexamic acid on death, disability, vascular occlusive events and other morbidities in patients with acute traumatic brain injury (CRASH-3): a randomised, placebo-controlled trial. Lancet 2019;394(10210):1713–23.
23. Bossers SM, Loer SA, Bloemers FW, et al. Association between pre-hospital tranexamic acid administration and outcomes of severe traumatic brain injury. JAMA Neurol 2021;78(3):338–45.
24. Rowell SE, Meier EN, McKnight B, et al. Effect of out-of-hospital tranexamic acid vs placebo on 6-month functional neurologic outcomes in patients with moderate or severe traumatic brain injury. JAMA 2020;324(10):961–74.
25. Bouma GJ, Muizelaar JP. Cerebral blood flow, cerebral blood volume, and cerebrovascular reactivity after severe head injury. J Neurotrauma 1992;9(Suppl 1): S333–48.
26. Bouma GJ, Muizelaar JP. Cerebral blood flow in severe clinical head injury. New Horiz Baltim Md 1995;3(3):384–94.
27. Muizelaar JP, Marmarou A, DeSalles AA, et al. Cerebral blood flow and metabolism in severely head-injured children. Part 1: Relationship with GCS score, outcome, ICP, and PVI. J Neurosurg 1989;71(1):63–71.
28. Tawil I, Stein DM, Mirvis SE, et al. Post-traumatic cerebral infarction: incidence, outcome, and risk factors. J Trauma 2008;64(4):849–53.
29. Liu S, Wan X, Wang S, et al. Post-traumatic cerebral infarction in severe traumatic brain injury: characteristics, risk factors and potential mechanisms. Acta Neurochir 2015;157(10):1697–704.
30. Stein NR, McArthur DL, Etchepare M, et al. Early cerebral metabolic crisis after TBI influences outcome despite adequate hemodynamic resuscitation. Neurocritical Care 2012;17(1):49–57.

31. Carrera E, Schmidt JM, Fernandez L, et al. Spontaneous hyperventilation and brain tissue hypoxia in patients with severe brain injury. J Neurol Neurosurg Psychiatry 2010;81(7):793–7.

32. Carney N, Totten AM, O'Reilly C, et al. Guidelines for the Management of Severe Traumatic Brain Injury, Fourth Edition. Neurosurgery. 2017;80(1):6-15. doi.

33. Juul N, Morris GF, Marshall SB, et al. Intracranial hypertension and cerebral perfusion pressure: influence on neurological deterioration and outcome in severe head injury. The Executive Committee of the International Selfotel Trial. J Neurosurg 2000;92(1):1–6.

34. Chesnut RM, Temkin N, Carney N, et al. A trial of intracranial-pressure monitoring in traumatic brain injury. N Engl J Med 2012;367(26):2471–81.

35. Gerber LM, Chiu YL, Carney N, et al. Marked reduction in mortality in patients with severe traumatic brain injury. J Neurosurg 2013;119(6):1583–90.

36. Farahvar A, Gerber LM, Chiu YL, et al. Increased mortality in patients with severe traumatic brain injury treated without intracranial pressure monitoring. J Neurosurg 2012;117(4):729–34.

37. Bernard F, Barsan W, Diaz-Arrastia R, et al. Brain Oxygen Optimization in Severe Traumatic Brain Injury (BOOST-3): a multicentre, randomised, blinded-endpoint, comparative effectiveness study of brain tissue oxygen and intracranial pressure monitoring versus intracranial pressure alone. BMJ Open 2022;12(3):e060188.

38. Godoy DA, Murillo-Cabezas F, Suarez JI, et al. "THE MANTLE" bundle for minimizing cerebral hypoxia in severe traumatic brain injury. Crit Care 2023;27(1):13.

39. Mellion SA, Bennett KS, Ellsworth GL, et al. High-dose barbiturates for refractory intracranial hypertension in children with severe traumatic brain injury. Pediatr Crit Care Med J Soc Crit Care Med World Fed Pediatr Intensive Crit Care Soc 2013; 14(3):239–47.

40. Roberts I, Sydenham E. Barbiturates for acute traumatic brain injury. Cochrane Database Syst Rev 2012;12(12):CD000033.

41. Hawryluk GWJ, Aguilera S, Buki A, et al. A management algorithm for patients with intracranial pressure monitoring: the Seattle International Severe Traumatic Brain Injury Consensus Conference (SIBICC). Intensive Care Med 2019;45(12): 1783–94.

42. Carney N, Totten AM, O'Reilly C, et al. Guidelines for the Management of Severe Traumatic Brain Injury. Brain Trauma Foundation https://static1.squarespace. com/static/63e696a90a26c23e4c021cee/t/640b5e97fa1baa040e5c59af/167846 6712870/Management_of_Severe_TBI_4th_Edition.pdf.

43. Torbic H, Forni AA, Anger KE, et al. Use of anti-epileptics for seizure prophylaxis after traumatic brain injury. Am J Health-Syst Pharm AJHP Off J Am Soc Health-Syst Pharm. 2013;70(9):759–66.

44. Inaba K, Menaker J, Branco BC, et al. A prospective multicenter comparison of levetiracetam versus phenytoin for early post-traumatic seizure prophylaxis. J Trauma Acute Care Surg 2013;74(3):766–71 [discussion: 771-773].

45. Cotton BA, Kao LS, Kozar R, et al. Cost-utility analysis of levetiracetam and phenytoin for post-traumatic seizure prophylaxis. J Trauma 2011;71(2):375–9.

46. Samuel S, Allison TA, Lee K, et al. Pharmacologic management of paroxysmal sympathetic hyperactivity after brain injury. J Neurosci Nurs J Am Assoc Neurosci Nurses 2016;48(2):82–9.

47. Meyfroidt G, Baguley IJ, Menon DK. Paroxysmal sympathetic hyperactivity: the storm after acute brain injury. Lancet Neurol 2017;16(9):721–9.

48. Cheng L, Cui G, Yang R. The impact of preinjury use of antiplatelet drugs on outcomes of traumatic brain injury: a systematic review and meta-analysis. Front Neurol 2022;13:724641.

49. Joseph B, Aziz H, Pandit V, et al. Low-dose aspirin therapy is not a reason for repeating head computed tomographic scans in traumatic brain injury: a prospective study. J Surg Res 2014;186(1):287–91.

50. Joseph B, Pandit V, Aziz H, et al. Clinical outcomes in traumatic brain injury patients on preinjury clopidogrel: a prospective analysis. J Trauma Acute Care Surg 2014;76(3):817–20.

51. Hecht JP, LaDuke ZJ, Cain-Nielsen AH, et al. Effect of preinjury oral anticoagulants on outcomes following traumatic brain injury from falls in older adults. Pharmacotherapy 2020;40(7):604–13.

52. Effect of intravenous corticosteroids on death within 14 days in 10 008 adults with clinically significant head injury (MRC CRASH trial): randomised placebo-controlled trial. Lancet 2004;364(9442):1321–8.

53. Final results of MRC CRASH, a randomised placebo-controlled trial of intravenous corticosteroid in adults with head injury—outcomes at 6 months. Lancet 2005;365(9475):1957–9.

54. Alali AS, Mukherjee K, McCredie VA, et al. Beta-blockers and traumatic brain injury: a systematic review, meta-analysis, and Eastern Association for the Surgery of Trauma Guideline. Ann Surg 2017;266(6):952–61.

55. Khalili H, Ahl R, Paydar S, et al. Beta-blocker therapy in severe traumatic brain injury: a prospective randomized controlled trial. World J Surg 2020;44(6):1844–53.

56. Giacino JT, Kalmar K, Eifert B, et al. Placebo-Controlled Trial of Amantadine for Severe Traumatic Brain Injury. N Engl J Med 2012. https://doi.org/10.1056/NEJMoa1102609.

57. Dougall D, Poole N, Agrawal N. Pharmacotherapy for chronic cognitive impairment in traumatic brain injury. Cochrane Dementia and Cognitive Improvement Group. Cochrane Database Syst Rev 2015. https://doi.org/10.1002/14651858.CD009221.pub2.

58. Gajewski BJ, Berry SM, Barsan WG, et al. Hyperbaric oxygen brain injury treatment (HOBIT) trial: a multifactor design with response adaptive randomization and longitudinal modeling. Pharmaceut Stat 2016;15(5):396–404.

59. Permenter CM, Fernández-de Thomas RJ, Sherman A I. Post-concussive Syndrome. In: StatPearls. StatPearls Publishing; 2023 Available at: http://www.ncbi.nlm.nih.gov/books/NBK534786/. Accessed May 9, 2023.

60. US Department of Health & Human Services; Centers for Disease Control (CDC); National Center for Injury Prevention and Control. Report to Congress on Mild Traumatic Brain Injury in the United States: Steps to Prevent a Serious Public Health Problem: (371602004-001). Published online 2003. doi:10.1037/e371602004-001.

61. Silverberg ND, Iaccarino MA, Panenka WJ, et al. Management of Concussion and Mild Traumatic Brain Injury: A Synthesis of Practice Guidelines. Arch Phys Med Rehabil 2020;101(2):382–93.

62. Zink BJ. Traumatic brain injury outcome: concepts for emergency care. Ann Emerg Med 2001;37(3):318–32.

63. Miller JD, Butterworth JF, Gudeman SK, et al. Further experience in the management of severe head injury. J Neurosurg 1981;54(3):289–99.

64. Brain Trauma Foundation. Early Indicators of Prognosis in Severe TBI. Available at: https://braintrauma.org/coma/guidelines/prognosis. Accessed May 9, 2023.

Management of Blunt Chest Trauma

Jared Griffard, MD, Lisa M. Kodadek, MD, FACS*

KEYWORDS

- Chest trauma • Blunt trauma • Thoracic injury • Rib fractures

KEY POINTS

- Blunt thoracic injury commonly includes rib fractures, sternal fracture, pneumothorax, hemothorax, and pulmonary contusions. Treatment is generally supportive with multimodal analgesia with or without tube thoracostomy.
- Tube thoracostomy may be safely deferred in patients with normal hemodynamics and simple pneumothorax less than or equal to 35 mm diameter on computed tomography imaging.
- Retained hemothorax should be treated early with video-assisted thoracoscopic surgery within 4 days of injury to reduce infectious complications and hospital length of stay.
- Extracorporeal membrane oxygenation may be safely and effectively used in select patients with blunt thoracic trauma and refractory hypoxia.
- Tracheobronchial injury, esophageal injury, diaphragmatic injury, blunt cardiac injury, and blunt aortic injury are less commonly seen after blunt thoracic trauma, but operative intervention is more frequently required.

INTRODUCTION

Blunt chest trauma constitutes a heterogeneous group of injuries and accounts for at least 10% of all hospital admissions for injury.[1] The most common mechanism leading to blunt chest trauma is motor vehicle collision (MVC), although ground-level falls are more common in older adults.[2] Blunt chest wall trauma carries a mortality of up to 25%,[3-5] and numerous injuries occurring in the thorax are life-threatening.[6]

Rib Fractures

Rib fractures may be categorized as simple, wedge, or complex fractures and are nondisplaced, offset, or displaced; ribs four through ten in the anterolateral region are most commonly injured.[7-9] Three or more contiguous ribs fractured in at least two locations are defined as a flail segment; paradoxical movement inward with respiration

Division of General Surgery, Trauma and Surgical Critical Care, Department of Surgery, Yale School of Medicine, 330 Cedar Street, Boardman Building 310, New Haven, CT 06510, USA
* Corresponding author.
E-mail address: lisa.kodadek@yale.edu

Surg Clin N Am 104 (2024) 343–354
https://doi.org/10.1016/j.suc.2023.09.007
0039-6109/24/© 2023 Elsevier Inc. All rights reserved.
surgical.theclinics.com

and outward with expiration is clinical flail chest.[10] Flail chest impedes thoracic expansion, decreases vital capacity, and is associated with significant underlying lung contusions. Flail segments are associated with extensive injuries and a mortality rate of 10% to 40%[11]; concomitant pulmonary contusions (PCs), pneumothorax, and hemothorax are common.[11,12] About 80% of patients with flail segments require intensive care unit (ICU) admission, with 60% requiring mechanical ventilation.[11]

Rib fractures can present with chest wall tenderness, ecchymosis, crepitus, or obvious deformity. Chest x-ray (CXR) diagnoses rib fractures with high specificity (84%–98%) but may miss almost 50% of fractures.[2,13] Computed tomography (CT) provides optimal sensitivity and specificity.[13,14]

Rib fracture treatment is primarily nonoperative, with multimodal pain management, respiratory therapy, and mobility as the mainstays of treatment. Incentive spirometry (IS) is recommended for patients $\geq$65 years old as a prognostic tool to determine the risk of pulmonary complications.[15] Spirometry use in a bundled protocol has been shown to reduce complications in all age groups.[16]

Multimodal analgesia is primarily used for treatment of pain associated with rib fractures.[17] Scheduled acetaminophen is well-tolerated with minimal side effects[18,19] and reaches peak effect within 1 hour.[20] non-steroidal anti-inflammatory drugs (NSAIDs) are used as an adjunct to acetaminophen.[21] Ketorolac decreases pneumonia risk and increases rate of ventilator-free and ICU-free days[22] without increasing rates of bleeding or acute kidney injury.[23] Intravenous (IV) ibuprofen and/or low-dose ketamine infusions may decrease overall narcotic use.[24,25] Opioids are effective but have unfavorable side effects: constipation, respiratory depression, somnolence, and addictive capacity. Prior opioid exposure significantly alters the treatment trajectory: opioid-naïve patients were prescribed a median of 16 days versus 36 days of treatment for those with prior opioid exposure.[26] The use of gabapentin for pain management is not strongly supported by evidence.[27]

Locoregional pain management is an important adjunct for treatment of rib fractures. Epidural catheters lead to lower subjective pain scores[28] and are conditionally recommended by the Eastern Association for the Surgery of Trauma (EAST).[29] In older patients, epidural catheters improved pain scores and are recommended.[30] Other locoregional pain management methods include serratus anterior blocks, paravertebral blocks, targeted intercostal nerve blocks, and erector spinae blocks. Paravertebral blocks can provide continuous analgesia and are non-inferior to epidural catheters.[28] Delirium in patients $\geq$65 years was decreased with regional analgesia in a multicenter cohort study.[31]

Consensus guidelines recommend surgical stabilization of rib fractures (SSRF) for patients with a flail segment.[30,32–34] SSRF can allow for better excursion of the chest wall, increased inspiratory volume[35] and increased lung volumes.[36] SSRF decreases mortality and is associated with improved outcomes including decreased need for tracheostomy.[30,32] Data suggest only minimal benefit in older patients.[37,38] The NON-FLAIL study showed decreased pain scores through 8 weeks of follow-up with reduced narcotic use after SSRF.[33]

Sternal Fractures

Sternal fracture (SF) occurs in 2% of patients with blunt trauma and 3.7% of patients injured in MVCs.[39,40] Only 22% to 26% of SFs are isolated; most have associated thoracic injuries.[41,42] SF can present with focal tenderness over the sternum or anterior chest wall ecchymosis.[6] CXR lacks specificity, with 81% to 93% of SFs visualized on CT only.[40,43] Bedside ultrasonography, while user-dependent, can also diagnose SFs.[43,44]

SFs are managed with multimodal analgesia, respiratory therapy, and early mobility. Despite the lack of strong supporting evidence, IS is often used as part of a bundled care set.[18,45] Operative fixation is used for unstable fractures, fracture displacement, respiratory insufficiency, and uncontrolled severe pain.[42,46] Sternal fixation improves pain scores with decreased opioid requirements, but long-term data are lacking.[46–48]

Pneumothorax

Pneumothorax, diagnosed in 40% to 50% of all patients with thoracic trauma, occurs when air accumulates between the parietal and visceral pleura.[49,50] Pneumothorax may be categorized as simple, open, tension, or occult. Simple pneumothoraces are secondary to lung parenchymal injury. Open pneumothoraces are contiguous with the atmosphere via wounds. In tension pneumothorax, air accumulates to pressures higher than atmospheric pressure with subsequent circulatory collapse from lack of venous return. Occult pneumothorax, a pneumothorax not clinically suspected or visualized on CXR but identified on CT scan, occurs in 22% of patients after blunt trauma.[2]

Signs of pneumothorax include unilateral decreased or absent breath sounds. CXR approaches 100% specificity but can miss 50% of pneumothoraces when compared with chest ultrasonography.[51] Ultrasonography is 91% to 99% sensitive; the absence of B-lines and lung sliding have a negative predictive value of 98% to 100%.[50,51] CT scan remains the gold standard for diagnosis. Large pneumothorax is defined as greater than 2 cm and greater than 3 cm by the British Thoracic Society and the American Thoracic Society, respectively.[2,52]

Pneumothorax is treated with tube thoracostomy to re-expand the lung and restore negative intrathoracic pressure.[6] Thoracostomy carries a complication rate of 19%; observation is safe for pneumothoraces ≤35 mm in diameter between visceral and parietal pleura on CT.[53–56] Observation of occult pneumothoraces with positive pressure ventilation is safe in hemodynamically normal patients.[57,58] Western Trauma Association (WTA) recommends tube thoracostomy for pneumothoraces greater than 35 mm on CT scan or greater than 20% on CXR in hemodynamically stable patients; thoracostomy tube is recommended regardless of size in hemodynamically unstable patients.[49] EAST and WTA recommend prophylactic antibiotics for thoracostomy to reduce the rate of empyema and pneumonia.[59,60]

Hemothorax

Hemothorax results from hemorrhage of the pulmonary parenchyma, intercostal vessels, pulmonary arteries, or pulmonary veins. Hemothorax or hemopneumothorax occurs in one-third of patients with chest trauma, with incidence increasing for each rib fractured.[5,61,62] Occult hemothorax is defined as hemothorax seen only on CT scan. Delayed hemothorax is the development or progression of hemothorax post-injury.[63,64] Retained hemothorax, an inadequately drained hemothorax, increases the risk of empyema, pneumonia, and further surgical intervention.[65]

Signs of hemothorax are nonspecific: decreased breath sounds, crepitus over ribs suggesting rib fractures, chest wall ecchymosis, and respiratory insufficiency. CXR can diagnose hemothoraces with 200 to 300 mL of blood required to visualize blunting of the costophrenic angles and almost 1000 mL is required for diagnosis on supine CXR.[2] Ultrasonography can be helpful in unstable patients, with 60% sensitivity and 98% specificity when evaluating for anechoic areas in the pleural spaces.[66] CT scan can detect small amounts of blood and is the gold standard for diagnosis.

Hemothoraces are treated with drainage, often with a thoracostomy tube. Small bore tubes (eg, 14 Fr pigtail catheters) are efficacious.[61,67–69] EAST conditionally recommends pigtail catheter usage with clinician-guided patient selection.[61] Thoracic irrigation via the thoracostomy tube, especially with ≥1000 mL, can reduce retained hemothorax rates and improve outcomes.[70–72] Occult hemothoraces can be observed, but volumes ≥300 mL and mechanical ventilation are risk factors for failure.[56] Delayed hemothorax may develop, especially in elderly patients.[63] Retained hemothorax may be treated with tissue plasminogen activator or streptokinase.[73] Thrombolytic regimens vary widely, however, and EAST conditionally recommends video-assisted thoracoscopic surgery (VATS) over thrombolysis in operative candidates.[61] If VATS is undertaken, it should be performed within 4 days of injury to reduce empyema rates and decrease hospital and ICU length of stay, ventilator days, and mortality.[61,74]

Pulmonary Contusions

PCs result from injury to lung parenchyma leading to edema and interstitial hemorrhage, with consequent loss of gas exchange, alveolar collapse, consolidation, and atelectasis.[10,75] Subsequent hypoxia is worsened by the increased shunting of blood through unventilated alveoli and decreased compliance of the lung. PCs occur in 20% to 35% of patients with blunt chest trauma and 70% are secondary to MVCs.[2,75,76] The severity of PCs can be quantified, but it does not completely explain the poor oxygenation seen in severe PC.[77] Increased CT scan utilization has led to increased incidence of PCs.[78]

Often, signs and symptoms of PCs develop hours to days post-injury as inflammation peaks ≥24 hours post-injury.[75] CXR can show moderate–severe PCs, with 73% of PCs seen on CT scan only.[78] PC treatment is supportive: supplemental oxygen, analgesia, IS, euvolemia, and observation. Severe PCs often require intubation to maintain oxygenation.[10] In refractory cases of hypoxia due to pulmonary contusions from trauma, extracorporeal membrane oxygenation (ECMO) may be considered for treatment.[79] Although patient selection is paramount, one study has shown a 74.1% survival to hospital discharge among patients requiring ECMO after blunt thoracic trauma.[80]

Tracheobronchial Injury

Tracheobronchial injuries are seen in 0.8% to 5% of injured patients.[10] Tracheobronchial injuries can present with respiratory distress and dyspnea, hoarseness, subcutaneous emphysema, pneumothorax, or hemoptysis.[81] Persistent air leak, pneumothorax, pneumomediastinum, or subcutaneous emphysema after thoracostomy tube placement should raise clinical suspicion for this diagnosis. CXR can show a "fallen lung sign" with atelectasis of the ipsilateral lung, absent hilum, and falling away of the lung toward the diaphragm. Chest CT scans can detect obvious disruptions, but the gold standard for diagnosis is bronchoscopy.[10,82]

Tracheobronchial injuries are treated operatively, with tracheal repair performed with absorbable sutures; simple lacerations can be repaired primarily, but extensive injuries often require debridement of necrotic tissue.[10] Lateral dissection is minimized to preserve blood supply for the trachea in the 3 and 9 o'clock positions. Repairs are buttressed with vascularized flaps of strap or intercostal muscles, pericardium, or pleura. Covered metal self-expanding tracheal stents are an efficacious alternative for poor surgical candidates.[82]

Esophageal Injury

Esophageal injury (EI) is rare (≤1% in blunt chest trauma) but carries a 9.8% mortality rate.[83] Signs of EI can include subcutaneous cervical air, hemoptysis, hoarseness, or neck hematoma. Fever, erythema, swelling, or airway distress can occur as mediastinitis develops. Contrast esophagography is the most useful diagnostic modality. CT esophagography can be used when fluoroscopy is unavailable with similar sensitivity and specificity.[84] When combined with contrast studies, diagnostic sensitivity of esophagoscopy approaches 90% to 100%.[84]

Broad spectrum antibiotics are initiated once EI is suspected.[85] Nonoperative management is indicated for hemodynamically stable patients with either a contained perforation or no contrast extravasation. Endoscopic interventions include endoscopic clipping, with 59% to 83% success, and covered esophageal stents.[85,86] Surgical management of EIs includes wide drainage with debridement of nonviable tissue and a two-layer closure with a vascularized tissue flap buttressing the repair; large esophageal perforations require esophageal diversion with end esophagostomy and distal enteral access placement.[10]

Diaphragmatic Injury

Traumatic diaphragmatic injury (TDI) incidence rate is 0.8% to 8%.[87] Most TDIs are initially asymptomatic or have nonspecific symptoms and most occur on the left. CXR has 27% to 62% sensitivity for left TDIs and 17% for right TDIs without visceral herniation.[88] CT scans are more sensitive (80%) and specific (98%) in detecting TDIs.[87] The gold standard for diagnosis is either open or minimally invasive surgical exploration.[88]

The treatment for TDIs is surgical: EAST conditionally recommends an abdominal approach for repair versus a thoracic approach, with laparoscopy considered for hemodynamically stable patients.[87,88]

Blunt Cardiac Injury

Blunt cardiac injury (BCI) is diagnosed in ≥70% of patients with high force blunt chest trauma.[89] BCI symptoms may be clinically absent and can develop over hours to days post-injury. Normal electrocardiogram (EKG) and troponin I levels rule out BCI.[89,90] A new right bundle branch block is the most common EKG abnormality.[91] High-sensitivity troponin T levels greater than 14 ng/L have been shown to correlate with worse outcomes.[92] Echocardiography is recommended in the presence of other abnormalities to provide diagnostic imaging and functional evaluation.[93] Transesophageal echocardiography may have higher specificity without obscured images from subcutaneous emphysema or hematomas.[94]

Most patients can be observed with admission and telemetry, but anatomic injuries warrant surgical evaluation to determine necessity of surgical repair. Arrhythmias may require pharmacologic intervention, and possibly, cardioversion and symptomatic heart block may require a pacemaker.[91,95]

Blunt Thoracic Aortic Injury

Blunt thoracic aortic injury (BTAI) can present with hemodynamic instability or nonspecific complaints: chest pain, interscapular pain, or difficulty breathing.[96] WTA recommends evaluating for BTAI after high-force mechanism of injury.[97] CXR findings may include widened mediastinum, left hemothorax, left apical cap, and loss of aortic knob.[15] CT angiography (CTA) is the gold standard, with a sensitivity of 95% to 100% and negative predictive value of almost 100%.[98] A standard CT scan with IV contrast will often capture BTAI, but a formal CTA is recommended if the diagnosis is uncertain.

Medical management of BTAI includes anti-impulse therapy with short-acting beta blockade with a goal of less than 100 mgHg systolic blood pressure and less than 100

BPM heart rate; calcium channel blockade can be added or used in place of beta-blockade. Grades I and II injuries can be managed medically with repeat CTA to assess stability.[96,97] Grades III and IV injuries should undergo surgical intervention, but Grade III injuries can be delayed safely for 48 to 72 hours if there are severe concomitant injuries. Endovascular repair is recommended due to its lower rates of morbidity and mortality.[98] Postoperative surveillance imaging is recommended, but ideal timing and length of surveillance are not established.[97]

CLINICS CARE POINTS

- Multimodal analgesia options for treatment of rib fractures may include acetaminophen, NSAIDs, ketamine infusion, epidural catheters, and locoregional pain management methods.
- Three or more contiguous ribs fractured in at least two locations are defined as a flail segment. Surgical stabilization of rib fractures may benefit select patient populations.
- Tube thoracostomy may be safely deferred in patients with normal hemodynamics and simple pneumothorax less than or equal to 35 mm diameter on computed tomography imaging.
- Prophylactic use of antibiotics for tube thoracostomy decreases the rate of pneumonia and empyema.
- Retained hemothorax should be treated early with video-assisted thoracoscopic surgery within 4 days of injury to reduce infectious complications and hospital length of stay.
- Extracorporeal membrane oxygenation may be safely and effectively used in select patients with blunt thoracic trauma and refractory hypoxia.
- Tracheobronchial injuries are diagnosed with bronchoscopy and treated operatively, with tracheal repair performed with absorbable sutures.
- A normal troponin I level along with a normal EKG rules out blunt cardiac injury.
- The initial management of blunt thoracic aortic injury include anti-impulse therapy with beta blockade.

AUTHORSHIP

Both authors meet authorship criteria as established by the International Committee on Medical Journal Editors' (ICMJE) Criteria.

DISCLOSURE

The authors have nothing to disclose.

REFERENCES

1. Dennis BM, Bellister SA, Guillamondegui OD. Thoracic Trauma. Surg Clin North Am 2017;97(5):1047–64.
2. Polireddy K, Hoff C, Kinger NP, et al. Blunt thoracic trauma: role of chest radiography and comparison with CT - findings and literature review. Emerg Radiol 2022;29(4):743–55.
3. Battle CE, Hutchings H, Evans PA. Risk factors that predict mortality in patients with blunt chest wall trauma: a systematic review and meta-analysis. Injury 2012;43(1):8–17.

4. Khandhar SJ, Johnson SB, Calhoon JH. Overview of thoracic trauma in the United States. Thorac Surg Clin 2007;17(1):1–9.

5. Lin FC, Li R, Tung Y, et al. Morbidity, mortality, associated injuries, and management of traumatic rib fractures. J Chin Med Assoc 2016;79(6):329–34.

6. American College of Surgeons. Advanced trauma life support: student manual. 10th edition. Chicago, IL: American College of Surgeons; 2018.

7. Bhavnagri SJ, Mohammed TL. When and how to image a suspected broken rib. Cleve Clin J Med 2009;76(5):309–14.

8. Harden A, Kang YS, Agnew A. Rib Fractures: Validation of an Interdisciplinary Classification System. Forensic Anthropology 2019;2(3):158–67.

9. Edwards JG, Clarke P, Pieracci FM, et al. Taxonomy of multiple rib fractures: Results of the chest wall injury society international consensus survey. J Trauma Acute Care Surg 2020;88(2):e40–5.

10. Feliciano DV MK, Moore EE. Trauma. 9th edition. New York, USA: McGraw Hill; 2020.

11. Dehghan N, de Mestral C, McKee MD, et al. Flail chest injuries: a review of outcomes and treatment practices from the National Trauma Data Bank. J Trauma Acute Care Surg 2014;76(2):462–8.

12. Getz P, Mommsen P, Clausen J, et al. Limited Influence of Flail Chest in Patients With Blunt Thoracic Trauma - A Matched-pair Analysis. In Vivo 2019;33(1):133–9.

13. Langdorf MI, Medak AJ, Hendey GW, et al. Prevalence and Clinical Import of Thoracic Injury Identified by Chest Computed Tomography but Not Chest Radiography in Blunt Trauma: Multicenter Prospective Cohort Study. Ann Emerg Med 2015;66(6):589–600.

14. Chapman BC, Overbey DM, Tesfalidet F, et al. Clinical Utility of Chest Computed Tomography in Patients with Rib Fractures CT Chest and Rib Fractures. Arch Trauma Res 2016;5(4):e37070.

15. Mukherjee K, Schubl SD, Tominaga G, et al. Non-surgical management and analgesia strategies for older adults with multiple rib fractures: A systematic review, meta-analysis, and practice management guideline from the Eastern Association for the Surgery of Trauma. J Trauma Acute Care Surg 2023;94(3):398–407.

16. Martin TJ, Eltorai AS, Dunn R, et al. Clinical management of rib fractures and methods for prevention of pulmonary complications: A review. Injury 2019; 50(6):1159–65.

17. Rogers FB, Larson NJ, Rhone A, et al. Comprehensive Review of Current Pain Management in Rib Fractures With Practical Guidelines for Clinicians. J Intensive Care Med 2023;38(4):327–39.

18. Witt CE, Bulger EM. Comprehensive approach to the management of the patient with multiple rib fractures: a review and introduction of a bundled rib fracture management protocol. Trauma Surg Acute Care Open 2017;2(1):e000064.

19. Wei S, Green C, Truong V, et al. Implementation of a multi-modal pain regimen to decrease inpatient opioid exposure after injury. Am J Surg 2019;218(6):1122–7.

20. Ayoub SS. Paracetamol (acetaminophen): A familiar drug with an unexplained mechanism of action. Temperature (Austin) 2021;8(4):351–71.

21. Harvin JA, Albarado R, Truong V, et al. Multi-Modal Analgesic Strategy for Trauma: A Pragmatic Randomized Clinical Trial. J Am Coll Surg 2021;232(3): 241–51.e3.

22. Yang Y, Young JB, Schermer CR, et al. Use of ketorolac is associated with decreased pneumonia following rib fractures. Am J Surg 2014;207(4):566–72.

23. Torabi J, Kaban JM, Lewis E, et al. Ketorolac Use for Pain Management in Trauma Patients With Rib Fractures Does not Increase of Acute Kidney Injury or Incidence of Bleeding. Am Surg 2021;87(5):790–5.

24. Bayouth L, Safcsak K, Cheatham ML, et al. Early Intravenous Ibuprofen Decreases Narcotic Requirement and Length of Stay after Traumatic Rib Fracture. Am Surg 2013;79(11):1207–12.

25. Carver TW, Kugler NW, Juul J, et al. Ketamine infusion for pain control in adult patients with multiple rib fractures: Results of a randomized control trial. J Trauma Acute Care Surg 2019;86(2):181–8.

26. Dalton MK, Chaudhary MA, Andriotti T, et al. Patterns and predictors of opioid prescribing and use after rib fractures. Surgery 2020;168(4):684–9.

27. Moskowitz EE, Garabedian L, Hardin K, et al. A double-blind, randomized controlled trial of gabapentin vs. placebo for acute pain management in critically ill patients with rib fractures. Injury 2018;49(9):1693–8.

28. Peek J, Smeeing DPJ, Hietbrink F, Hietbrink F, et al. Comparison of analgesic interventions for traumatic rib fractures: a systematic review and meta-analysis. Eur J Trauma Emerg Surg 2019;45(4):597–622.

29. Galvagno SM, Smith CE, Varon AJ, et al. Pain management for blunt thoracic trauma: A joint practice management guideline from the Eastern Association for the Surgery of Trauma and Trauma Anesthesiology Society. J Trauma Acute Care Surg 2016;81(5):936–51.

30. Brasel KJ, Moore EE, Albrecht RA, et al. Western Trauma Association Critical Decisions in Trauma: Management of rib fractures. J Trauma Acute Care Surg 2017; 82(1):200–3.

31. O'Connell KM, Patel KV, Powelson E, et al. Use of regional analgesia and risk of delirium in older adults with multiple rib fractures: An Eastern Association for the Surgery of Trauma multicenter study. J Trauma Acute Care Surg 2021;91(2): 265–71.

32. Kasotakis G, Hasenboehler EA, Streib EW, et al. Operative fixation of rib fractures after blunt trauma: A practice management guideline from the Eastern Association for the Surgery of Trauma. J Trauma Acute Care Surg 2017;82(3):618–26.

33. Pieracci FM, Leasia K, Bauman Z, et al. A multicenter, prospective, controlled clinical trial of surgical stabilization of rib fractures in patients with severe, nonflail fracture patterns (Chest Wall Injury Society NONFLAIL). J Trauma Acute Care Surg 2020;88(2):249–57.

34. Sawyer E, Wullschleger M, Muller N, et al. Surgical Rib Fixation of Multiple Rib Fractures and Flail Chest: A Systematic Review and Meta-analysis. J Surg Res 2022;276:221–34.

35. Prins JTH, Van Lieshout EMM, Overtoom HCG, et al. Long-term pulmonary function, thoracic pain, and quality of life in patients with one or more rib fractures. J Trauma Acute Care Surg 2021;91(6):923–31.

36. Campbell D, Arnold N, Wake E, et al. Three-dimensional volume-rendered computed tomography application for follow-up fracture healing and volume measurements pre-surgical rib fixation and post-surgical rib fixation. J Trauma Acute Care Surg 2021;91(6):961–5.

37. Hoepelman RJ, Beeres FJP, Heng M, et al. Rib fractures in the elderly population: a systematic review. Arch Orthop Trauma Surg 2022;143(2):887–93.

38. Chen Zhu R, de Roulet A, Ogami T, et al. Rib fixation in geriatric trauma: Mortality benefits for the most vulnerable patients. J Trauma Acute Care Surg 2020;89(1): 103–10.

39. Yeh DD, Hwabejire JO, DeMoya MA, et al. Sternal fracture–an analysis of the National Trauma Data Bank. J Surg Res 2014;186(1):39–43.

40. Perez MR, Rodriguez RM, Baumann BM, et al. Sternal fracture in the age of panscan. Injury 2015;46(7):1324.

41. Doyle JE, Diaz-Gutierrez I. Traumatic sternal fractures: a narrative review. Mediastinum 2021;5:34.

42. Klei DS, de Jong MB, Oner FC, et al. Current treatment and outcomes of traumatic sternal fractures-a systematic review. Int Orthop 2019;43(6):1455–64.

43. Schellenberg M, Inaba K, Bardes JM, et al. The combined utility of extended focused assessment with sonography for trauma and chest x-ray in blunt thoracic trauma. J Trauma Acute Care Surg 2018;85(1):113–7.

44. Racine S, Drake D. BET 3: Bedside ultrasound for the diagnosis of sternal fracture. Emerg Med J 2015;32(12):971–2.

45. Macheel C, Reicks P, Sybrant C, et al. Clinical Decision Support Intervention for Rib Fracture Treatment. J Am Coll Surg 2020;231(2):249–256 e2.

46. Bauman ZM, Todd SJ, Raposo-Hadley A, et al. Impact of sternal fixation on patient outcomes: A case matched review. J Trauma Acute Care Surg 2023;94(4):573–7.

47. Harston A, Roberts C. Fixation of sternal fractures: a systematic review. J Trauma 2011;71(6):1875–9.

48. Bauman ZM, Yanala U, Waibel BH, et al. Sternal fixation for isolated traumatic sternal fractures improves pain and upper extremity range of motion. Eur J Trauma Emerg Surg 2022;48(1):225–30.

49. de Moya M, Brasel KJ, Brown CVR, et al. Evaluation and management of traumatic pneumothorax: A Western Trauma Association critical decisions algorithm. J Trauma Acute Care Surg 2022;92(1):103–7.

50. Tran J, Haussner W, Shah K. Traumatic Pneumothorax: A Review of Current Diagnostic Practices And Evolving Management. J Emerg Med 2021;61(5):517–28.

51. Chan KK, Joo DA, McRae AD, et al. Chest ultrasonography versus supine chest radiography for diagnosis of pneumothorax in trauma patients in the emergency department. Cochrane Database Syst Rev 2020;7(7):CD013031.

52. Citak N, Ozdemir S. Which pneumothorax volume/size measurement method can best predict surgical indication in primary spontaneous pneumothorax patients? A comparison of six different methods. Gen Thorac Cardiovasc Surg 2022;70(10):871–9.

53. Bou Zein Eddine S, Boyle KA, Dodgion CA, et al. Observing pneumothoraces: The 35-millimeter rule is safe for both blunt and penetrating chest trauma. J Trauma Acute Care Surg 2019;86(4):557–64.

54. Walker SP, Barratt SL, Thompson J, et al. Conservative Management in Traumatic Pneumothoraces: An Observational Study. Chest 2018;153(4):946–53.

55. Beattie G, Cohan CM, Tang A, et al. Observational management of penetrating occult pneumothoraces: Outcomes and risk factors for interval tube thoracostomy placement. J Trauma Acute Care Surg 2022;92(1):177–84.

56. Gilbert RW, Fontebasso AM, Park L, et al. The management of occult hemothorax in adults with thoracic trauma: A systematic review and meta-analysis. J Trauma Acute Care Surg 2020;89(6):1225–32.

57. Brasel KJ, Stafford RE, Weigelt JA, et al. Treatment of occult pneumothoraces from blunt trauma. J Trauma 1999;46(6):987–90, discussion 990-1.

58. Kirkpatrick AW, Rizoli S, Ouellet J, et al. Occult pneumothoraces in critical care: a prospective multicenter randomized controlled trial of pleural drainage for

mechanically ventilated trauma patients with occult pneumothoraces. J Trauma Acute Care Surg 2013;74(3):747–54, discussion 754-5.

59. Ayoub F, Quirke M, Frith D. Use of prophylactic antibiotic in preventing complications for blunt and penetrating chest trauma requiring chest drain insertion: a systematic review and meta-analysis. Trauma Surg Acute Care Open 2019;4(1):e000246.

60. Freeman JJ, Asfaw SH, Vatsaas CJ, et al. Antibiotic prophylaxis for tube thoracostomy placement in trauma: a practice management guideline from the Eastern Association for the Surgery of Trauma. Trauma Surg Acute Care Open 2022;7(1):e000886.

61. Patel NJ, Dultz L, Ladhani HA, et al. Management of simple and retained hemothorax: A practice management guideline from the Eastern Association for the Surgery of Trauma. Am J Surg 2021;221(5):873–84.

62. Liman ST, Kuzucu A, Tastepe AI, et al. Chest injury due to blunt trauma. Eur J Cardio Thorac Surg 2003;23(3):374–8.

63. Choi J, Anand A, Sborov KD, et al. Complication to consider: delayed traumatic hemothorax in older adults. Trauma Surg Acute Care Open 2021;6(1):e000626.

64. Choi J, Villarreal J, Anderson W, et al. Scoping review of traumatic hemothorax: Evidence and knowledge gaps, from diagnosis to chest tube removal. Surgery 2021;170(4):1260–7.

65. Prakash PS, Moore SA, Rezende-Neto JB, et al. Predictors of retained hemothorax in trauma: Results of an Eastern Association for the Surgery of Trauma multi-institutional trial. J Trauma Acute Care Surg 2020;89(4):679–85.

66. Staub LJ, Biscaro RRM, Kaszubowski E, et al. Chest ultrasonography for the emergency diagnosis of traumatic pneumothorax and haemothorax: A systematic review and meta-analysis. Injury 2018;49(3):457–66.

67. Bauman ZM, Kulvatunyou N, Joseph B, et al. Randomized Clinical Trial of 14-French (14F) Pigtail Catheters versus 28-32F Chest Tubes in the Management of Patients with Traumatic Hemothorax and Hemopneumothorax. World J Surg 2021;45(3):880–6.

68. Kulvatunyou N, Bauman ZM, Edine SBZ, et al. The small (14 Fr) percutaneous catheter (P-CAT) versus large (28-32 Fr) open chest tube for traumatic hemothorax: A multicenter randomized clinical trial. J Trauma Acute Care Surg 2021;91(5):809–13.

69. Beeton G, Ngatuvai M, Breeding T, et al. Outcomes of Pigtail Catheter Placement versus Chest Tube Placement in Adult Thoracic Trauma Patients: A Systematic Review and Meta-Analysis. Am Surg 2023;89(6):2743–54.

70. Crankshaw L, McNickle AG, Batra K, et al. The Volume of Thoracic Irrigation Is Associated With Length of Stay in Patients With Traumatic Hemothorax. J Surg Res 2022;279:62–71.

71. Kugler NW, Carver TW, Milia D, et al. Thoracic irrigation prevents retained hemothorax: A prospective propensity scored analysis. J Trauma Acute Care Surg 2017;83(6):1136–41.

72. Kugler NW, Carver TW, Paul JS. Thoracic irrigation prevents retained hemothorax: a pilot study. J Surg Res 2016;202(2):443–8.

73. Hendriksen BS, Kuroki MT, Armen SB, et al. Lytic Therapy for Retained Traumatic Hemothorax: A Systematic Review and Meta-analysis. Chest 2019;155(4):805–15.

74. Ziapour B, Mostafidi E, Sadeghi-Bazargani H, et al. Timing to perform VATS for traumatic-retained hemothorax (a systematic review and meta-analysis). Eur J Trauma Emerg Surg 2020;46(2):337–46.

75. Rendeki S, Molnar TF. Pulmonary contusion. J Thorac Dis 2019;11(Suppl 2): S141–51.
76. Miller C, Stolarski A, Ata A, et al. Impact of blunt pulmonary contusion in poly-trauma patients with rib fractures. Am J Surg 2019;218(1):51–5.
77. Zingg SW, Gomaa D, Blakeman TC, et al. Oxygenation and Respiratory System Compliance Associated With Pulmonary Contusion. Respir Care 2022;67(9):1100–8.
78. Rodriguez RM, Friedman B, Langdorf MI, et al. Pulmonary contusion in the pan-scan era. Injury 2016;47(5):1031–4.
79. Hamera J, Menne A. Extracorporeal Life Support for Trauma. Emerg Med Clin North Am 2023;41(1):89–100.
80. Jacobs JV, Hooft NM, Robinson BR, et al. The use of extracorporeal membrane oxygenation in blunt thoracic trauma: A study of the Extracorporeal Life Support Organization database. J Trauma Acute Care Surg 2015;79(6):1049–53.
81. Shemmeri E, Vallieres E. Blunt Tracheobronchial Trauma. Thorac Surg Clin 2018; 28(3):429–34.
82. Grewal HS, Dangayach NS, Ahmad U, et al. Treatment of Tracheobronchial In-juries: A Contemporary Review. Chest 2019;155(3):595–604.
83. Raff LA, Schinnerer EA, Maine RG, et al. Contemporary management of traumatic cervical and thoracic esophageal perforation: The results of an Eastern Associa-tion for the Surgery of Trauma multi-institutional study. J Trauma Acute Care Surg 2020;89(4):691–7.
84. Norton-Gregory AA, Kulkarni NM, O'Connor SD, et al. CT Esophagography for Evaluation of Esophageal Perforation. Radiographics 2021;41(2):447–61.
85. Khaitan PG, Famiglietti A, Watson TJ. The Etiology, Diagnosis, and Management of Esophageal Perforation. J Gastrointest Surg 2022;26(12):2606–15.
86. Schraufnagel DP, Mubashir M, Raymond DP. Non-iatrogenic esophageal trauma: a narrative review. Mediastinum 2022;6:23.
87. Reitano E, Cioffi SPB, Airoldi C, et al. Current trends in the diagnosis and man-agement of traumatic diaphragmatic injuries: A systematic review and a diag-nostic accuracy meta-analysis of blunt trauma. Injury 2022;53(11):3586–95.
88. McDonald AA, Robinson BRH, Alarcon L, et al. Evaluation and management of traumatic diaphragmatic injuries: A Practice Management Guideline from the Eastern Association for the Surgery of Trauma. J Trauma Acute Care Surg 2018;85(1):198–207.
89. Shoar S, Hosseini FS, Naderan M, et al. Cardiac injury following blunt chest trauma: diagnosis, management, and uncertainty. Int J Burns Trauma 2021; 11(2):80–9.
90. Clancy K, Velopulos C, Bilaniuk JW, et al. Screening for blunt cardiac injury: an Eastern Association for the Surgery of Trauma practice management guideline. J Trauma Acute Care Surg 2012;73(5 Suppl 4):S301–6.
91. Nair L, Winkle B, Senanayake E. Managing blunt cardiac injury. J Cardiothorac Surg 2023;18(1):71.
92. Keskpaik T, Starkopf J, Kirsimagi U, et al. The role of elevated high-sensitivity car-diac troponin on outcomes following severe blunt chest trauma. Injury 2020;51(5): 1177–82.
93. Huis In 't Veld MA, Craft CA, Hood RE. Blunt Cardiac Trauma Review. Cardiol Clin 2018;36(1):183–91.
94. Scagliola R, Seitun S, Balbi M. Cardiac contusions in the acute care setting: His-torical background, evaluation and management. Am J Emerg Med 2022;61: 152–7.

95. El-Andari R, O'Brien D, Bozso SJ, et al. Blunt cardiac trauma: a narrative review. Mediastinum 2021;5:28.
96. Mazzaccaro D, Righini P, Fancoli F, et al. Blunt Thoracic Aortic Injury. J Clin Med 2023;12(8):2903.
97. Brown CVR, de Moya M, Brasel KJ, et al. Blunt thoracic aortic injury: A Western Trauma Association critical decisions algorithm. J Trauma Acute Care Surg 2023; 94(1):113–6.
98. Davis KA. Blunt thoracic aortic injury diagnosis and management: two decades of innovation from Memphis. Trauma Surg Acute Care Open 2023;8(Suppl 1): e001084.

Damage Control Laparotomy and Management of the Open Abdomen

Jennifer Serfin, MD*, Christopher Dai, DO,
James Reece Harris, DO, Nathan Smith, DO

KEYWORDS

- Damage control laparotomy • Open abdomen management
- Intra-abdominal hypertension

KEY POINTS

- Open abdomen management is safe and effective for a select group of patients.
- There are multiple techniques that can be used to reduce fluid loss, maintain abdominal sterility, and improve possibility of closure.
- Delayed closure of the abdominal cavity is sometimes the best option in patients who are unstable, do not have complete control of their original pathology, or would have negative outcomes because of abdominal closure.

INTRODUCTION AND HISTORY OF THE OPEN ABDOMEN

Open abdomen management (OAM) was initially described during World War II as an option to control the "burst abdomen" after abdominal war wounds.[1] Dr Ogilvie described the multitude of challenges that these injuries posed. For one, they were normally composed of multiple wounds, which destabilized the abdominal wall. These wounds would be associated with contamination leading to adhesions in the early setting, which would be denser and more numerous than in a nontraumatic setting. Finally, he described the challenge of being the second surgeon as the initial operation was likely performed by another. Given these challenges and the large abdominal wall defect not amenable to primary closure, OAM was introduced. Dr Ogilvie's attempts at temporary management included a canvas soaked in Vaseline sutured to the fascial edges as a bridging mesh. This would prevent further retraction of fascial edges and would bolster the abdominal wall enough to allow use of respiratory muscles.[1]

As his experience in the theater of war increased, he enhanced his management of combat wounds. He extrapolated his experience to non-wartime injuries. With his and

Good Samaritan Regional Medical Center, 3600 NW Samaritan Drive Suite H407, Corvallis, OR 97330, USA
* Corresponding author. Good Samaritan Regional Medical Center, 3600 NW Samaritan Drive, Corvallis, OR 97330.
E-mail address: jserfin@samhealth.org

Surg Clin N Am 104 (2024) 355–366
https://doi.org/10.1016/j.suc.2023.09.008
0039-6109/24/© 2023 Elsevier Inc. All rights reserved.

surgical.theclinics.com

past surgeon's experience, immediate primary closure had fallen out of practice in traumatic wounds and delayed closure prevailed as the standard of care. He believed that this standard of care should also be extended to non-traumatic pathology citing the prevalence of abdominal incision infections in appendicitis and duodenal perforations. He proposed closure of abdominal wounds 4 days after the index operation to decrease the future possibility of incisional infection.[2]

OAM continued to be refined for the next few decades mostly in the setting of intra-abdominal sepsis. Intra-abdominal sepsis had a high mortality rate and keeping an abdomen open served to treat the abdominal cavity essentially as an abscess cavity. Dr Steinberg described a temporary closure over gauze packs in suppurative peritonitis. This allowed a second look in 48 to 72 hours after the index operation and delayed closure.[3] At about the same time, surgeons in Belgium tested planned re-laparotomies 2 to 3 days after the initial laparotomy for peritonitis. This technique demonstrated a mortality of approximately 29%, which was an improvement from the previously observed 73% in the general surgery population. Planned re-laparotomies gained traction as an accepted procedure and were continued until the abdomen could no longer be closed. At that point, the abdomen was temporarily closed, packed with soaked gauze or with placement of a nonabsorbable mesh to retain abdominal contents.[4]

Initial techniques of OAM and temporary closure exposed many of the complications that we know today. These included insensible fluid loss, entero-atmospheric fistulae, and loss of domain. Continued morbidity associated with OAM and temporary closure drove the development of new techniques to avoid these complications. Absorbable mesh, plastic bags, Velcro, and zipper techniques were refined into the temporary abdominal closure (TAC) devices that we use today. As the techniques expanded so did the indications for the use of TAC. What was initially recognized solely as a strategy to manage intra-abdominal sepsis now included intra-abdominal hypertension and damage control surgery.

DISCUSSION
Indications for Open Abdomen Management

OAM is indicated in abdominal compartment syndrome (ACS), intra-abdominal sepsis, or damage control surgery for hemorrhage and traumatic injury. Although it initially gained traction in the realm of intra-abdominal sepsis, the landscape of OAM in surgery changed. With the increasing prevalence of damage control surgery and established treatment guidelines for intra-abdominal hypertension and ACS, OAM use became more common.

Intra-Abdominal Hypertension/Abdominal Compartment Syndrome

ACS as a clinical entity is defined as intra-abdominal pressure greater than 20 mm Hg and new end-organ failure.[5] The pathophysiology of ACS is related to both direct and indirect effects on intra-abdominal organs as well as systemic effects. The increased abdominal pressure leads to decreased venous return to the heart, decreased end-organ perfusion, and decreased diaphragmatic excursion, leading to the commonly seen signs in ACS.

Theories relating to ACS have been documented as early as the nineteenth century.[6] Although there were many early descriptions, including its effects on solid organs, its effect on preload and the descriptions of "burst abdomen" after the closure of an abdomen under tension, its place as a clinical entity was not yet fully recognized. In 2013, the consensus guidelines of intra-abdominal hypertension and ACS were updated by the World Society of the Abdominal Compartment Syndrome. In their guidelines, they recommend decompressive laparotomy in two settings: primary ACS with associated organ failure or secondary ACS with progressive worsening or end-organ function. Primary ACS is ACS due to "injury or disease in the abdominopelvic region," whereas secondary ACS is due to systemic disease not originating in the abdominal cavity.[5]

Intra-Abdominal Sepsis

Intra-abdominal sepsis is one of the original indications for OAM. In the setting of severe peritonitis, continued reinspections allowed for control of infection essentially treating the abdomen as a large abscess cavity. Historically, some investigators advocated for continued re-laparotomies until the abdomen could no longer be closed. Current techniques allow for continued "re-looks" while safely controlling intra-abdominal contents and fluid losses while treating intra-abdominal sepsis. The goal in these situations would be to continue OAM until the infection is controlled or until further sources of infection within the peritoneal cavity are no longer identified.

Damage Control Laparotomy

In the setting of severe injury, whether traumatic or pathologic, laparotomy can be aimed to immediately control the injury while allowing the patient to physiologically respond to the insult. This is usually indicated in the instances of significant hemorrhage requiring packing, need for large volume resuscitation, correction of physiologic parameters such as acidosis or hypothermia or need for staged reinspection and repair of destructive injuries. In these situations, the care of these patients is performed in phases.

Phase 0 comprises the initial presentation and triage until initial laparotomy (**Fig. 1**). Phase 1 is focused on limiting operative time while controlling the cause of the

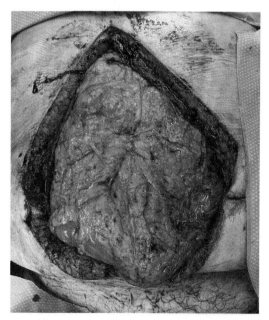

Fig. 1. Open abdomen with omentum covering majority of bowel.

physiologic insult. This includes hemorrhage and contamination control while ensuring perfusion to end organs and extremities. Phase 2 involves resuscitation of the patient before definitive repair in phase 3. OAM is a vital component of phases 1 and 2 of damage control surgery, OAM allows for time to adequately resuscitate the patient before definitive management and/or closure.[7]

TYPES OF TEMPORARY ABDOMINAL CLOSURE FOR OPEN ABDOMEN MANAGEMENT

TAC is a cornerstone in the management of OAM. TAC is a method in which the viscera is protected while managing an open abdomen, allows expedited reexploration of the abdomen in subsequent procedures, and can aid in preventing repeat damage to abdominal fascia.[8] As OAM has progressed and evolved so have methods of TAC.

Primary Skin Approximation

In an emergent setting, need for expeditious departure from operating room (OR) to intensive care unit (ICU) for resuscitation, or in a resource poor setting, TAC can be obtained by simply suturing closed the skin of the abdomen. Using towel clips to close abdominal skin is another similar method. This is the simplest, oldest, and one of the fastest forms of TAC but does have drawbacks. It should not be used in ACS and used with caution in intra-abdominal sepsis. It does not aid in preventing fascial retraction. A small single-center study has recently suggested similar clinical outcomes and complications comparing simple whipstitch suture closure and ABTHERA Open Abdomen Negative Pressure Therapy in the setting of blunt or penetrating trauma.[9] This method is also a cost saving and may be good option in a resource poor setting.

Silo or Bogota Bag

This method involves suturing a sterile plastic bag (can be a 3L saline bag) to the fascial edges to achieve TAC. This is a cost-effective option for TAC. Because this method provides a tension-free closure, it will not aid in ease of fascial re-approximation. Additional negative aspects of the silo or Bogota Bag are the inability to drain peritoneal fluid and it has been linked to higher intestinal fistula rate.[8] On the other hand, this method can be an advantage when OAM is used for ACS and devitalized bowel is a concern because it allows direct inspection of the bowel through the clear plastic.

Barker's Vacuum Pack Method

Before current negative pressure wound therapy (NPWT) devices, this technique was an inexpensive and easy to apply method of TAC. First described by Barker and colleagues in the 1990s, this method consists of applying a perforated polyethylene sheet under the fascia, covering the viscera, followed by moist surgical towels, two 10F flat silicone suction drains laid on the top of the towels, and covered with an adhesive iodophor-impregnated drape.[10] Drains are connected to continuous suction. This technique can be performed with commonly used surgical materials and applied quickly. Despite it being the original method of vacuum pack TAC, it has now been replaced with newer and improved NPWT TAC devices.

Negative Pressure Wound Therapy

This is one of the most common TAC methods used in the United States.[9,11] One example of this is the ABTHERA Open Abdomen Negative Pressure Therapy (**Figs. 2–4**). This method removes peritoneal fluid which can help to reduce bowel edema, provides negative pressure which can decrease fascial retraction, protects abdominal contents, and

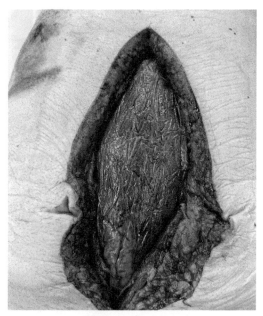

Fig. 2. Plastic-covered inner portion of ABTHERA Open Abdomen Negative Pressure Therapy.

can be applied and taken down quickly. Another benefit is the lack of fascial sutures required for this method, so it decreases direct fascial injury in OAM. NPWT TAC has been associated with higher rates of successful abdominal closure and decreased fistula rates compared with non-NPWT methods in OAM for peritonitis or ACS.[12,13] New data

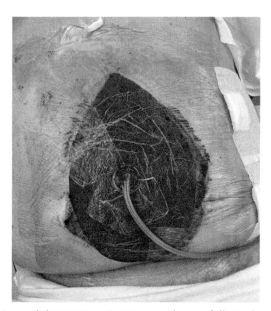

Fig. 3. ABTHERA Open Abdomen Negative Pressure Therapy fully in place after exploratory laparotomy.

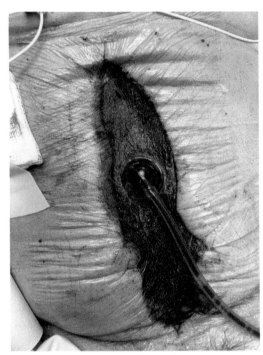

Fig. 4. ABTHERA Open Abdomen Negative Pressure Therapy after second look with reduce skin separation.

are showing even better outcomes regarding fascial closure and decreased complications when NPWT is combined with fascial traction systems.[11,14]

Wittmann Patch

This is a method incorporates Velcro sheets that are sutured to the edges of the fascia to help re-approximate the fascia. It is a fascial traction system that can aid in re-approximating fascia in the setting of OAM. The patch can be peeled apart for abdominal reentry, and as intra-abdominal swelling decreases, the patch can be re-approximated tighter in a subsequent manner. There are other products/techniques similar to this such as the abdominal re-approximation anchor (ABRA) or the vacuum and mesh-mediated fascial traction, mesh-mediated fascial traction, and so forth. Many studies have showed the benefits of combining the Wittmann patch (or ABRA) with NPWT regarding successful fascial closure, reduced time to fascial closure, and reduced complication rates.[13–16] The idea is similar to serial placement of retention sutures to aid in fascial closure without the downside of fascial trauma by repeatedly replacing the sutures. In the newest practice management guidelines from the Eastern Association for the Surgery of Trauma, there is a conditional recommendation to use fascial traction systems combined with NPWT due to the improved rate of primary fascial closure without worsening mortality or fistula formation.[11]

OPEN ABDOMEN MANAGEMENT IN THE ICU
Ongoing Resuscitation and Sepsis Control

The indication for OAM will help direct the postoperative ICU management. Despite the inciting insult or injury, resuscitation and correction of physiologic abnormalities should be top priority. Correcting the lethal triad of hypothermia, acidosis, and coagulopathy should be first.[17] Common end points for resuscitation should be used such as improving vital signs, urine output goals, base deficit correction, and clearing of serum lactate levels. Hypothermia can worsen both coagulopathy and acidosis. Increased heat loss can be assumed in a patient with an open abdomen, so maintaining normothermia is paramount. Coagulopathy should be corrected with blood products based on laboratory values and or viscoelastic tests (thromboelastography [TEG] or rotational thromboelastometry [ROTEM]). Acid–base deficits corrected with fluid resuscitation, ventilator manipulation, and addressing the underlying cause. To continue broad spectrum antibiotics in the setting of intra-abdominal sepsis, the course will be dictated based on source control and the specific clinical scenario. If OAM is for a non-sepsis reason, then prophylactic antibiotics can be discontinued after 24 hours.[18]

Fluid Status

Fluid loss, electrolyte loss, and protein loss are dramatically increased in the setting of OAM.[19,20] Fluid resuscitation will be needed, but over resuscitation with fluids also brings challenges such as bowel edema, increasing risk for ACS (yes, even in the setting of an open abdomen with a TAC), volume overload, pulmonary edema, and acute respiratory distress syndrome. Volume overload has been linked to decrease in primary fascial closure rates along with its other known complications.[17,19] The goal of volume resuscitation is a balanced resuscitation to euvolemia with attempts to minimize the sequela of volume overload.[17–19] Diuresis has been proposed as a way of decreasing bowel edema but the literature on this is mixed and no formal recommendations can be made at this time for this indication.[11,17] The use of NPWT can aid in decreasing bowel edema, and some devices like the ABTHERA can help monitor peritoneal fluid losses for accurate measurements.[12,13,18]

Nutrition

It has already been discussed above that protein loss is a significant factor in the open abdomen. During critical illness, the body enters a catabolic state. Nutritional support is essential during this time. Traditional nitrogen balance calculations, which are the most common way to determine protein requirements, do not account for protein loss from the open abdomen.[20] A study looking at abdominal fluid nitrogen and losses from an open abdomen state determined that there is approximately 1.9 ± 1.1 g of nitrogen lost per liter of abdominal fluid.[20] Another study estimates this loss at 2 to 4.6 g of nitrogen lost per liter of abdominal fluid depending on the type of TAC.[17] Given this, nutritional supplementation in the patient undergoing OAM is critical and has been shown to improve the rates of abdominal closure and decrease complications associated with the open abdomen. Enteral feeding, when appropriate given bowel continuity and other clinical factors, is the optimal way for nutritional support in the setting of an open abdomen and has been proven safe and beneficial. Immediate enteral feeding in patients who underwent damage control laparotomy (DCL) had no effect on abdominal closure rate and was associated with decrease in pneumonia rates.[21] Early enteral feeding in the setting of open abdomen is also associated with higher rates of earlier primary abdominal closure, lower fistula rates, lower hospital charges, and decreased mortality.[17,22,23] In 2012, the Western Trauma Association published a large multicenter trial comparing OAM patients who received enteral nutrition versus patients kept nil per os or nothing by mouth (NPO) before abdominal closure and found that the enteral nutrition group had increased fascial closure rates, decreased mortality, and decreased complication rates.[23] Given these findings, nutritional support with enteral feedings is strongly supported in the patient undergoing OAM when possible.

Direct Peritoneal Resuscitation

Direct peritoneal resuscitation (DPR) is another developing technique used for resuscitation of patients undergoing OAM. Even after the initial insult has been managed, secondary injury from ischemic reperfusion injury (IRI) through various physiologic mechanisms related to imbalances of vasoconstrictive to vasodilatory mediators and loss of endothelial mechanisms to vasodilate occur.[24] DPR with glucose-based peritoneal dialysis (PD) solution is suspected to reduce and combat IRI secondary to microvascular visceral vasoconstriction by increased vasodilation from adenosine and nitric oxide release from glucose and its degradation product.[24] This increase in visceral blood flow is thought to decrease inflammatory mediators through improved clearance of inflammatory mediators, and the hypertonicity of the PD solution could help reduce intra-abdominal edema. The Eastern Association for the Surgery of Trauma's systematic review with meta-analysis and practice guidelines on management of the open abdomen addresses DPR and the three leading studies for DPR by Smith and colleagues. Although results are compelling for improved primary closure rates as well as other benefits, more independent studies are needed to provide further support of this strategy.[11,25–27] The studies by Smith and colleagues demonstrated increase in primary fascial closure rates for OAM patients undergoing DPR as well as decreased intra-abdominal complications from OAM (likely due to time to fascial closure), improved visceral blood flow, and reduction in circulating inflammatory cytokines but mentions that there was no difference in volume of resuscitation in first 24 hours, no difference in injury severity score, and no difference in morbidity or mortality.[24–27] Another article published in the Surgical Infections journal in 2022 retrospectively analyzed patients undergoing DCL and DPR versus DCL without DPR and concluded that infection complications and mechanical failure of the closure technique were similar in the two groups and the DPR + patients had a longer time to final closure.[28] DPR should be used with hesitancy until more independent studies and conclusive data are available.[11]

RISKS OF OPEN ABDOMEN MANAGEMENT

We have described above many potential risks and sequelae of the open abdomen, such as fluid losses, electrolyte imbalances, increased nutritional need, and infection. Some more challenging risks and complications include fistulas and loss of domain in patients undergoing OAM. Early closure of the abdominal wall and fascia is the most effective way to reduce complications of the open abdomen.

Loss of Domain

Throughout the duration of the open abdomen, the fascia of the abdominal wall retracts laterally, making primary closure significantly more difficult as time goes on. Traditional OAM was with planned ventral hernia formation and delayed abdominal wall reconstruction.[16] Since then, with the progression of better TAC techniques and more effective ways to optimize patients for earlier primary closure, this traditional method is becoming less common. The best way to prevent loss of domain is earlier closure of the abdominal fascia. As discussed above, the use of newer TACs such as NPWT, Wittmann patch, other dynamic fascial traction techniques, or combination of these, will aid in earlier closure of the abdomen.

Fistulas

Fistula formation in the setting of OAM is one of the more serious complications due to their difficulty to control and repair.[19] No method of TAC has been independently associated with decrease in fistula formation.[11] TAC with NPWT has been shown to decrease fistula formation rate by reducing the time to primary fascial closure.[12,13] The only way to definitively decrease fistula formation is closure of the abdominal wall as soon as it can be safely done. If a fistula does form, this can complicate abdominal wall reconstruction in the future. Traditional fistula management should be trialed to aid in spontaneous closure before abdominal wall reconstruction. If the fistula persists, timing of fistula takedown with concomitant or delayed abdominal wall reconstruction will need to be well planned.

TIMING OF TAKE BACK TO OR

The timing of taking a patient back to the OR for a second-look operation varies in each unique surgical scenario. It is recommended that the patient is resuscitated in the ICU before returning to the OR and is usually recommended to occur between 24 and 72 hours after initial operation.[8] Generally though, return to the OR should ideally take place between 24 and 48 hours. There is a delicate balance between making sure that the patient is adequately resuscitated to safely return to the OR while also limiting the amount of time between surgeries to decrease OAM complications. The patient may need to be taken back multiple times depending on the clinical scenario, but the goal of each operation includes progressing toward definitive closure of the abdomen.

CLOSURE OF THE OPEN ABDOMEN

Once ongoing resuscitation efforts are complete and the cause of OAM has been addressed, early fascial and abdominal closure should be the next strategy of management.[8] Primary fascial closure is the ideal option. If this is not possible, there is high tension of the fascia when brought together, or there is concern for development of intra-abdominal hypertension/ACS, then delayed closure of the fascia leading to expected ventral hernia can be considered.

Closure Without Mesh

In some circumstances, if the fascia cannot be approximated after OAM, then planned granulation followed by skin grafting may be required to cover intra-abdominal contents until definitive abdominal wall reconstruction is possible. Another option is the use of hydrocolloid dressings which can be a simple, effective, and cost-efficient choice for management and coverage of long-term open abdomen patients.[29] Before abdominal wall reconstruction, it is recommended to obtain a CT scan for preoperative planning. Abdominal wall reconstruction options include modified Rives-Stoppa technique, component release procedures, transversus abdominis release technique, or combination techniques.

Closure with Mesh

There are positive benefits to mesh use at the time of initial laparotomy closure for high-risk hernia patients. The PRImary Mesh closure of Abdominal midline wounds (PRIMA) trial was an international, double-blinded randomized controlled trial comparing onlay reinforcement, sublay reinforcement, and primary suture after midline laparotomy and found that onlay mesh reinforcement had a significant reduction in hernia prevention as well as no increase in surgical site infection.[30] A 2-year follow-up study of the PRIMA trial published in 2017 showed a significant reduction in incisional hernias with onlay mesh reinforcement compared with sublay mesh reinforcement and primary suture only.[31] In regard to hernia repair after OAM, data are very limited on prophylactic mesh use during delayed primary fascial closure. A small trial of 10 patients looking at prophylactic onlay mesh (of either long-term absorbable alloplastic or nonabsorbable mesh) implantation during definitive fascial closure after open abdomen therapy showed promising results with no hernia formation at 12.4 $\pm$ 10.8 months.[32] Again, the data for mesh use at the time of closure after OAM are very limited and need further studies before more official recommendations can be made.

CONCLUSION AND RECOMMENDATIONS

The management of the open abdomen is a tool that all general and trauma surgeons should have in their armamentarium as all will encounter patients who require DCL and OAM. As technology and understanding continue to advance, the domain of open abdominal management will continue to evolve. Early fascial closure, when appropriate, is always the goal. When this is not possible, NPWT is the preferred method of management given decreased trauma to fascial edges and decreased fistula formation until definitive abdominal closure can be accomplished.

CLINIC CARE POINTS

- Use open abdomen management (OAM) when patient is too unstable for completion of surgery, needs a second look, or is anatomically unable to be closed at the time of index operation.
- Chose the technique of OAM that is best for the patient with the resources available of your institution.
- Plan final abdominal closure to provide the best opportunity for closure with lowest risk of ventral hernia when possible.

DISCLOSURE

The authors have nothing to disclose.

REFERENCES

1. Ogilvie WH. The late complications of abdominal war-wounds. Lancet 1940; 236(6105):253–7.
2. Ogilvie WH. Surgical Lessons of War applied to Civil Practice. BMJ 1945;1(4400): 619–23.
3. Steinberg D. On leaving the peritoneal cavity open in acute generalized suppurative peritonitis. Am J Surg 1979;137(2):216–20.
4. Penninckx FM, Kerremans RP, Lauwers PM. Planned relaparotomies in the surgical treatment of severe generalized peritonitis from intestinal origin. World J Surg 1983;7(6):762–6.
5. Kirkpatrick AW, Roberts DJ, de Waele J, et al. Intra-abdominal hypertension and the abdominal compartment syndrome: updated consensus definitions and clinical practice guidelines from the World Society of the Abdominal Compartment Syndrome. Intensive Care Med 2013;39(7):1190–206.
6. Gracias VH. Abdominal compartment syndrome in the open abdomen. Arch Surg 2002;137(11):1298.
7. Johnson JW, Gracias VH, Schwab CW, et al. Evolution in damage control for exsanguinating penetrating abdominal injury. J Trauma Inj Infect Crit Care 2001; 51(2):261–71.

8. Coccolini F, Roberts D, Ansaloni L, et al. The open abdomen in trauma and non-trauma patients: WSES guidelines. World J Emerg Surg 2018;13(1):7.
9. Collins R, Dhanasekara CS, Morris E, et al. Simple suture whipstitch closure is a reasonable option for many patients requiring temporary abdominal closure for blunt or penetrating trauma. Trauma Surg Acute Care Open 2022;7(1):e000980.
10. Barker DE, Kaufman HJ, Smith LA, et al. Vacuum pack technique of temporary abdominal closure: a 7-year experience with 112 patients. J Trauma 2000; 48(2):201–6 [discussion: 206-7].
11. Mahoney EJ, Bugaev N, Appelbaum R, et al. Management of the open abdomen: a systematic review with meta-analysis and practice management guideline from the Eastern Association for the Surgery of Trauma. J Trauma Acute Care Surg 2022;93(3):e110–8.
12. Perez D, Wildi S, Demartines N, et al. Prospective evaluation of vacuum-assisted closure in abdominal compartment syndrome and severe abdominal sepsis. J Am Coll Surg 2007;205(4):586–92.
13. Atema JJ, Gans SL, Boermeester MA. Systematic review and meta-analysis of the open abdomen and temporary abdominal closure techniques in non-trauma patients. World J Surg 2015;39(4):912–25.
14. Quyn AJ, Johnston C, Hall D, et al. The open abdomen and temporary abdominal closure systems - historical evolution and systematic review. Colorectal Dis 2012; 14(8):e429–38.
15. Nemec HM, Benjamin Christie D, Montgomery A, et al. Wittmann Patch : Superior Closure for the Open Abdomen. Am Surg 2020;86(8):981–4.
16. Wang Y, Alnumay A, Paradis T, et al. Management of Open Abdomen After Trauma Laparotomy: A Comparative Analysis of Dynamic Fascial Traction and Negative Pressure Wound Therapy Systems. World J Surg 2019;43(12):3044–50.
17. Chabot E, Nirula R. Open abdomen critical care management principles: resuscitation, fluid balance, nutrition, and ventilator management. Trauma Surg Acute Care Open 2017;2(1):e000063.
18. Regner JL, Kobayashi L, Coimbra R. Surgical strategies for management of the open abdomen. World J Surg 2012;36(3):497–510.
19. Demetriades D. Total management of the open abdomen. Int Wound J 2012;9: 17–24.
20. Cheatham ML, Safcsak K, Brzezinski SJ, et al. Nitrogen balance, protein loss, and the open abdomen. Crit Care Med 2007;35(1):127–31.
21. Dissanaike S, Pham T, Shalhub S, et al. Effect of immediate enteral feeding on trauma patients with an open abdomen: protection from nosocomial infections. J Am Coll Surg 2008;207(5):690–7.
22. Collier B, Guillamondegui O, Cotton B, et al. Feeding the open abdomen. J Parenter Enteral Nutr 2007;31(5):410–5.
23. Burlew CC, Moore EE, Cuschieri J, et al. Who should we feed? Western Trauma Association multi-institutional study of enteral nutrition in the open abdomen after injury. J Trauma Acute Care Surg 2012;73(6):1380–7 [discussion 1387-8].
24. Pera SJ, Schucht J, Smith JW. Direct Peritoneal Resuscitation for Trauma. Adv Surg 2022;56(1):229–45.
25. Smith JW, Garrison NR, Matheson PJ, et al. Direct Peritoneal Resuscitation Accelerates Primary Abdominal Wall Closure after Damage Control Surgery. J Am Coll Surg 2010;210(5):658–64.
26. Smith JW, Neal Garrison R, Matheson PJ, et al. Adjunctive treatment of abdominal catastrophes and sepsis with direct peritoneal resuscitation. J Trauma Acute Care Surg 2014;77(3):393–9.

27. Smith JW, Matheson PJ, Franklin GA, et al. Randomized Controlled Trial Evaluating the Efficacy of Peritoneal Resuscitation in the Management of Trauma Patients Undergoing Damage Control Surgery. J Am Coll Surg 2017;224(4): 396–404.

28. Edwards JD, Quinn SA, Burchette M, et al. Direct peritoneal resuscitation in trauma patients results in similar rates of intra-abdominal complications. Surg Infect 2022;23(2):113–8.

29. Valderrama OM, Goldstein AL, del Carmen Monteza Gallardo S, et al. Successful management of the open abdomen with hydrocolloid dressing in a resource-constrained setting. Hernia 2021;25(6):1519–27.

30. Nieuwenhuizen J, Eker HH, Timmermans L, et al. A double blind randomized controlled trial comparing primary suture closure with mesh augmented closure to reduce incisional hernia incidence. BMC Surg 2013;13:48.

31. Jairam AP, Timmermans L, Eker HH, et al. Prevention of incisional hernia with prophylactic onlay and sublay mesh reinforcement versus primary suture only in midline laparotomies (PRIMA): 2-year follow-up of a multicentre, double-blind, randomised controlled trial. Lancet 2017;390(10094):567–76.

32. Schaaf S, Schwab R, Güsgen C, et al. Prophylactic Onlay Mesh Implantation During Definitive Fascial Closure After Open Abdomen Therapy (PROMOAT): Absorbable or Non-absorbable? Methodical Description and Results of a Feasibility Study. Front Surg 2020;7:578565.

Management of Pelvic Trauma

Jennifer E. Baker, MD[a], Nicole L. Werner, MD, MS[b],
Clay Cothren Burlew, MD[c],*

KEYWORDS

- Pelvic fractures • Pelvic trauma • Preperitoneal pelvic packing • Angioembolization
- Resuscitative endovascular balloon occlusion of the aorta • Open pelvis fracture

KEY POINTS

- Pelvic fractures occur in 3% to 8% of trauma patients with a mortality of 5% to 14%. Patients that present in shock have a mortality of greater than 30% in modern series.
- The pelvic vasculature and viscera are in close continuity with the bony pelvis; therefore, high-energy pelvic ring disruptions are often associated with significant hemorrhage.
- Preperitoneal pelvic packing with external fixation has been demonstrated to decrease mortality in patients with pelvic fractures presenting in shock.
- Angioembolization is highly effective at controlling arterial hemorrhage; highly selective embolization using gelfoam is advocated over empiric bilateral internal iliac artery embolization with coils.
- A protocolized approach to patients with hemodynamically unstable pelvic fractures reduces mortality; in the exsanguinating patient a multidisciplinary approach incorporating several different techniques (binders, external fixation, pelvic packing, REBOA, or angioembolization) to arrest hemorrhage should be utilized.

INTRODUCTION

Pelvic trauma and pelvic fractures are common traumatic injuries. Patients present on a spectrum from clinically insignificant fractures to pelvic ring disruptions with life-threatening exsanguination. Pelvic fractures are associated with hemorrhage because the neurovascular complexes intimately neighbor the bony structures. Hemorrhagic shock from a pelvic fracture can be challenging to detect in the trauma bay as it is often unappreciable on physical examination or focused assessment with sonography

[a] Division of GI, Trauma, and Endocrine Surgery, Department of Surgery, University of Colorado Anschutz Medical Campus, 12631 East 17th Avenue, Aurora, CO 80045, USA; [b] Division of Acute Care and Regional Surgery, Department of Surgery, University of Wisconsin School of Medicine and Public Health, 600 Highland Avenue H4/367, Madison, WI 53792, USA; [c] Division of GI, Trauma, and Endocrine Surgery, Department of Surgery, University of Colorado Anschutz Medical Campus, 12631 E 17th Avenue, Box C313, Aurora, CO 80045, USA
* Corresponding author.
E-mail address: clay.burlew@cuanschutz.edu

Surg Clin N Am 104 (2024) 367–384
https://doi.org/10.1016/j.suc.2023.10.001
0039-6109/24/© 2023 Elsevier Inc. All rights reserved.

surgical.theclinics.com

for trauma (FAST). While a pelvic radiograph may suggest the diagnosis, a high clinical suspicion for pelvic sources of hemorrhage lies with the clinician.

Optimal care of patients with pelvic fractures remains a significant challenge. Most management approaches involve a multidisciplinary team. In the exsanguinating patient, hemorrhage control remains the top priority and may be achieved with a combination of external stabilization (pelvic binding or external skeletal fixation), resuscitative endovascular balloon occlusion of the aorta (REBOA), preperitoneal pelvic packing (PPP), and/or angioembolization (AE). The choice of intervention and the order of intervention remains an area of active research to determine the optimal strategy.

EPIDEMIOLOGY

The incidence of pelvic ring fractures has been previously estimated at 23 cases per 100,000 persons per year, with prehospital deaths occurring in 3 cases per 100,000 persons per year. There is equal incidence of lower energy and high-energy pelvic ring fractures at 10 cases per 100,000 persons per year.[1] Following trauma it is estimated that approximately 3.0% to 8.0% of patients suffer a pelvic fracture, with an all-cause mortality of 5% to 14% in all pelvic fracture patients.[1–4] The patient cohort who is hemodynamically unstable due to pelvic fracture related bleeding comprises only 7% to 13% of all pelvic fracture patients, however mortality reaches over 30%.[3,5,6]

RELEVANT ANATOMY

The bony pelvic anatomy is composed of the sacrum and 2 innominate bones (composed of ilium, ischium, and pubis); this is known as the pelvic ring. The pubic symphysis forms the anterior fusion point between the innominate bones; posteriorly, the sacrum, and innominate bones are joined. If one aspect of the bony pelvis is injured, heightened suspicion should be raised for an injury to the opposite side. The strength of the pelvic ring, however, comes from the significant ligamentous attachments with multiple anterior and posterior attachments (**Fig. 1**).

The arterial and venous structures of the pelvis are closely associated with the pelvic bones. At L5, the aorta divides into the common iliac arteries; further division into the external and internal iliac arteries (IIA) occurs just anterior to the sacroiliac joints. The internal iliac artery then dives into the pelvis and branches along the lateral wall of the innominate bones (**Fig. 2**). Venous analogs run beside named arterial branches. Additionally, there are venous plexuses adjacent to the pelvic viscera and sacrum that are especially vulnerable to shear injury.[7] In pelvic hemorrhage, only 10% to 15% of bleeding is arterial, with most bleeding occurring from venous and bony sources. Arterial bleeding in pelvic fractures often have injuries to the pudendal artery and superior gluteal artery.[8] In addition to the vasculature, the bony pelvis also protects the abdominal viscera.[9,10] The intrapelvic viscera at risk of being injured are the distal third of the sigmoid colon, rectum, urinary bladder, vagina, and proximal urethra.

TAXONOMY OF PELVIC FRACTURES

There are 3 primary classification systems for pelvic fractures (**Table 1**). The Tile classification relies upon the mechanical stability of the pelvis, grouping injuries into one of 3 types: Type A: stable, Type B: rotationally unstable, vertically stable, and Type C: rotationally and vertically unstable.[11,12] The Young and Burgess classification is based on the type of force applied to the pelvis and includes 4 types of injuries: lateral compression (LC), anteroposterior compression (APC), vertical shear (VS), and combined mechanism injury (**Fig. 3**A-G). The World Society of Emergency Surgery

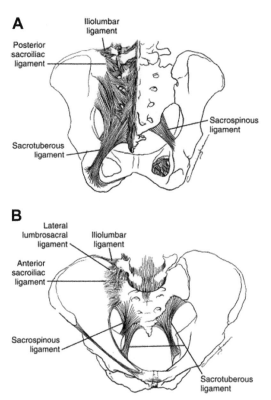

Fig. 1. Ligament and bony pelvis anatomy. (From Tile M, editor: Fractures of the Pelvis and Acetabulum, 3rd ed. Baltimore, Williams and Wilkins, 2003.). Copyright © 2003 Marvin Tile.

(WSES) classification system combines the patient's hemodynamic status with the Young and Burgess classification system, assigning injuries as mild, moderate, or severe.[13] Validation studies of the WSES classification have demonstrated that it is predictive of mortality, whereas the other 2 classification systems are not.[14,15]

PATIENT EVALUATION

The initial assessment and management of a patient with concern for a pelvic injury should follow the Advanced Trauma Life Support (ATLS) principles.[16] Priority should be placed on the ABCs (airway, breathing, circulation). Large bore intravenous access should be obtained, and early blood product resuscitation initiated for hemodynamically unstable patients. Expeditious investigation with trauma bay specific imaging should be performed; a chest radiograph, pelvis radiograph, and FAST are routinely employed to triage areas of possible hemorrhage in hemodynamically unstable patients. While the FAST examination is not sensitive enough to exclude pelvic bleeding, it remains accurate to detect significant intraperitoneal hemorrhage in patients with pelvic fractures.[17,18] In patients with hemodynamic instability and concern for a pelvic fracture based on mechanism or examination findings, external stabilization with a pelvic binder or sheet should be immediately performed, even before pelvic radiographs are taken.

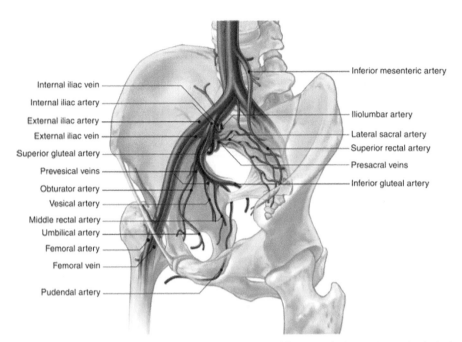

Fig. 2. Vascular anatomy of the pelvis. Geeraerts, T., Chhor, V., Cheisson, G. et al. Clinical review: Initial management of blunt pelvic trauma patients with haemodynamic instability. Crit Care 11, 204 (2007). https://doi.org/10.1186/cc5157.

Assessment for contusions, lacerations, and ecchymosis/hematomas over the iliac wings, pubis, perineum, labia, and scrotum should be standard during the secondary examination. Open pelvic fractures have a higher mortality rate and require antibiotic administration and often operative washout with or without fecal diversion. Palpation of the pelvis should be performed by applying gentle rotational, anteroposterior, and superoinferior stress to the iliac crests. Patients without pain during these maneuvers are unlikely to have an unstable pelvic fracture; the sensitivity and specificity of pain are 100% and 93%, respectively.[19] The urethral meatus should be inspected to clinically assess for a urethral injury/transection. In addition to blood at the urethral meatus, other findings suggestive of a urethral injury include scrotal or perineal bruising or a "high riding" prostate. If a urethral injury is suspected, 1 pass of a foley catheter may be attempted by the team but if urine is not rapidly encountered or if there is any resistance, foley placement should be abandoned until a retrograde urethrogram or suprapubic catheter can be completed. A digital rectal examination should be completed to assess for the presence of blood and concomitant rectal injury. In women, blood at the vaginal introitus or on digital/speculum examination heralds a vaginal injury and an open fracture.

Laboratory evaluation including hemoglobin/hematocrit, lactate, blood gas, and coagulation profile should be performed to assess for physiologic derangements and coagulopathy. Foley placement permits an evaluation for hematuria signaling a bladder injury. If gross hematuria is not present, urinalysis should be performed, and microscopic hematuria should trigger further evaluation with a computed tomography (CT) cystogram. In hemodynamically stable patients, multiphasic CT scan of the pelvis with intravenous contrast delineates pelvic geometry and associated pelvic

Table 1
Pelvic fracture classifications

Young and Burgess			Tile Classification		World Society of Emergency Surgery	
LC	Transverse pubic rami fracture	Type A^a	Stable		Minor^a	Hemodynamically and mechanically stable
LC I^a	Ipsilateral sacral compression	A1	Not involving the pelvic ring; avulsion injuries		Grade 1	APC I and LC I
LC II^b	Ipsilateral iliac wing	A2	Stable, minimal displacement of the ring		Moderate^b	Hemodynamically stable, mechanically unstable
LC III^b	Ipsilateral LC I or LC II; contralateral APC injury	A3	Transverse sacrum/coccyx fracture		Grade II	APC II/III and LC II/III
APC	Symphyseal diastasis or longitudinal rami fracture	Type B^b	Rotational instability, vertical stability		Grade III	VS and CM
APC I^a	Pubic symphysis widening <2.5cm or SI joint widening (intact ligaments)	B1	External rotation instability, open book		Severe^b	Hemodynamically unstable lesions independently of mechanical status
APC II^b	Pubic symphysis widening >2.5cm; widened SI joint (intact posterior SI ligaments, disrupted anterior SI ligaments)	B2	LC injury: Internal instability; ipsilateral only		Grade IV	Any
		B3	LC injury; bilateral rotational instability, open book			
APC III^b	Complete SI joint disruption with lateral displacement (disrupted ligaments)	Type C^b	Rotational and vertical instability			
		C1	Unilateral vertically unstable			
VS**	Symphyseal diastasis or vertical displacement (anterior and posterior)	C2	Bilateral, one side rotationally unstable, other side vertically unstable			
CMI**	Combination of any injury patterns	C3	Bilateral, both sides rotationally and vertically unstable			

The Young and Burgess classification, the Tile classification, and the World Society for Emergency Surgery classification for traumatic pelvic fractures.
Abbreviations: APC, anteroposterior compression; CMI, combined mechanism injury; LC, lateral compression; VS, vertical shear.
^a stable fracture pattern
^b unstable fracture pattern

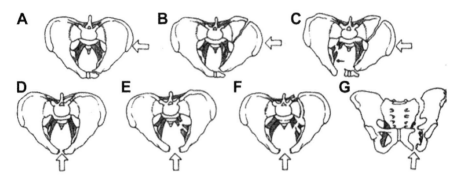

Fig. 3. Young and burgess classification. (*A*): LC I, (*B*): LC II, (*C*): LC III, (*D*): APC I, (*E*): APC II, (*F*): APC III, (*G*): VS. Reproduced with permission from Beaty JH (ed): Orthopaedic Knowledge Update 6. American Academy of Orthopaedic Surgeons; 1998: 427-239.

hematomas. CT scans that do not demonstrate intravenous contrast extravasation (ie, arterial bleeding) have negative predictive values of 98.0% to 99.8% for requiring angiography; positive predictive values of contrast extravasation on CT range from 69.2% to 90%.[20] Additional adjuncts such as CT cystography and CT ureterogram may be performed with suspicion for a urinary system injury.

PENETRATING PELVIC TRAUMA MANAGEMENT

Evaluation of a patient with penetrating pelvic trauma follows ATLS principles.[16] Care should be taken to thoroughly evaluate the perineum, buttocks, and genitalia for wounds or expanding hematomas. Radiographic imaging should be performed to identify retained ballistics. Patients with hemodynamic instability, peritonitis, evisceration, or gross blood per rectum/vagina should then be taken to the operating room for exploration and control of hemorrhage and intraabdominal injuries. Patients with intraperitoneal free air, a large volume of free fluid, or other findings consistent with intraperitoneal bowel or bladder injury also necessitate operative exploration.

If a patient does not have immediate indications for operative exploration, CT imaging can be performed to evaluate the tract of the gunshot wound or stab wound. This scan should include intra-rectal water-soluble contrast, as this has demonstrated a 95% sensitivity and 96% specificity for rectal trauma. If rectal contrast is not used, rigid sigmoidoscopy may be necessary as the sensitivity of CT drops to 36%.[21,22] CT cystography and delayed phased imaging can be performed to look for renal collecting system and bladder injuries. When bowel, intraperitoneal bladder, ureter, vaginal, or scrotal injuries are found on evaluation, operative intervention is indicated. When vascular injuries are identified with IV contrast, the location and extent of injury will determine operative accessibility and the utility of an endovascular approach. Extraperitoneal bladder injuries can be safely managed conservatively with bladder drainage for 10 to 14 days, however data are pooled between blunt and penetrating trauma.[23,24]

Nonoperative management can be trialed in hemodynamically stable patients who remain awake and cooperative with abdominal examinations.[25,26] Serial monitoring of vital signs, hemoglobin/white blood cell count values, and abdominal examinations are required. Treatment failure and operative intervention occurs if the patient develops peritonitis, hemodynamic instability, fever/leukocytosis, or a transfusion requirement of more than 2 units.[25]

BLUNT PELVIC TRAUMA MANAGEMENT
Hemodynamically Stable

Hemodynamically stable patients with pelvis fractures should be managed in a multidisciplinary fashion with orthopedic surgeons, physical therapy, occupational therapy, and trauma surgeons. There is controversy on the use of AE in hemodynamically stable patients with intravenous contrast extravasation on CT imaging. The need for AE should be evaluated on an individual patient basis.[20] Operative fixation and timing will be based on fracture geometry, geometric stability, patient mobility, and other existing injuries.

Hemodynamically Unstable

Multiple treatment options exist for the management of the hemodynamically unstable pelvic fracture patient. These include pelvic binding, external fixation, REBOA, PPP, AE, or often, a combination of these techniques. There continues to be debate regarding the optimal care of these complex patients, and care should be individualized based upon patient presentation. A protocolized approach toward management should be implemented at each institution based upon local resources and expertise (**Fig. 4**).

Pelvic binding

The posterior venous plexus and fractured bony surfaces are most often the source of bleeding in patients with a pelvic fracture.[7] The intent of a pelvic binder is to reduce the pelvic fractures into a more anatomic position and decrease fracture motion, thus slowing bleeding. It also decreases the pelvic volume, increases pelvic stability, and promotes stability in clot formation.[7,27–29] In a single institution study, patients with pelvic binders had significantly fewer blood transfusions (9.9 units) as compared to patients who underwent immediate, operative anterior pelvic fixation (21.5 units).[27] However, pelvic binders have not been shown to impact mortality.[27,29,30]

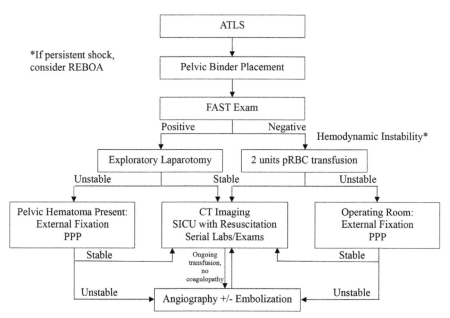

Fig. 4. Algorithm for hemodynamically unstable pelvic fracture patients.

The WSES, Western Trauma Association (WTA), and the Eastern Association for the Surgery of Trauma (EAST) all advocate for the empiric placement of pelvic binders in hemodynamically unstable patient with suspected pelvic truama.[13,20,31] However, care must be taken to place pelvic binders correctly as 40% to 45% are suboptimally placed. Placement should ideally be at the level of the greater trochanters with just enough force to close any pubic diastasis (**Fig. 5**).[32] Perfect alignment of fracture elements is not the goal as gentle reduction will attain stabilization and prevention of further movement and tearing of pelvic vasculature. Many different binders are available commercially, offering clear instructions and convenient fasteners for maintaining closure. Alternatively, a folded sheet situated at the greater trochanters secured with large clamps or penetrating towel clips is equally effective (**Fig. 6**).[33]

Resuscitative endovascular balloon occlusion of the aorta

REBOA (Prytime Medical, Boerne, Texas) evolved from endovascular techniques of occlusion balloons in emergent aortic surgery. Intra-aortic balloon occlusion was used in the Korean War for traumatic hemorrhage, and was revisited in civilian trauma patients in 2013.[33]

REBOA placement is achieved by accessing the common femoral artery with ultrasound guidance and placing a 7 Fr access sheath. The REBOA catheter is then advanced through the sheath to zone I (supraceliac) or zone III (infrarenal) of the aorta.[34,35] The catheter tip position should first be confirmed with portable abdominal radiography; the balloon is then inflated with diluted contrast to again confirm positioning of the balloon with plain radiography (**Fig. 7**A and B). The balloon should remain inflated until definitive pelvic hemorrhage control is obtained.

There have been a variety of published reports touting the utility of REBOA as a temporizing measure or a bridge to definitive hemorrhage control.[36–38] Specific reports addressing the role of REBOA in complex pelvic fracture patients indicate that REBOA may have a role in temporarily increasing the patient's blood pressure *en route* to the operative room for pelvic packing. A single study publication reported one of the lowest mortality rates for patients in refractory shock due to pelvic fracture related hemorrhage when REBOA was utilized.[39]

To determine which patients may benefit from REBOA placement, the American Association for the Surgery of Trauma created the Aortic Occlusion for Resuscitation in Trauma and Acute Care Surgery (AORTA) registry[40]; future research should focus on delineating the patient population that would most benefit from this invasive intervention. Within the WTA and WSES guidelines, REBOA is included as an adjunct to

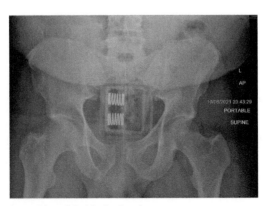

Fig. 5. Pelvic reduction with pelvic binder in place.

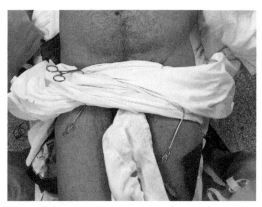

Fig. 6. Pelvic binding utilizing sheet technique.

prolong survival until definitive management; however, the exact role remains debated.[13,31] EAST is developing practice management guidelines for the use of REBOA in hemorrhage control.

The most feared complication following REBOA remains arterial access related limb ischemic complications (ARLICs); utilizing the AORTA database, 8.6% of patients were found to have sustained ARLICs. ARLICs are associated with unstable pelvic fractures, administration of tranexamic acid, and severe shock.[41]

External fixation

External fixation (EF) is a surgical procedure to stabilize pelvic fractures. Its rationale is the same as an external pelvic binder; it decreases the pelvic volume and provides

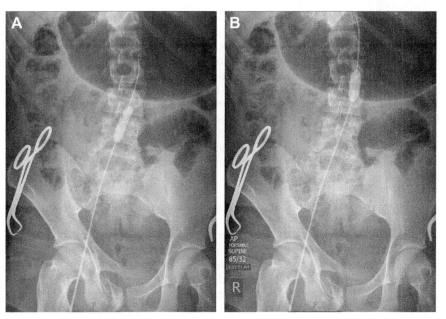

Fig. 7. (A) REBOA radiography confirming malposition in iliac artery and (B) repositioning in zone III of the aorta.

pelvis stability, thereby limiting additional trauma and bleeding. Unlike a binder, it has improved access to the groin vasculature and may be utilized for several weeks without the risks of skin breakdown that are known to occur when binders remain in place for prolonged periods of time.[13,29,42,43]

Multiple EF types exist including traditional anterior EF frames with Schanz pins placed into the iliac crests. This is typically used in damage control settings and for APC II/APC III and LC II/LC III fracture patterns. A lateral C-clamp may be used for VS type injuries in which vertical stability is necessary. However, this technique is more technically challenging and is less often utilized.[13,29] When EF is performed in tandem with PPP or laparotomy, it is important to communicate with the orthopedic surgeon on placement of the crossbars for adequate exposure. With isolated PPP, the crossbar may be located high near the umbilicus. If both laparotomy and PPP are to be performed, the crossbar should be oriented below the pubic symphysis.[44]

EF can be used as a sole intervention for pelvic fracture hemorrhage. The use of EF alone has demonstrated decreased mortality and complications compared to patients that have not undergone EF.[45,46] EF is also commonly performed in tandem with PPP, as the first step to stabilize the pelvis to permit efficacious packing against a rigid frame.

Definitive fixation of the pelvis should be delayed until after the initial resuscitation of the patient is complete and adverse physiology is corrected. Fewer complications and improved outcomes have been demonstrated if definitive pelvic fixation is performed within 24 to 36 hours of admission.[47,48] However, in severely injured patients with marked physiologic derangements, delaying definitive fixation of more than 4 days may be appropriate.[49] Timing of pelvic fixation should be determined through a thoughtful, multidisciplinary approach.

Preperitoneal pelvic packing

Preperitoneal pelvic packing (PPP) is an open surgical technique in which one packs laparotomy pads into the preperitoneal space along the pelvic ring.[44,50] The packs tamponade bleeding from both venous and bony bleeding sources. PPP is typically performed in patients with continued hemodynamic instability despite placement of a pelvic binder and transfusion of 2 units of packed red blood cells. It is commonly performed after the pelvis has been stabilized by EF (**Fig. 8**A and B). To perform PPP, a lower midline incision is made just above the pubic symphysis, typically 4 to 8 cm in length. The fascia is then incised while leaving the peritoneum intact. The bladder is subsequently retracted to one side, and 3 laparotomy pads are packed deep into the pelvis; this is then repeated on the other side (**Fig. 9**). The fascia and skin are then closed (**Fig. 10**). Laparotomy pads should be removed in 24 to 48 hours and the entire preperitoneal space should be evaluated for bleeding and hemostasis achieved.[44]

There remains a significant morbidity and mortality rate in these complex pelvic fracture patients. However, the cohort undergoing EF/PPP is a relatively small number of the total injured patients with pelvic fractures, only approximately 8%. The most common complication after PPP is infection in the pelvic space, which can range from 4% to 21%.[5,51,52] This typically occurs in the setting of open fractures, concomitant bowel or bladder injuries, and perineal degloving injuries. There is also an association between pelvic space infection and repeat packing[5]; therefore, patients should not return to the operating room for pelvic unpacking until their coagulopathy and hypothermia are addressed. Additionally, when unpacking the pelvis, careful attention to hemorrhage control is paramount; small areas of bleeding

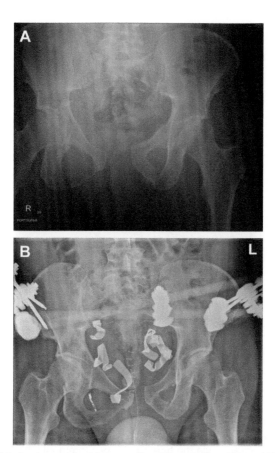

Fig. 8. APC III pelvic fracture before intervention (*A*) and after PPP and EF (*B*).

may require suture ligation, clips, electrocautery, or topical hemostatic agents for control. Interestingly, repacking the pelvis is noted to increase infection rates, but there is no association between how long the packs are left in place and infectious morbidity.[52]

Overall mortality in a hemodynamically unstable patient treated with a PPP first approach for pelvic fracture hemorrhage is 21%.[5] Compared to a modern day, multi-center evaluation of pelvic fracture management, patients presenting in shock had a 32% mortality rate.[53] This demonstrates that protocolizing PPP/EF in a single institution as a first line intervention for hemodynamically unstable patients reduced deaths from hemorrhage by 30%.[54] When compared to AE, PPP demonstrated a shorter time to intervention and overall a lower mortality in patients with pelvic fracture-related hemorrhage.[5] When compared to REBOA alone, PPP has decreased 24 hour (18% vs 32%) and in hospital (37% vs 52%) mortality in a single series.[55]

Angioembolization

Angioembolization (AE) for pelvic trauma and hemorrhage was first described in 1972 by Margolies and colleagues[56]. In 1985, a small series by Pannetta and colleagues found that AE successfully controlled hemorrhage in 85% of patients with hemody-namically unstable pelvic fractures, which resulted in a 36% mortality reduction.[57]

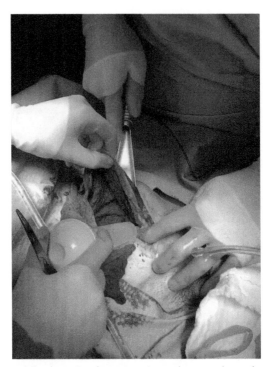

Fig. 9. Laparotomy pads deep in the preperitoneal space (seen here at the time of unpacking).

For arterial bleeding in the pelvis, AE is quite effective for hemorrhage control. AE involves selective embolization of bleeding vessels identified within the pelvis on digital subtraction angiography via the femoral artery. Commonly the IIA or its branches are the identified source of bleeding and can be targeted with either gelfoam or coils (**Fig. 11**A-E).[58] In some hemodynamically unstable patients, nonselective bilateral IIA embolization is selected as the only remaining option and may be effective in decreasing inflow into the pelvic vasculature. Ischemic complications of the perineum and pelvic organs with this technique do occur but are rarely reported. These

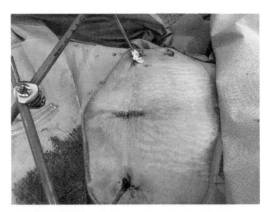

Fig. 10. Preperitoneal pelvic packing incision with external fixation.

devastating complications serve as a cautionary tale and may direct the physician to options other than empiric bilateral IIA embolization.[5,59]

Perhaps not surprisingly, AE is not without its own downsides. While AE is very effective for arterial bleeding, venous and bony bleeding sources may not be impacted. AE has a longer time to intervention with some studies describing median times of up to 6 hours before hemorrhage control is achieved.[60,61] The reason for this wide range of time is likely due to the variability of interventional radiology (IR) availability. In a survey sent to ACS verified level 1 trauma centers, 54% reported that 24-h IR coverage was available; 71% of centers reported IR teams were able to arrive within 20 to 30 minutes of activation.[62] Finally, AE is an invasive modality with access related complications reported.

AE is a complementary intervention in patients undergoing EF/PPP, as up to 13% will have persistent transfusion requirements heralding possible ongoing arterial hemorrhage in the pelvis.[6] For those patients with (1) greater than 4u red cell transfusion requirements, (2) in the 12 hours after PPP, (3) once the patient's coagulopathy is corrected, diagnostic angiography should be performed. If a bleeding source is identified, selective AE is performed; empiric embolization is not routinely advocated. AE may also be utilized as a primary hemorrhage control technique in patients who have a REBOA placed in the ED as a bridging technique. Outcomes comparing REBOA as a bridging technique to either PPP or AE are an ongoing area of study.[63]

Open Pelvic Fractures

Open pelvic fractures are characterized by direct communication between the fracture and the external environment (through the skin, rectum, vagina, or urogenital tract). Only 2% to 4% of all pelvic fractures are considered open but they have an estimated mortality of up to 50%.[64,65] Mortality is attributable to the pelvic fracture and associated hemorrhage in 30% to 50%, but mortality from pelvic sepsis occurs in 33%.[66] Bleeding in open pelvic fracture patients can be controlled with PPP, despite some reports to the contrary.[67] AE is often performed in these patients and has a reported success rate of 89% in controlling hemorrhage. Associated anorectal injuries were present in 33% of cases and urogenital injuries were found in 33% of injuries.[64]

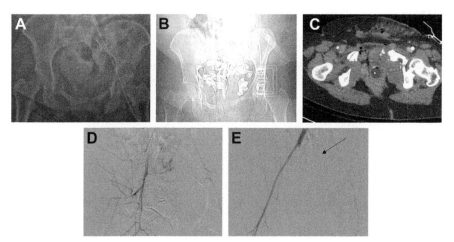

Fig. 11. LC III pelvic fracture (A), after pelvic packing and pelvic binder (B), arterial extravasation on CT imaging (C), angiogram with arterial extravasation from multiple branches of internal iliac artery (D), angiogram after gelfoam embolization of internal iliac artery (E).

Management of open fractures includes the basic principles or fracture washout, antibiotics, and limiting the source of contamination. Fecal diversion has been proposed as a mechanism to control contamination of large skin defects that communicate with pelvic fractures and potential hardware. Faringer and colleagues described a selective approach of diversion when the wound in the perineum extended from the lower abdominal wall to the sacrum and extends to the anus or close to the anus where closure/vacuum seal is not possible.[68] However, it remains unclear if this prevents infections; 27% of diverted patients developed infection, while 29% of patients without fecal diversion developed an infection.[66]

There is a high incidence of bladder, urethra, and ureteral trauma with open pelvis fractures. Bladder ruptures may be managed with foley catheterization for extraperitoneal injuries and with direct repair in 2 layers for intraperitoneal injuries. Urethral injuries are often managed with suprapubic catheter placement or repair over a foley catheter (delayed or immediate) when feasible.[69] Ureteral repair may be performed in the immediate hospitalization or in a delayed fashion. In hemodynamically unstable patients, ligation of the ureter may be performed with percutaneous nephrostomy tube placement in the ipsilateral kidney.

SUMMARY

Pelvic trauma remains a unique challenge for clinicians, particularly in complex, multisystem trauma patients that present with hemodynamic instability. A multidisciplinary approach to treatment of pelvic trauma and hemorrhage is required for optimal patient care. While each trauma center will adapt their protocol for treatment based upon local resources and clinician expertise, familiarity with the techniques of pelvic binding, REBOA, EF, PPP, and AE is paramount.[29] Each of these may be utilized based upon patient presentation, injury mechanism, admission physiology, and resources.

DISCLOSURE

The authors received no financial support for this publication. The authors have no commercial or financial conflicts of interest to disclose.

REFERENCES

1. Balogh Z, King KL, Mackay P, et al. The epidemiology of pelvic ring fractures: A population-based study. J Trauma 2007;63:1006–73.
2. Giannoudis PV, Grotz MRW, Tzioupis C, et al. Prevalence of pelvic fractures, associated injuries, and mortality: The united kingdom perspective. J Trauma 2007;63:875–83.
3. Constantini TW, Coimbra R, Holcomb JB, et al. Current management of hemorrhage from severe pelvic fractures: results of an American Association for the Surgery of Trauma multi-institutional trial. J Trauma Acute Care Surg 2016;80(5):717–25.
4. Pohlemann T, Stengel D, Tosounidis G, et al. Survival trends and predictors of mortality in severe pelvic trauma: estimates from the German Pelvic Trauma Registry Initiative. Injury 2011;42:997–1002.
5. Burlew CC, Moore EE, Stahel PF, et al. Preperitoneal pelvic packing reduces mortality in patients with life-threatening hemorrhage due to unstable pelvic fractures. J Trauma Acute Care Surg 2017;82(2):233–42.
6. Burlew CC, Moore EE, Smith WR, et al. Preperitoneal pelvic packing/external fixation with secondary angioembolization: Optimal care for life-threatening hemorrhage from unstable pelvic fractures. J Am Coll Surg 2011;212(4):628–35.

7. White CE, Hsu JR, Holcomb JB. Haemodynamically unstable pelvic fractures. Injury 2009;40(10):1023–30.
8. O'Neill P, Riina j, Sclafani S, et al. Angiographic findings in pelvic fractures. Clin Orthop Relat Res 1996;329:60–7.
9. Becker I, Woodley SH, Stringer MD. The adult human pubic symphysis: a systemic review. J Anat 2010;217(5):475–87.
10. Mahadevan V. Anatomy of the pelvis. Surg 2018;36(7):333–8.
11. Pennal GF, Tile M, Waddell JP, et al. Pelvic disruption: assessment and classification. Clin Orthop Relat Res 1980;151:12–21.
12. Young JW, Burgess AR, Brumback RJ, et al. Pelvic fractures: value of plain radiography in early assessment and management. Radiology 1986;160(2):445–51.
13. Coccolini F, Stahel PF, Montori G, et al. Pelvic trauma: WSES classification and guidelines. World J Emerg Surg 2017;12:5.
14. Li PH, Hsu TA, Kuo YC, et al. The application of the WSES classification system for open pelvic fractures – validation and supplement from a nationwide data bank. World J Emerg Surg 2022;17:29.
15. Wang SH, Fu CY, Bajani F, et al. Accuracy of the WSES classification system for pelvic ring disruptions: An international validation study. World J Emerg Surg 2021;16:54.
16. Committee of trauma of ACS. Advanced trauma life support (ATLS) student manual. 10th edition. Chicago: ACS; 2012.
17. Schwed AC, Wagenaar A, Reppert AE, et al. Trust the FAST: Confirmation that the FAST examination is highly specific for intra-abdominal hemorrhage in over 1,200 patients with pelvic fractures. J Trauma Acute Care Surg 2021;90(1):137–42.
18. Chaijareenont C, Krutsri C, Sumpritparadit P, et al. FAST accuracy in major pelvic fractures for decision-making of abdominal exploration: systemic review and meta-analysis. Ann Med Surg 2020;60:175–81.
19. Shlamovitz GZ, Mower WR, Bergman J, et al. How (un)useful is the pelvic ring stability examination in diagnosing mechanically unstable pelvic fractures in blunt trauma patients? J Trauma 2009;66(3):815–20.
20. Cullinane DC, Schiller HJ, Zielinski MD, et al. Eastern Association for the Surgery of Trauma practice management guidelines for hemorrhage in pelvic fracture – update and systemic review. J Trauma 2011;71(6):1850–68.
21. Hornez E, Monchal T, Boddaert G, et al. Penetrating pelvic trauma: Initial assessment and surgical management in emergency. J Visc Surg 2016;153:79–90.
22. Trust MD, Veith J, Brown CVR, et al. Traumatic rectal injuries: Is the combination of computed tomography and rigid proctoscopy sufficient. J Trauma Acute Care Surg 2018;85(6):1033–7.
23. Anderson RE, Keilhani S, Moses RA, et al. Current management of extraperitoneal bladder injuries: Results from the multi-institutional genito-urinary trauma study (MiGUTS). J Urol 2020;204(3):538–44.
24. Urry RJ, Clarke DL, Bruce JL, et al. The incidence, spectrum and outcomes of traumatic bladder injuries within the Pietermaritzburg metropolitan trauma service. Injury 2016;47:1057–63.
25. Navsari PH, Edu S, Nicol AJ. Nonoperative management of pelvic gunshot wounds. Am J Surg 2011;201:784–8.
26. Velmahos GC, Demetriades D, Cornwell EE 3rd. Transpelvic gunshot wounds: Routine laparotomy or selective management? World J Surg 1998;22(10):1034–8.
27. Croce MA, Magnotti LJ, Savage SA, et al. Emergent pelvic fixation in patients with exsanguinating pelvic fractures. J Am Coll Surg 2007;204(5):935–42.

28. Dreizin D, Bodanapally U, Mascarenhas D, et al. Quantitative MDCT assessment of binder effects after pelvic ring disruptions using segmented pelvic haematoma volumes and multiplanar caliper measurements. Euro Rad 2018;28:3953–62.

29. DuBose JJ, Burlew CC, Joseph B, et al. Pelvic fracture-related hypotension: a review of contemporary adjuncts for hemorrhage control. J Trauma Acute Care Surg 2021;91(4):e93–103.

30. Agri F, Bourgeat M, Becce F, et al. Association of pelvic fracture patterns, pelvic binder use and arterial angioembolization with transfusion requirements and mortality rates; a 7-year retrospective cohort study. BMC Surg 2017;17:103.

31. Tran TL, Brasel KJ, Karmy-Jones R, et al. Western Trauma Association critical decision in trauma: Management of pelvic fracture with hemodynamically instability – 2016 updates. J Trauma Acute Care Surg 2016;81(6):1171–4.

32. Williamson F, Coulthard LG, Hacking C, et al. Identifying risk factors for suboptimal pelvic binder placement in major trauma. Injury 2020;51:971–7.

33. Prasarn ML, Conrad B, Small J, et al. Comparison of circumferential pelvic sheeting versus the T-POD on unstable pelvic injuries: A cadaveric study of stability. Injury Int J Care Injured 2013;44:1756–9.

34. Stokes SC, Theodorou CM, Zakaluzny SA, et al. REBOA in combat causalities: The past, present, and future. J Trauma Acute Care Surg 2021;91(2):S56–64.

35. Prytime Medical. The ER-REBOATM catheter quick reference guide: 6 REBOA steps: ME-FIIS (Pronounced ME-FIZZ) Available at: http://prytimemedical.com/wp-content/uploads/2017/08/ER-REBOA-Catheter-Quick-Reference-Guide-wall-poster.pdf. Accessed July 17, 2023.

36. Brenner M, Teeter W, Hoehn, et al. Use of resuscitative endovascular balloon occlusion of the aorta for the proximal aortic control in patients with severe hemorrhage and arrest. JAMA Surg 2018;153(2):130–5.

37. Cannon J, Morrison J, Lauer C, et al. Resuscitative endovascular balloon occlusion of the aorta (REBOA) for hemorrhagic shock. Mil Med 2018;183:55–9.

38. Castellini G, Gianola S, Biffl A, et al. Resuscitative endovascular balloon occlusion of the aorta (REBOA) in patients with major trauma and uncontrolled haemorrhagic shock: a systemic review with meta—analysis. World J Emerg Surg 2021;15:41.

39. Werner NL, Moore EE, Hoehn M, et al. Inflate and pack! Pelvic packing combined with REBOA deployment prevents hemorrhage related deaths in unstable pelvic fractures. Injury 2022 Oct;53(10):3365–70.

40. DuBose JJ, Scalea TM, Brenner M, et al. The AAST prospective Aortic Occlusion for Resuscitation in Trauma and Acute Care Surgery (AORTA) registry: Data on contemporary utilization and outcomes of aortic occlusion and resuscitative balloon occlusion of the aorta (REBOA). J Trauma Acute Care Surg 2016;81(3):409–19.

41. Laverty RB, Treffalls RN, McEntire SE, et al. Life over limb: arterial access-related limb ischemic complications in 48-hour REBOA survivors. J Trauma Acute Care Surg 2021;92(4):723–8.

42. Hoch A, Zeidler S, Pieroh P, et al. Trends and efficacy of external emergency stabilization of pelvic ring fractures: Results from the German Pelvic Trauma Registry. Euro J Trauma Emerg Surg 2021;47:523–5313.

43. Prasarn ML, Horodyski M, Schneider PS, et al. Comparison of skin pressure measurements with the use of pelvic circumferential compression devices on pelvic ring injuries. Injury Int J Care Injured 2016;47:717–20.

44. Burlew CC. Preperitoneal pelvic packing: A 2018 EAST master class video presentation. J Trauma Acute Care Surg 2018;85(1):224–8.

45. Schmall H, Larsen MS, Stuby F, et al. Effectiveness and complications of primary C-clamp stabilization or external fixation for unstable pelvic fractures. Injury 2019; 50(11):1959–65.

46. Ohmori T, Kitamura T, Nishida T, et al. The impact of external fixation on mortality in patients with an unstable pelvic ring fracture: A propensity-matched cohort study. Bone Joint Lett J 2018;100(2):233–41.

47. Vallier HA, Cureton BA, Ekstein C, et al. Early definitive stabilization of unstable pelvis and acetabulum fractures reduces morbidity. J Trauma 2010;69(3):677–84.

48. Vallier HA, Moore TA, Como JJ, et al. Complications are reduced with a protocol to standardize timing of fixation based on response to resuscitation. J Orthop Surg Res 2015;10:155.

49. Pape H, Stalp M, Griensven Mv, et al. Optimal timing for secondary surgery in polytrauma patients: an evaluation of 4,314 serious-injury cases. Chirurg 1999; 70(11):1287–93.

50. Burlew CC. Preperitoneal packing for exsanguinating pelvic fractures. Int Orthop 2017;41:1825–9.

51. Anand T, El-Qawaqzeh, Nelson A, et al. Association between hemorrhage control interventions and mortality in US trauma patients with hemodynamically unstable pelvic fractures. JAMA Surg 2023;158(1):63–71.

52. Shim H, Jang JY, Kim JW, et al. Effectiveness and postoperative wound infection of preperitoneal pelvic packing in patients with hemodynamic instability caused by pelvic fracture. PLoS One 2018 Nov 5;13(11):e0206991.

53. Costantini TW, Coimbra R, Holcomb JB, et al. Current management of hemorrhage from severe pelvic fractures: results of an American Association for the Surgery of Trauma multi-institutional trail. J Trauma Acute Care Surg 2016;80(5): 717–25.

54. Parry JA, Smith WR, Moore EE, et al. The past, present, and future management of hemodynamic instability in patients with unstable pelvic ring injuries. Injury 2021;52(10):2693–6.

55. Mikdad S, van Erp IAM, Moheb ME, et al. Preperitoneal pelvic packing for early hemorrhage control reduces mortality compared to resuscitative endovascular balloon occlusion of the aorta in severe blunt pelvic trauma patients: a nationwide analysis. Injury 2020;51(8):1834–9.

56. Margolies MN, Ring EJ, Waltman AC, et al. Arteriography in the management of hemorrhage from pelvic fractures. New Engl J Med 1972;287(7):317–21.

57. Panetta T, Sclafani SJ, Goldstein AS, et al. Percutaneous transcatheter embolization for massive bleeding from pelvic fractures. J Trauma 1985;25(11):1021–9.

58. Vaidya R, Waldron J, Scott A, et al. Angiography and embolization in the management of bleeding pelvic fractures. J Am Acad Ortho Surg 2018;26(4):e68–76.

59. Bonde A, Velmahos A, Kalva S, et al. Bilateral internal iliac artery embolization for pelvic trauma: Effectiveness and safety. Am J Surg 2020;220:454–8.

60. Schwartz DA, Medina M, Cotton BA, et al. Are we delivering two standards of care for pelvic trauma? Availability of angioembolization after hours and on weekends increases time to therapeutic intervention. J Trauma Acute Care Surg 2013; 76(1):134–9.

61. Tesoriero RB, Bruns BR, Narayan M, et al. Angiographic embolization for hemorrhage following pelvic fracture: Is it "time" for a paradigm shift? J Trauma Acute Care Surg 2016;82(1):18–26.

62. Jarvis S, Orlando A, Blondeau B, et al. Variability in the timeliness of interventional radiology availability for angioembolization of hemodynamically unstable pelvic

fractures: A prospective survey among US level 1 trauma centers. Patient Saf Surg 2019;13:23.

63. Brenner M, Moore L, Zakhary B, et al. Scalpel or sheath? Outcomes comparison between preperitoneal pelvic packing and angioembolization for definitive hemorrhage control after REBOA. J Endovasc Resusc Trauma Management 2020; 4(1):49–55.

64. Mi M, Kanakaris NK, Wu X, et al. Management and outcomes of open pelvic fractures: an update. Injury 2021;52:2738–45.

65. Hermans E, Edwards MJR, Goslings JC, et al. Open pelvic fracture: The killing fracture? J Orthop Surg Res 2018;13:83.

66. Woods RK, O'Keefe G, Rhee P, et al. Open pelvic fracture and fecal diversion. Arch Surg 1998;133:281–6.

67. Moskowitz EE, Burlew CC, Moore EE, et al. Preperitoneal pelvic packing is effective for hemorrhage control in open pelvic fractures. Am J Surg 2018;215(4): 675–7.

68. Faringer PD, Mullins RJ, Feliciano PD, et al. Selective fecal diversion in complex open pelvic fractures from blunt trauma. Arch Surg 1994;129:958–64.

69. Wu K, Posluszny JA, Branch J, et al. Trauma to the pelvis: injuries to the rectum and genitourinary organs. Cur Trauma Rep 2015;1:8–15.

Management of the Mangled Extremity

Erin Farrelly, MD*, Rae Tarapore, MD[1], Sierra Lindsey, MD[1],
Mark D. Wieland, MD[1]

KEYWORDS

- Mangled extremity • Amputation • Orthopedic trauma • Limb salvage

KEY POINTS

- Mangled extremities are one of the most complex injuries encountered in the trauma setting. Successful treatment requires both general protocols and individualized plans based on the patient and injury with coordination between multiple services.
- Several classification systems of mangled extremities have been developed in an attempt to standardize the management of patients and to facilitate communication among physicians; these include the Gustilo-Anderson classification for open fractures and the Mangled Extremity Severity Score.
- Initial treatment incorporates an initial trauma survey, extremity-focused history, physical examination, assessment of vascular and neurologic status, antibiotic administration, tetanus prophylaxis, and control of blood loss.
- Following the initial management, surgical management follows in the form of either primary amputation or attempts at limb salvage.
- Although both amputation and limb salvage have been associated with chronic disability, new surgical techniques and evolving rehabilitation options offer hope for the future.

INTRODUCTION/CLASSIFICATION AND DEFINITION

Mangled extremities are one of the most complex injuries encountered in the trauma setting. Successful treatment requires both general protocols and individualized plans based on the patient and the injury and coordination between multiple services. Mangled extremities are an indicator of a high-energy mechanism of injury and should alert emergency physicians to the need for a full trauma survey.

This article will provide an overview of the mangled extremity, including the classifications commonly used, important steps for initial management, definitive treatment options, and long-term outcomes. Successful development and application of treatment protocols can be life-altering for patients affected by these devastating injuries.

Department of Orthopaedic Surgery, MedStar Orthopaedic Institute, Union Memorial Hospital, Baltimore, MD, USA
[1] Present address. 201 E. University Parkway, Baltimore, MD 21218, USA
* Corresponding author. 277 Rancheros Drive, Suite 101, San Marcos, CA 92069.
E-mail address: Erin.Farrelly@gmail.com

Surg Clin N Am 104 (2024) 385–404
https://doi.org/10.1016/j.suc.2023.10.006
0039-6109/24/© 2023 Elsevier Inc. All rights reserved.
surgical.theclinics.com

There are multiple ways to define the mangled extremity. One definition commonly used is any limb that has sustained an injury to at least 3 out of 4 of the following: soft tissue, nerves, bones, and blood vessels.[1] The term mangled extremity has also been applied to injuries that are proximal to the hindfoot or radiocarpal joint and requires either amputation or complex reconstruction (complex reconstruction includes procedures such as bone grafting, soft tissue coverage, nerve or vascular repair, or fasciotomies).[2] Other authors have used more general descriptions, such as an at-risk or threatened limb, meaning that there is a significant risk of amputation.

These injuries most often occur because of high-energy accidents. Some common mechanisms include ballistic injuries, motorcycle and motor vehicle accidents, and accidents involving industrial machinery. The mechanism of injury and force required to cause a mangled extremity put the patient at high risk for associated injuries. It is imperative that every patient with these injuries has a full primary trauma survey and ongoing secondary and tertiary surveys. It is easy to become distracted by a mangled extremity.

The extent of injury to the limb may not be immediately apparent. This causes challenges regarding triage, initial management, surgical planning, and long-term management. Ongoing evaluations of function and inspection of the wound in the operating room are necessary to fully define the injury.

Several classification systems of mangled extremities have been developed in an attempt to standardize the management of patients and to facilitate communication among physicians. A variety of systems have been proposed to categorize mangled extremities based on the degree of soft tissue damage, anatomic defects, and the presence or absence of associated injuries. Some of these include the Gustilo-Anderson classification, Mangled Extremity Severity Score (MESS), Orthopedic Trauma Association Classification, and the Predictive Salvage Index.

The Gustilo-Anderson classification categorizes open fractures by the extent of soft tissue damage present. This provides guidance regarding surgical management and antibiotic use. In contrast with the classifications that aim to prognosticate injuries, this classification is limited to guiding initial management (**Table 1**). Despite its limited interobserver reliability and fairly narrow scope, this classification remains commonly used among traumatologists.[3] Thus, it remains important for traumatologists to be familiar with this system because it aids in communication and guides initial management. The classification is intended to be applied during the evaluation in the operating room because it is not possible to fully evaluate the extent of injury in the trauma bay without risking increased contamination and pain.[4]

The predictive salvage index (PSI) was created in 1987 by Howe and colleagues.[5] This score was based on a small retrospective cohort including 21 injured extremities. It included criteria such as the time from injury to arrival in the operating room, the level of arterial injury, and the quantitative degree of muscle, bone, and skin injury (**Table 2**). This system has been challenged in the literature during the past several decades due to the limited patient sample size that it was based on. Still, although some have argued that it has a limited sensitivity and specificity,[6] others have described the PSI as having acceptable diagnostic value when used in conjunction with other scoring systems and patient factors.[7]

The MESS was proposed in 1990 by Johansen and colleagues[8] and incorporates factors including patient age, limb ischemia, presence/absence of shock, and skeletal/soft tissue injury (**Table 3**). This classification aims to provide objectivity in prognosticating the probability of limb salvage. The MESS score has received criticism in the literature during the past few decades because of its low ability to predict whether a limb is salvageable.[9] However, it continues to be used in lower extremity trauma literature, in part, because it is familiar to most surgeons.[10]

Table 1
Gustilo-Anderson classification

Fracture Type	Description	Antibiotic Management
I	Clean wound <1 cm in diameter, simple fracture pattern. Low energy	First-generation cephalosporin
II	Laceration >1 cm, <10 cm without significant soft tissue crushing. Moderately contaminated, medium energy	First-generation cephalosporin
III	Extensive soft tissue injury >10 cm. High energy, significant contamination. Subdivided into 3 types	First-generation cephalosporin *and* aminoglycoside
IIIA	Adequate soft tissue coverage despite high energy and large wound	First-generation cephalosporin *and* aminoglycoside
IIIB	Inadequate soft tissue coverage, periosteal stripping	First-generation cephalosporin *and* aminoglycoside
IIIC	Associated with vascular injury that requires repair	First-generation cephalosporin *and* aminoglycoside

From: Gustilo RB, Mendoza RM, Williams DN. Problems in management of type III (severe) open fractures: a new classification of type III open fractures. J Trauma. 1984;24:742–746. https://doi. org/10.1097/00005373-198408000-00009.

The limb salvage index (LSI) was established in 1991 by Russell and colleagues,[11] and it aims to help guide clinical decision-making regarding whether to attempt heroic limb-saving procedures or primarily amputate (**Table 4**). The LSI requires intraoperative evaluation in order to be applicable.[11] Thus, it cannot be applied in the emergency department. However, it is a useful tool because it features more extensive criteria than many other scoring systems. Recent analysis shows that it maintains acceptable diagnostic accuracy in modern care for mangled extremities.[7]

The Nerve injury, Ischemia, Soft-tissue contamination, Skeletal injury, Shock, and Age (NISSSA) scoring system was introduced in 1994 by McNamara and colleagues.[12]

Table 2
Predictive salvage index—absolute indication for amputation greater than 8

Level of arterial injury	Suprapopliteal	1
	Popliteal	2
	Infrapopliteal	3
Degree of bone injury	Mild	1
	Moderate	2
	Severe	3
Degree of muscle injury	Mild	1
	Moderate	2
	Severe	3
Interval from time of injury to operating room	<6 h	1
	6–12 h	2
	>12 h	3

From: Howe HR, Jr, Poole GV, Jr, Hansen KJ, Clark T, Plonk GW, Koman LA, Pennell TC. Salvage of lower extremities following combined orthopedic and vascular trauma. A predictive salvage index. Am Surg. 1987;53:205–208.

Table 3 Mangled Extremity Severity Score—absolute indication for amputation greater than 7 points		
Energy	Low	1
	Medium	2
	High	3
	Very High	4
Ischemia	Perfused	1
	Pulseless, decreased capillary refill	2
	Cold, insensate, numb, paralyzed (score doubled for ischemia >6 h)	3
Shock	Systolic BP > 90 consistently	1
	Transient hypotensive	2
	Persistent hypotension	3
Age	<30	1
	30–50	2
	>50	3

Abbreviations: BP, blood pressure.
Data from Johansen K, Daines M, Howey T, Helfet D, Hanson ST., Jr Objective criteria accurately predict amputation following lower extremity trauma. J Trauma. 1990;30:568–572. https://doi.org/10.1097/00005373-199005000-00007.

This classification (**Table 5**) is a complex modification of the MESS classification, which is described above. This score was established based on a small retrospective cohort of 24 patients. The authors touted that it was an improvement on the MESS in terms of sensitivity and specificity. However, in modern literature and among physicians, the MESS classification tends to be used more commonly.[13]

All of the aforementioned classifications have varying utility that has been broadly debated in trauma literature. A 2015 systematic review of all scoring systems compared the MESS, PSI, LSI, and NISSSA scores. This review concluded that the MESS seems to be more accurate than the LSI in terms of predicting limb salvage, whereas the NISSSA demonstrates low sensitivity and specificity in most studies. The LSI shows more accuracy when applied to Gustilo Type III tibia fractures, and the PSI has a very high sensitivity when used to predict successful limb salvage.[13] Similarly, a study in 2008 compared the MESS, PSI, NISSSA, and Hannover Fracture Scale-98. None reliably predicted the Sickness Impact Profile of patients 6 or 24 months after limb salvage.[9]

Each above-described classification and scoring system has strengths and weaknesses. Although useful when describing injuries, a single scoring system cannot be used in isolation when deciding to amputate or pursue limb salvage. The extent of injury varies greatly among patients with mangled extremities. Concomitant injuries and preexisting medical conditions also affect prognosis. Many patients hold strong preferences for limb salvage versus amputation. Treatment of a mangled extremity requires multidisciplinary care among physicians, as well as shared decision-making with the patient and their support system.

Successful long-term care of these patients depends on continued coordinated care. Emergency and trauma physicians, orthopedics, plastics and vascular surgeons are typically needed for acute management of patients with mangled extremities. Patients with mangled extremities require urgent attention, given the severity of skin, soft tissue, vascular, nervous, and osseous damage present and the potential for long-term disability. As treatment progresses, involvement of reconstructive surgeons, rehabilitation teams, social work, psychologists, and pain management specialists is necessary for successful management.

Table 4		
Limb salvage index—absolute indication for amputation greater than 6		
Artery	0	Contusion, intimal tear, partial laceration, or avulsion (pseudo-aneurysm) with no distal thrombosis and palpable pedal pulses; complete occlusion of 1 of 3 shank vessels or profunda
	1	Occlusion of 2 or more shank vessels, complete laceration, avulsion, or thrombosis of femoral or popliteal vessels without palpable pedal pulses
	2	Complete occlusion of femoral, popliteal, or 3 of 3 shank vessels with no distal runoff available
Nerve	0	Contusion or stretch injury; minimal clean laceration of femoral, peroneal, or tibial nerve
	1	Partial transection or avulsion of sciatic nerve; complete or partial transection of femoral, peroneal, or tibial nerve
	2	Complete transection or avulsion of sciatic nerve; complete transection or avulsion of both peroneal and tibial nerves
Bone	0	Closed fracture 1 or 2 sites; open fracture without comminution or with minimal displacement; closed dislocation without fracture; open joint without foreign body; fibula fracture
	1	Closed fracture at 3 or more sites on same extremity; open fracture with comminution or moderate-to-large displacement; segmental fracture; fracture dislocation; open joint with foreign body; bone loss <3 cm
	2	Bone loss >3 cm; Type III-B or III-C fracture (open fracture with periosteal stripping, gross contamination, extensive soft tissue injury-loss)
Skin	0	Clean laceration, single or multiple, or small avulsion injuries, all with primary repair; first-degree burn
	1	Clean laceration, single or multiple, or small avulsion injuries, all with primary repair; first-degree burn
Muscle	0	Laceration or avulsion involving a single compartment or single tendon
	1	Laceration or avulsion involving 2 or more compartments; complete laceration or avulsion of 2 or more tendons
	2	Crush injury
Deep Vein	0	Contusion, partial laceration, or avulsion; complete laceration or avulsion if alternate route of venous return is intact; superficial vein injury
	1	Complete laceration, avulsion, or thrombosis with no alternate route of venous return
WIT	0	<6 h
	1	6–9 h
	2	9–12 h
	3	12–15 h
	4	>15 h

From: Russell WL, Sailors DM, Whittle TB, Whittle TB, Fisher DF, Jr, Burns RP. Limb salvage versus traumatic amputation. A decision based on a seven-part predictive index. Ann Surg. 1991;213:473–480. https://doi.org/10.1097/00000658-199105000-00013.

INITIAL TREATMENT

Advanced trauma life support protocol should be initiated for all patients with a mangled extremity. These injuries can easily be distracting from more subtle life-threatening injuries. Each patient should be worked up using the ABCDE's of the initial trauma assessment. It is critical to assess for injuries to major organ systems. It is vital that the care team is not diverted by the severe appearance of a mangled extremity at the expense of this thorough initial trauma assessment.[14] Mangled extremities are frequently caused by high-energy trauma with associated polytrauma. The patient must be fully assessed for other injuries, preexisting comorbidities, and vascular status.[15]

Table 5
Nerve injury, Ischemia, Soft-tissue contamination, Skeletal injury, Shock, and Age—absolute indication for amputation greater than 11

Category	Score		
Nerve injury	0	Sensate	No nerve injury
	1	Dorsal	DPN, SPN, or femoral nerve injury
	2	Plantar partial	Tibial nerve injury
	3	Plantar complete	Sciatic nerve injury
Ischemia	0	None	Good to fair pulses
	1	Mild	Reduced pulses, normal perfusion
	2	Moderate	No pulses, Doppler present, prolonged capillary refill
	3	Severe	Pulseless, cool, no Doppler pulses
Soft tissue/contamination	0	Low	Gustilo Type I
	1	Medium	Gustilo type II
	2	High	Gustilo type IIIA
	3	Severe	Gustilo type IIIB
Skeletal	0	Low Energy	Spiral/oblique fracture, minimal displacement
	1	Medium energy	Transverse fracture, minimal comminution, low energy GSW
	2	High energy	Moderate displacement, moderate comminution, butterfly fragment(s), high-energy GSW
	3	Severe energy	Segmental, severe comminution, bony loss
Shock	0	Normotensive	Systolic BP consistently >90
	1	Transient hypotension	Systolic BP transiently <90
	2	Persistent hypotension	Systolic BP persistently <90
Age	0	Young	<30 y
	1	Middle aged	30–50 y
	2	Old	>50 y

Abbreviations: DPN, deep peroneal nerve; GSW, gun shot wound; SPN, superficial peroneal nerve.

From: McNamara MG, Heckman JD, Corley FG. Severe open fractures of the lower extremity: a retrospective evaluation of the mangled extremity severity score (MESS) J Orthop Trauma. 1994;8:81–87. https://doi.org/10.1097/00005131-199404000-00001.

Once the initial trauma survey is complete, an extremity-focused history and physical examination is performed. When possible, this includes determining the mechanism of injury, patient's past medical and surgical history, social history (including vocation, smoking status, prior ambulatory status, handedness, and social support system) and a thorough physical examination. This is typically an ongoing process. The patient may not be able to initially provide all information due to their clinical status.

As the patient is being resuscitated, the initial management of the extremity begins. Antibiotics are administered. The wound is assessed, photographed, irrigated, and dressed. Once a dressing is in place, it is typically not removed until the operating room. This avoids ongoing blood loss and contamination. Vascular status is assessed. Fractures are reduced and temporarily stabilized by splints or traction. Patients with mangled extremities often arrive at the emergency department with a tourniquet in place. Unless hemorrhage is severe, this can be replaced with a pressure dressing during the trauma survey to avoid prolonged ischemia times. Vascular status should be evaluated before and after bony manipulation. Vascular assessment begins with pulse palpation and is followed sequentially by the use of bedside Doppler assessment and Ankle-Brachial Index (ABI) or Brachial-Brachial indices. There are many factors that can influence the accuracy of ABI. If pulses or ABI are abnormal, further assessment of vascular status by CTA or angiogram is necessary.

Duration of ischemia is a significant prognostic factor. Vascular status is assessed by the evaluation of peripheral pulses, skin color, and capillary refill.[15] Injuries that are highly associated with vascular injury include supracondylar femur fractures, knee dislocations, proximal tibia fractures, and penetrating injuries of the posterior and medial thigh. If there is evidence of vascular injury (decreased pulses compared to the contralateral side), CTA or angiogram should be obtained and vascular surgery should be consulted.[15] However, the assessment of distal perfusion should not take precedence over assessment of life-threatening injuries such as brain trauma or truncal hemorrhage.[14]

A thorough sensory and motor examination is necessary to evaluate for potential nerve injuries. The mechanism of injury is an important prognostic factor in nerve injuries. Mechanisms that involve contamination, torsion, and crush injuries have a worse prognosis than sharp and clean injuries. Motor and sensory nerve function should also be assessed (**Table 6** of Peripheral Nerve Injury Findings adapted from **Table 4** in Scalea Western Trauma).

Many trauma centers have treatment protocols for patients with open fractures and limb-threatening injuries. This facilitates a standardized approach and decreases the risk of missed injuries. A good example of this is the algorithmic approach proposed by the Western Trauma Association.

During the initial survey, members of the team control blood loss by manual pressure, pressure dressing, or use of a tourniquet. Exploration of the wound in the emergency department is not recommended because it can worsen bleeding and cause wound contamination.[1] If bleeding cannot be controlled via these methods, the patient should be taken to the operating room to control bleeding.[14]

Antibiotics and tetanus prophylaxis should be administered.[1] Time to antibiotics is the only factor consistently associated with decreased infection in the setting of open fractures.[16] The preferred antibiotic regimen for a mangled extremity is typically a first-generation cephalosporin, aminoglycoside, and gentamicin. Individual risk factors should be considered when choosing antibiotics. Farming, industrial, and war injuries can involve contamination with atypical organisms.[15] Penicillin and metronidazole may be given when there is concern for anaerobic bacterial contamination.[15] Antibiotics may be adjusted if the patient has a known history of methicillin resistant staph

Table 6	
Peripheral nerve injury—motor and sensory findings	
Nerve	**Findings**
Femoral nerve	Motor: unable to perform knee extension Sensory: numbness over distal one-third of anteromedial aspect of thigh
Common peroneal nerve	Motor: foot drop—weakness or inability to dorsiflex foot and toes; inability to evert foot
Deep peroneal nerve	Motor: weakness or inability to dorsiflex foot and toes Sensory: diminished or absent sensation dorsal web space between first and second toes
Superficial peroneal nerve	Motor: inability to evert foot Sensory: diminished or absent sensation dorsal foot (with exception of dorsal web space between first and second toes)
Tibial nerve	Motor: weakness or absence of toe plantarflexion Sensory: numbness over sole and heel of foot
Median nerve	Motor: weakness or inability to flex thumb and index finger IP joints against resistance Sensory: decreased or absent sensation on volar surface of thumb, index, and middle fingers
Radial nerve	Motor: weak or absent dorsiflexion of wrist and/or thumb Sensory: decreased or absent sensation in dorsal web space between thumb and index fingers
Ulnar nerve	Motor: weak or absent finger abduction and adduction Sensory: decreased or absent sensation little finger and ulnar half of ring finger

Abbreviations: IP, proximal and distal interphalangeal joints.

From: Scalea TM, DuBose J, Moore EE, West M, Moore FA, McIntyre R, Cocanour C, Davis J, Ochsner MG, Feliciano D. Western Trauma Association critical decisions in trauma: management of the mangled extremity. J Trauma Acute Care Surg. 2012 Jan;72(1):86-93. https://doi.org/10.1097/TA.0b013e318241ed70. PMID: 22310120

aureus (MRSA) or if there is a high risk of atypical organisms (such as an injury with marine contamination or in certain desert settings).

Once the trauma evaluation is completed, surgical management begins. This consists of either primary amputation or attempts at limb salvage. Uncontrollable hemodynamic instability caused by an extremity injury and near complete traumatic amputation are absolute indications for primary amputation. Relative indications for primary amputation were proposed in 1989. They include nerve disruption, warm ischemia time (WIT) of more than 6 hours, and crush injury to the ipsilateral foot.[17] These have become more relative because treatment has advanced. Loss of plantar sensation is no longer considered an indication for primary amputation because this may resolve with time (**Fig. 1**).

Surgical management of the mangled extremity is staged. Surgical management begins with thorough irrigation and debridement. Notably, Pollak and colleagues found that the time from open lower extremity injury to debridement is not a significant independent predictor of the risk of infection.[2] Rather, thorough debridement and immediate administration of antibiotics are more critical in preventing infection. In most cases, the wound is extended proximally and distally to gain full exposure. In some cases, such as injury to the antero-medial leg where soft tissues are poor, a separate incision is made.[18] Ideally, the approach that is anticipated for definitive fixation is used. It is not unusual to discover intraoperatively that the zone of injury and contamination extends beyond what is visualized in the trauma bay. Adequate exposure is

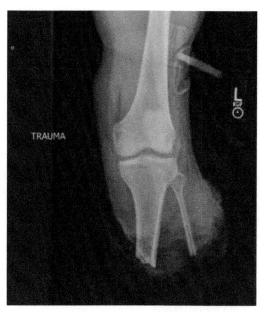

Fig. 1. Example of a case where limb salvage was not an option.

necessary to thoroughly clean the wound. A systematic debridement is performed, beginning deep and working to superficial. The bone ends are exposed and the medullary canal is inspected and cleaned using a curette.

The wound is irrigated with normal saline solution using a low-pressure system such as cystoscopy tubing. High-pressure lavage has not been shown to provide any reduction in rates of reoperation compared with low-pressure irrigation and should be avoided because it risks decreased early bone healing, pushing bacteria into the intramedullary canal, and creating fissures in cortical bone. Additives to saline have not been shown to be beneficial.[16] During the initial irrigation and debridement, foreign material and devitalized tissue are removed while preserving healthy and vital tissues. Muscle may sometimes improve over time, particularly if a tourniquet was used. Therefore, muscle that is of questionable viability at the initial debridement is maintained. If there is evidence of acute compartment syndrome or impending compartment syndrome, fasciotomies should be performed.[15]

In the setting of major soft tissue compromise, external fixation is used for provisional stabilization.[15] Ideally, all pins are placed outside of the anticipated incisions. A small frag plate can be used to temporarily supplement external fixation. This can greatly increase stability. It is typically removed at the time of definitive fixation. This has not been shown to increase the rate of infection or flap failure (**Figs. 2** and **3**).[19]

Provisional stabilization should be performed quickly to allow for resuscitation of the patient. This is particularly true if there is evidence of vascular injury. Provisional stabilization provides a stable limb for vascular surgeons to perform revascularization. In the setting of arterial disruption to the extremity, an intraluminal shunt should be used if salvage is an option.[1] Fasciotomies are performed in all cases of revascularization due to the high risk of compartment syndrome and reperfusion injury. Nerves are inspected for evidence of injury.

Mangled extremities typically require multiple debridements. The principles of damage control orthopedics are adhered to throughout these procedures.[20] The primary

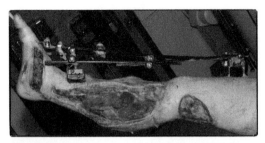

Fig. 2. External fixation outside of the zone of injury.

debridement and provisional stabilization is done rapidly, and the patient is returned to the intensive care unit for resuscitation. Compression dressings are typically placed during the initial surgery to avoid excessive blood loss.

Once the patient's overall clinical status has improved, they return to the operating room (OR) for a repeat debridement, removing any nonviable tissue. Antibiotic bead pouches and wound vacs may be used to decrease infection.[21] There is evidence that topical vancomycin powder at the wound of compound fractures may also decrease the risk of infection.[22] If the need for soft tissue reconstruction is anticipated, it is helpful for plastic surgery to be present at debridements to assess the soft tissue injury and begin planning for coverage.

Once the wound seems clean and well perfused and the patient is able to tolerate longer procedures, definitive management is undertaken. In treatment of mangled extremities, this typically requires coordination between multiple surgical subspecialties. Orthopedic treatment classically consists of converting external fixation to internal

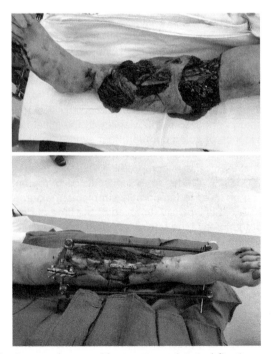

Fig. 3. External fixation supplemented by temporary internal fixation.

fixation using plates and screws or intramedullary devices. There is evidence that soft tissue coverage within 48 hours of final implant placement greatly reduces the risk of infection. Many trauma centers have moved to a model of "fix and flap" by an ortho-plastic team because of this.[23] Vascular grafts and treatment of nerve injuries by microsurgery teams may be needed.

Limb Salvage Versus Amputation

Long-term treatment options include limb salvage and amputation. The classic adage of life over limb remains true. In cases of hemodynamic instability that cannot other-wise be controlled, primary amputation is necessary in order to save a patient's life. In cases without absolute contraindications to limb salvage, the decision to either amputate or attempt limb salvage remains complex. Advancements in microsurgery and orthopedic surgery have made it possible to preserve limbs that previously would not have been salvageable. However, complex limb salvage is associated with signif-icant risks.[24]

Whether or not limb salvage should be attempted is an ongoing question that needs to be revisited with the patient and multidisciplinary team as the patient is resuscitated and additional injuries are identified. Salvage of a mangled extremity typically entails multiple, complex surgeries and may require prolonged anesthesia time and be asso-ciated with significant blood loss. In patients with severe abdominal or cardiothoracic injuries, those who are consistently hemodynamically unstable, or those with major neurologic injury, the patient may not be able to tolerate the multiple surgical interven-tions that are necessary for complex limb reconstruction.[24] In these cases, amputation can be lifesaving.

The decision to proceed with amputation or limb salvage is a difficult one. This may be made even more complicated by additional injuries, particularly if these prevent the patient from participating in the conversation. Multiple attempts have been made to develop a scoring system that correlates with prognosis in order to guide manage-ment. Unfortunately, as discussed above, none of the current scoring systems has been shown to reliably predict the ultimate need for amputation.

Except in cases of in extremis, the decision for limb salvage versus amputation in-volves shared decision-making between the patient and physicians. The treatment course taken depends on the patient's goals, preinjury activity level, comorbidities, age, and occupation.

Amputation

Amputation offers some advantages over limb salvage, particularly in the short term. Amputation typically leads to definitive management with fewer procedures (on average 3.5 compared to 8), less operative time, and shorter hospital stays compared to limb salvage. Shorter rehabilitation (12 vs 30 months) and faster return to work have also been reported.[25]

The most significant predictor for the ultimate need for amputation seems to be the degree of soft tissue injury. Patients with substantial soft tissue injury should be coun-seled that limb salvage may not be successful. A risk of limb loss up to 50% has been reported for Gustilo type III injuries. However, this system has highly variable interob-server reliability, limiting its ability for use as a prognostic tool.[20] Higher MESS scores indicate an increased risk of amputation, particularly scores over 7.[1] Additionally, WIT should be considered in the risk of limb loss. WIT refers to the time that the injured body part remains at core temperature after blood supply has been compromised prior to the extremity cooling and revascularization. WIT should not exceed 6 hours in the lower extremity and 8 hours in the upper extremity.[24] If the WIT exceeds these limits, the MESS score is automatically doubled. This is typically an absolute contra-indication to limb salvage (**Figs. 4** and **5**).[11]

Risks associated with amputation include residual limb and wound complications, neuroma formation, chronic pain, phantom limb pain, and prosthesis-related issues.[25] Phantom limb pain is common, occurring in up to 50% of patients after amputation. Ulcerations are also common, occurring in 24% to 50% of patients. Typically, patients visit their prosthetist approximately 4 times per year for adjustments and require a new prosthesis on average every 2 years.[26]

Patients should be counseled that although recovery from amputation is typically quicker than limb salvage, it is still not a quick recovery. Typical time to final prosthesis fitting is more than 6 months.[25] Rehospitalization is common (29%), often for residual limb complications. Falls are also common, particularly in the first year after amputation. Approximately 14% of patients require revision surgery (often for wound complications or heterotopic ossification).[26]

Currently, the most common prosthesis is a socket-fitting prosthesis. This type of prosthetic uses a custom molded socket. Residual limb complications, such as ulcerations, are common with these type of prosthetics and may lead to the need for additional procedures.

When an amputation is performed, the focus is on providing a residual limb that maximizes rehab potential. In the setting of trauma, amputations are typically performed in a staged manner to maximize the length of the residual limb and decrease the risk of infection and dehiscence. The initial procedure consists of amputating only the portion of the limb that is clearly not salvageable. Thorough irrigation and

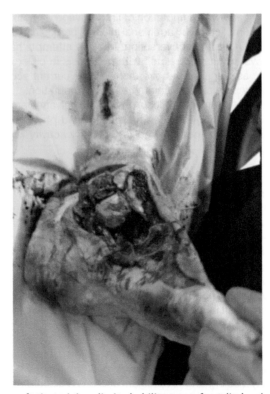

Fig. 4. Cases where soft tissue injury limited ability to perform limb salvage.

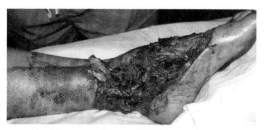

Fig. 5. Cases where soft tissue injury limited ability to perform limb salvage.

debridement of nonviable tissue is performed. Serial irrigation and debridements are performed until the remaining tissue seems clean and well perfused. Antibiotic beads and wound vacs may be used to maximize healing and decrease bacterial load.

Once the residual limb seems to be free of contamination and ischemic tissue, the definitive amputation is performed. All nerves are traced out and sharply incised. They are allowed to retract into the muscle to decrease the risk of neuroma formation. All vessels are tied off proximal to the amputation site with several nonabsorbable ties and/or clips. The bone is beveled to a smooth, round end to decrease the risk of pressure points. Myodesis and myoplasty secure muscle tension. Rotational flaps may be used to create robust coverage of the bone. Once the amputation is completed, the tourniquet is deflated to ensure hemostasis. Compression dressings are placed. These are later exchanged for shrinkers.[27,28]

Efforts are made to make the most distal amputation possible while maintaining enough bone to support a prosthetic and enough soft tissue to adequately cover the residual bone and provide shock absorption. Ideally, the amputation is performed outside of the zone of injury. This decreases the risk of heterotopic ossification. Studies have shown that patients have a better ambulatory status and are more likely to use prosthetics with more distal amputations. Patients with below knee amputations have improved ability to navigate uneven ground and require less energy expenditure when walking than patients with above knee amputations.[26] Sometimes, an amputation is performed through the zone of injury to maximize the likelihood of successful rehabilitation. When this is necessary, the area should be thoroughly debrided and the wound should not be closed primarily (**Fig. 6**).

There have been significant developments in prosthetic technology in the last decade. This is due, in part, to the many extremity injuries sustained during Operation Enduring Freedom. Recent advances include osseointegrated prostheses, which connect the prosthesis directly to the residual bone. This technique has been used in cases where a more proximal amputation is needed (such as high above knee

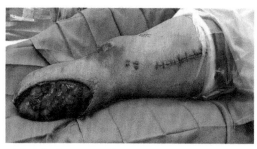

Fig. 6. Amputation through the zone of injury. Below knee amputation was preserved through multiple procedures.

amputations). By allowing the prosthesis to connect directly to bone, it is hypothesized that there is better stability in cases where prosthetic wear would be otherwise impractical. This also allows simpler donning of the prosthetic. It may avoid some of the risks of wound complications because there is less friction. There has been an improved rate of prosthetic use in these cases with few deep infections.[29]

Bone bridge technique (also referred to as synostosis, osteomyoplasty, or the Ertl technique) involves using a bone bridge (typically fibula from the amputated segment) to bridge between the residual tibia and fibula. It has been proposed that this provides better distribution of weight, decreasing the risks of prosthetic complications. However, complications have been seen with this procedure, frequently involving healing of the bone bridge. Most studies did not show improved outcomes with this technique.[30,31] A more recent study among military members did show a higher return to duty in patients treated with this procedure. This may indicate a subtle improvement in function.[32]

Electrodes are sometimes integrated into the musculature to assist with mechanical movement of the limb. Targeted muscle reinnervation involves using transected nerves to innervate muscles in the distal aspect of the residual limb in order to control myoelectric prosthetics. Myoelectric prosthetics are of particular interest for the upper extremity, where prosthetics have previously been disappointing.[28] Hand transplants have also been successfully performed for carefully selected patients.[33,34]

Unfortunately, prosthetics are expensive. Many patients have limited access to even basic prosthetics. The lifetime cost of amputation is actually 3 times higher than that of limb salvage due to the cost of prosthetics.[35] There are resources available through organizations such as the Amputee Coalition and Challenged Athletes Foundation, which help patients to access prosthetics.

Limb Salvage

Limb salvage techniques have advanced significantly in the last few decades. Techniques such as vascularized flaps, microsurgery, and bone regeneration have made limb salvage possible for injuries that previously would have required amputation. These interventions require a multidisciplinary approach with plastic surgery, orthopedics, vascular, and general surgery teams. Ideally, members of the rehab and pain management teams should be involved early in the process to maximize outcomes.

Some patients have a strong preference for limb salvage. They should be counseled that limb salvage is a lengthy, unpredictable undertaking. On average, patients undergoing limb salvage and reconstruction have a significantly longer hospitalization compared to amputees.[24] Rehospitalizations are common. Limb salvage often requires multiple procedures, including washouts, soft tissue coverage, and bone stabilization.

Limb salvage is described as a reconstructive ladder. Emergent management consists of a thorough debridement, provisional stabilization, and reestablishing perfusion. As the patient's overall clinical status improves, more complex procedures are performed.

Primary closure can be performed if there is no gross contamination and the skin can be approximated without tension.[36] In these cases, there does not seem to be an increased risk of deep infection rate.[37] This criterion may be met for isolated Type IIIA open fractures but is uncommon in cases of mangled extremities.

When primary closure is not possible, the patient returns to the OR every few days for serial debridements. Any contamination and nonviable tissue is removed, attempting to maintain all vital structures. Once hemostasis has been achieved, wound vacs can be used to decrease bacterial load and increase granulation tissue.[38,39] Antibiotic beads and topical vancomycin can also decrease bacterial load.[40]

Once the wound seems clean and tissues seem viable, definitive fixation is performed. Antibiotic-coated intramedullary nails and implants may reduce the risk of infection.[41] Ideally, soft tissue coverage is performed at the same time as definitive fixation. Multiple studies have shown that this decreases the risk of infection.[23,42]

It is common for later procedures to be necessary to achieve bone union. These secondary procedures may be planned, such as the Masquelet technique. This technique is a 2-staged procedure. An antibiotic-impregnated cement spacer is used to temporarily fill a bone defect. This is later exchanged for bone graft. Procedures may also be necessary to address nonunion. These include auto and allografting and revision of fixation. Bone transport may be used to address bone defects. This can be achieved using a ringed fixator or specialized intramedullary nails. The risk of nonunion increases with bone defects larger than 2.5 cm.[43]

Soft tissue coverage options include allograft, split thickness skin grafting, pedicled flaps, rotational flaps, and free flaps. The plastic surgery team determines which type of soft tissue coverage is most likely to succeed based on the individual scenario. This considers the size of the soft tissue defect, the need for additional procedures through the graft, the anticipated rehabilitation of the patient, and the patient's comorbidities and smoking status.[44] The risks associated with the recommended graft should be discussed with the patient so they are able to make an informed decision between limb salvage and amputation.

Free flaps are powerful tools for achieving soft tissue coverage. The increased blood supply to the bone provided by a successful flap can also improve bone healing. However, placement of a free flap requires sacrificing another muscle (such as the latissimus dorsi or rectus abdominis). There is a risk of failure of the flap to take, which may lead to the need for delayed amputation. Some patients may feel that this risk is not worth taking, particularly given that they may be more dependent on these muscles for ambulation if they ultimately need an amputation or have a limb with decreased function after limb salvage.

The ultimate goal of limb salvage is to give the patient the best chance at having a functional limb. In the past, surgeons spoke of limb salvage patients whose limbs were saved but their lives were ruined. They referenced patients who became depressed, disabled, drug-dependent, and even divorced in the process of saving their severely injured extremities. Advances during the last few decades have made it possible to more successfully salvage limbs. However, this requires significant resources. The patient's individual goals and preferences should be at the forefront of all decision-making (**Fig. 7**).

LONG-TERM OUTCOMES

Long-term outcomes of patients with mangled extremities are variable. Unfortunately, a significant amount of long-term disability has been reported with both limb salvage and amputation. Postoperative patient satisfaction scoring and functional scoring vary depending on population and management.[45]

Follow-up studies of patients who have undergone amputations show that phantom limb pain, degenerative changes of adjacent joints, and low back pain are common.[46,47] In long-term follow-up, more patients with amputations are used, compared to patients with limb salvage. Return to work is also faster among patients with amputations. However, the rate of unemployment in both groups is high and many require a vocational change. Depression and post traumatic stress disorder (PTSD) are common after limb-threatening injuries.[48]

Compared to amputation, limb salvage is associated with longer hospital stays, increased number of operations, increased morbidity and mortality, and an increased risk of overall complications.

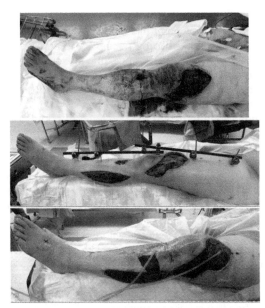

Fig. 7. A mangled extremity with severe contamination that was treated with limb salvage. The patient healed without infection and resumed ambulating.

The lower extremity assessment project (LEAP) study is one of the most commonly referenced studies looking at outcomes of patients with limb-threatening injuries. It is a multicenter retrospective study focusing on lower extremity trauma in the United States. In this study, the researchers found no significant difference in functional outcome measures between amputation and limb salvage.[26,49] The LEAP study showed that patients had overall poor outcomes at both the 2-year and 7-year follow-ups, regardless of intervention chosen.

In contrast, the military extremity trauma amputation/limb salvage (METALS) study found different results among military personnel. In this study, researchers found that service members had better functional outcomes (higher return to duty, increased likelihood of participating in sports, and lower risk of PTSD) with amputation compared to limb salvage. Investigators recognized that their cohort may have a selection bias (more patients with amputations responded than limb salvage recipients). In addition, this data may not be applicable to the general population. Military personnel tend to be younger and healthier than civilians and may have better access to prosthetics.[50]

In several studies, including LEAP and METALS, patients who sustained limb-threatening injuries had high rates of psychological effects, including depression, PTSD, and acute stress disorder. This was true regardless of whether limb salvage or amputation was pursued. This is closely related to physical and overall functional results. The LEAP study found that at 3 months after injury, anxiety, pain, and depression were correlated with an overall poorer outcome.[49] These patients were less likely to return to work or previous activity level.[27]

Some factors are associated with improved outcomes. For example, patients with higher self-efficacy scores were found to have better outcome scores and a higher likelihood of returning to work.[27] A strong social support network seems to correlate with an improved patient-reported outcome.

All studies should be interpreted with caution. Outcomes are highly dependent on the characteristics of the individual patient and no 2 injuries are identical.

In addition, outcomes may not be as dismal currently as they seemed at the times of earlier studies. Newer research has shown improved outcomes when patients begin earlier rehab.[51] This was exemplified by the military's Return to Run program.[52] Promising results have also been seen in the military with the use of a customized orthosis that was developed based on the principles of prosthetics ExoSym (a custom makde hybrid prosthetic-orthotic device) (IDEO).[53] This is now available to civilians as well (Exosym). Further studies are needed to assess its impact on return to activity in civilian patients who have undergone limb salvage.

SUMMARY

Mangled extremities represent one of the most challenging traumatic injuries. They indicate the need for a comprehensive trauma assessment to rule out coexisting injuries. Treatment options include amputation and attempts at limb salvage. Although both have been associated with chronic disability, new surgical techniques and evolving rehabilitation options offer hope for the future.

CLINICS CARE POINTS

- Advanced trauma life support (ATLS) protocol should be initiated for all patients presenting with a mangled extremity.
- Initial management of mangled extremities in the trauma bay includes immediate administration of antibiotics, reduction, splinting, provisional wound care, and vascular examination.
- Initial management in the operating room consists of thorough debridement, rapid provisional stabilization of skeletal injuries, reestablishing perfusion, and fasciotomies.
- Limb preservation should never be attempted at the expense of survival.
- The decision between limb salvage and amputation must be individualized based on the patient's overall clinical status, specific injury, and goals.
- No currently available scoring system accurately predicts outcome.
- Definitive management typically requires multiple procedures and requires coordination between the trauma team and multiple surgical subspecialties.
- Whenever possible, definitive fixation and soft tissue coverage should be performed within 48 hours of each other.
- Patients and their support networks should be counseled that both limb salvage and amputation have a high risk of complications, including need for multiple procedures, long-term physical disability, and a high risk of depression and PTSD.

DISCLOSURE

The authors have no disclosures to report.

REFERENCES

1. Prasarn ML, Helfet DL, Kloen P. Management of the mangled extremity. Strategies Trauma Limb Reconstr 2012;7(2):57–66.
2. Pollak AN, Jones AL, Castillo RC, et al, LEAP Study Group. The relationship between time to surgical debridement and incidence of infection after open high-energy lower extremity trauma. J Bone Joint Surg Am 2010;92(1):7–15.

3. Kim PH, Leopold SS. In brief: gustilo-anderson classification. [corrected]. Clin Orthop Relat Res 2012;470(11):3270–4. Erratum in: Clin Orthop Relat Res. 2012 Dec;470(12):3624. Erratum in: Clin Orthop Relat Res. 2019 Oct;477(10):2388.

4. Gustilo RB, Mendoza RM, Williams DN. Problems in management of type III (severe) open fractures: a new classification of type III open fractures. J Trauma 1984;24:742–6.

5. Howe HR Jr, Poole GV Jr, Hansen KJ, et al. Salvage of lower extremities following combined orthopedic and vascular trauma. a predictive salvage index. Am Surg 1987;53:205–8.

6. Bonanni F, Rhodes M, Lucke JF. The futility of predictive scoring of mangled lower extremities. J Trauma 1993;34:99–104.

7. Lee CH, Chang YJ, Li TS, et al. Vascular trauma in the extremities: factors associated with the outcome and assessment of amputation indexes. Acta Cardiol Sin 2022;38(4):455–63.

8. Johansen K, Daines M, Howey T, et al. Objective criteria accurately predict amputation following lower extremity trauma. J Trauma 1990;30:568–72.

9. Thuan V, Ly MD, Thomas G, Travison PhD, et al, the LEAP Study Group. Ability of lower-extremity injury severity scores to predict functional outcome after limb salvage. J Bone Joint Surg Am 2008;90:1738–43.

10. Abdo EM, Farouk N, Elimam SE, et al. Mangled extremity severity score in the assessment of extremity injuries - is it reliable? Vasc Endovascular Surg 2023; 57(5):445–50.

11. Russell WL, Sailors DM, Whittle TB, et al. Limb salvage versus traumatic amputation. a decision based on a seven-part predictive index. Ann Surg 1991;213: 473–80.

12. McNamara MG, Heckman JD, Corley FG. Severe open fractures of the lower extremity: a retrospective evaluation of the mangled extremity severity score (MESS). J Orthop Trauma 1994;8:81–7.

13. Schirò GR, Sessa S, Piccioli A, et al. Primary amputation vs limb salvage in mangled extremity: a systematic review of the current scoring system. BMC Musculoskelet Disord 2015;16:372.

14. Scalea TM, DuBose J, Moore EE, et al. Western trauma association critical decisions in trauma: management of the mangled extremity. J Trauma Acute Care Surg 2012;72(1):86–93.

15. Bumbaširević M, Matić S, Palibrk T, et al. Mangled extremity- modern concepts in treatment. Injury 2021;52(12):3555–60.

16. Bhandari M, Jeray KJ, Petrisor BA, et al. A trial of wound irrigation in the initial management of open fracture wounds. N Engl J Med 2015;373(27):2629–41.

17. Lange RH. Limb reconstruction versus amputation decision making in massive lower extremity trauma. Clin Orthop Relat Res 1989;243:92–9.

18. Marecek GS, Nicholson LT, Auran RT, et al. Use of a defined surgical approach for the debridement of open tibia fractures. J Orthop Trauma Volume 2018; 32(1):e1–5.

19. Fowler T, Whitehouse M, Riddick A, et al. A Retrospective Comparative Cohort Study Comparing Temporary Internal Fixation to External Fixation at the First Stage Debridement in the Treatment of Type IIIB Open Diaphyseal Tibial Fractures. J Orthop Trauma 2019;33(3):125–30.

20. Rush RM Jr, Beekley AC, Puttler EG, et al. The mangled extremity. Curr Probl Surg 2009;46:851–926.

21. Henry SL, Ostermann PA, Seligson D. Prophylactic use of antibiotic impregnated beads in open fractures. J Trauma 1990;30(10):1231–8.

22. Qadir Rabah, Costales T, Coale M, et al. Vancomycin powder use in fractures at high risk of surgical site infection. J Orthop Trauma 2021;35(1):23–8.

23. Kuripla C, Tornetta P 3rd, Foote CJ, et al. Timing of Flap Coverage With Respect to Definitive Fixation in Open Tibia Fractures. J Orthop Trauma 2021;35(8):430–6.

24. Okereke I, Abdelfatah E. Limb Salvage Versus Amputation for the Mangled Extremity: Factors Affecting Decision-Making and Outcomes. Cureus 2022;14(8): e28153.

25. Hertel R, Strebel N, Ganz R. Amputation versus reconstruction in traumatic defects of the leg: Outcome and costs. J Orthop Trauma 1996;10(4):223–9.

26. Dillingham TR, Pezzin LE, MacKenzie EJ, et al. Use and satisfaction with prosthetic devices among persons with trauma-related amputations: A long-term outcome study. Am J Phys Med Rehabil 2001;80(8):563–71.

27. Ellen J, MacKenzie 1, Bosse Michael J, Castillo Renan C, et al. Functional outcomes following trauma-related lower-extremity amputation. J Bone Joint Surg Am 2004;86(8):1636–45.

28. Tintle SM, Baechler MF, Nanos GP, et al. Traumatic and trauma-related amputations: general priniciples and lower-extremity amputations. J Bone Joint Surg Am 2010;92:2852–68.

29. Brånemark R, Berlin O, Hagberg K, et al. A novel osseointegrated per- cutaneous prosthetic system for the treatment of patients with transfe- moral amputation: a prospective study of 51 patients. Bone Joint Lett J 2014;96-B:106–13.

30. Keeling JJ, Shawen SB, Forsberg JA, et al. Comparison of functional outcomes following bridge synostosis with non-bone-bridging transtibial combat-related amputations. J Bone Joint Surg Am 2013;95:888–93.

31. Pinzur MS, Beck J, Himes R, et al. Distal tibiofibular bone-bridging in transtibial amputation. J Bone Joint Surg Am 2008;90:2682–7.

32. Plucknette BF, Krueger CA, Rivera JC, et al. Combat-related bridge synostosis versus traditional transtibial amputation: comparison of military-specific outcomes. Strateg Trauma Limb Reconstr 2015;11:5–11.

33. Hebe D, Kvernmo, Gorantla Vijay S, Gonzalez Ruben N, et al. Hand transplantation. Acta Orthop 2005;76(1):14–27.

34. Georgescu AV, Battiston B. Mangled upper extremity. Injury 2021;52(12): 3588–604.

35. MacKenzie EJ, Jones AS, Bosse MJ, et al. Health-care costs associated with amputation or reconstruction of a limb-threatening injury. J Bone Joint Surg Am 2007;89:1685–92.

36. Rajasekaran S. Early versus delayed closure of open fractures. Injury 2007;38: 890–5.

37. Scharfenberger, Alabassi K, Smith S, et al. Primary wound closure after open fracture: a prospective cohort study examining nonunion and deep infection. J Orthop Trauma 2017;31(3):121–6.

38. Stannard JP, Volgas DA, Stewart R, et al. Negative pressure wound therapy after severe open fractures: A prospective randomized study. J Orthop Trauma 2009; 23(8):552–7.

39. Blum ML, Esser M, Richardson M, et al. Negative pressure wound therapy reduces deep infection rate in open tibial fractures. J Orthop Trauma 2012;26(9): 499–505.

40. Caroom C, et al. Intrawound vancomycin powder reduces bacterial load in contaminated open fracture model. J Orthop Trauma: October 2018;32(10): 538–41.

41. Tatman Lauren, Gajari V, Obremskey WT. Tibia antibiotic intramedullary nail. J Orthop Trauma 2021;35:S46–8.
42. Pincus Daniel, Byrne JP, Nathens AB, et al. Delay in flap coverage past 7 days increases complications for open tibia fractures: a cohort study of 140 north american trauma centers. J Orthop Trauma Volume 2019;33(4):161–9.
43. Obremskey, Tornetta P, Luly J, et al. Outcomes of patients with large versus small bone defects in open tibia fractures treated with an intramedullary nail: a descriptive analysis of a multicenter retrospective study. J Orthop Trauma Volume 2022; 36(8):388–96.
44. Parrett BM, Bou-Merhi JS, Buntic RF, et al. Refining outcomes in dorsal hand coverage: consideration of aesthetics and donor-site morbidity. Plast Reconstr Surg 2010;126(5):1630–8.
45. Bosse MJ, MacKenzie EJ, Kellam JF, et al. An analysis of outcomes of reconstruction or amputation after leg- threatening injuries. N Engl J Med 2002;347: 1924–31.
46. Norvell DC, Czerniecki JM, Reiber GE, et al. The prevalence of knee pain and symptomatic knee osteoarthritis among veteran traumatic amputees and non-amputees. Arch Phys Med Rehabil 2005;86:487–93.
47. Smith DG, Ehde DM, Legro MW, et al. Phantom limb, residual limb, and back pain after lower extremity amputations. Clin Orthop Relat Res 1999;361:29–38.
48. McCarthy ML, MacKenzie EJ, Edwin D, et al, LEAP study group. Psychological distress associated with severe lower-limb injury. J Bone Joint Surg Am 2003; 85:1689–97.
49. Higgins TF, Klatt JB, Beals TC. Lower extremity assessment project (LEAP)–the best available evidence on limb-threatening lower extremity trauma. Orthop Clin North Am 2010;41(2):233–9.
50. Doukas WC, Hayda RA, Frisch HM, et al. The military extremity trauma amputation/limb salvage (METALS) study: outcomes of amputation versus limb salvage following major lower-extremity trauma. J Bone Joint Surg Am 2013;95(2):138–45.
51. Bedigrew KM, Patzkowski JC, Wilken JM, et al, Skeletal Trauma Research Consortium STReC. Can an integrated orthotic and rehabilitation program decrease pain and improve function after lower extremity trauma? Clin Orthop Relat Res 2014;472:3017–302.
52. Owens JG, Blair JA, Patzkowski JC, et al, Skeletal Trauma Research Consortium. Return to running and sports participation after limb preservation. J Trauma 2011; 71:S120–4.
53. Blair JA, Patzkowski JC, Blanck RV, et al, Skeletal Trauma Research Consortium STReC. Return to duty after integrated orthotic and rehabilitation initiative. J Orthop Trauma 2014;28:e70–4.

Nutritional Support in Critically Ill Trauma Patients

Renaldo Williams, MD, Daniel Dante Yeh, MD, MHPE*

KEYWORDS

- Enteral nutrition - Parenteral nutrition - Post-pyloric feeding - Volume-based feeding

KEY POINTS

- Enteral nutrition should be initiated within 24 to 48 hours of injury.
- Patients should receive 80% of estimated calorie requirements in the first week of critical illness.
- Modified Nutritional Risk in the Critically Ill score assessment should be used to identify patients at high nutritional risk.
- Parenteral nutrition is safe and not associated with increased infectious complications.
- Perioperative nutrition may be continued in patients with a controlled airway.

INTRODUCTION

Critically ill trauma patients present a challenge for clinicians attempting to optimize nutritional support. Features unique to trauma patients include gastrointestinal discontinuity (secondary to damage control surgery), and inability to obtain accurate weights due to external fixator hardware and missing limbs (for example after traumatic amputation). Hypermetabolism after severe injury, previously felt to be universal in previous eras, is highly variable and difficult to predict.

Although nutritional interventions have been investigated for decades, older studies are plagued by methodological flaws and outdated practices that are no longer relevant in a modern intensive care unit. Practices such as early goal-directed therapy,[1] restrictive blood transfusion,[2] lung protective ventilation,[3] catheter care bundles,[4] moderate glycemic control,[5] and conscientious fluid therapy[6] have completely changed the delivery of critical care and therefore the results of any trials conducted prior to routine implementation of these practices cannot be extrapolated into practice. To further add confusion, recent high-impact randomized trials have reported ambiguous and sometimes conflicting results. "Negative" critical care trials are common when enrolling heterogenous populations and specifically in nutritional intervention trials, the inclusion of low-risk patients dilutes any potential signal of benefit.

Department of Surgery, Denver Health Medical Center, University of Colorado, Ernest E. Moore Shock Trauma Center, MC0206, 777 Bannock Street, Denver, CO 80204-4507, USA
* Corresponding author.
E-mail address: dante.yeh@dhha.org

Surg Clin N Am 104 (2024) 405–421
https://doi.org/10.1016/j.suc.2023.10.002
0039-6109/24/© 2023 Elsevier Inc. All rights reserved.

Additionally, critically ill patients have a multitude of complex interacting factors and a blunt outcome such as mortality, while easy to measure, is often confounded by non-nutritional factors including limitations of treatment due to changing goals of care. For nutrition trials in critical care, it is challenging to measure a mechanistically plausible and meaningful endpoint and to enroll sufficient subjects to demonstrate a minimum clinically important difference. One limitation inherent to all recently published trials is the low number of enrolled surgical and trauma patients. Therefore, most recommendations and practices are extrapolated from medical intensive care unit (ICU) patients. This review will summarize our current understanding of nutritional therapy for critically injured patients specifically regarding whom to feed, when to feed, how much to feed, and by which route to feed.

PATIENT SELECTION—WHOM TO FEED?

Critically ill patients are at high risk for morbidity and mortality and iatrogenic malnutrition will only further increase these risks if not addressed early. However, not every ICU patient requires early and aggressive nutritional intervention. For example, previously healthy and well-nourished patients with low disease acuity expected to have a short ICU stay are likely to do well regardless of ICU nutritional support. Therefore, nutritional status should be assessed upon ICU arrival to determine which patients would benefit from supplementation. Baseline nutrition status is often difficult to ascertain due to inability to obtain a history from an obtunded or sedated patient and fluid resuscitation causing tissue edema obscuring accurate weight and physical examination for clinical signs of malnutrition. Reliance on biomarkers such as albumin and transthyretin (prealbumin) is discouraged due to confounding by the acute phase reaction (inflammation) and is not currently recommended for purposes of nutritional assessment or monitoring.[7,8]

While the majority of nutrition screening tools have been developed in healthy populations, the Nutritional Risk in the Critically Ill (NUTRIC) score was developed and externally validated specifically in critically ill populations.[9] The original NUTRIC score included IL-6, which is very infrequently measured in usual clinical practice, and therefore the subsequent *modified NUTRIC (mNUTRIC)* omits IL-6 and has been shown to be valid.[10] This mNUTRIC is calculated using age, severity of illness scores (Acute Physiology and Chronic Health Evaluation [APACHE II] and Sequential Organ Failure Assessment [SOFA]), medical comorbidities, and pre-ICU nutritional status (**Table 1**). Pre-ICU nutritional status is inferred from number of hospital days prior to ICU admission, with the assumption that oral intake on the wards is usually poor. Patients with mNUTRIC score ≥ 5, are at higher risk of complications (including mortality)[10] and it is this population that may benefit most from aggressive and eary and aggressive nutritional intervention. Interestingly, those with a mNUTRIC score 0 to 5 did not demonstrate any survival benefit across a wide range of calories received (**Fig. 1**). Thus, the Society of Critical Care Medicine (SCCM), American Society for Parenteral and Enteral Nutrition (ASPEN), and European Society for Clinical Nutrition and Metabolism (ESPEN) all recommend using the mNUTRIC score to identify patients most likely to benefit from early and aggressive nutritional intervention.[7,11]

TIMING OF NUTRITIONAL SUPPORT INITIATION—WHEN TO FEED?

After selecting the appropriate patients for nutritional intervention, the next most important question is timing of initiation of enteral nutrition (EN), parenteral nutrition (PN), or both. Meta-analyses of randomized controlled trials (RCTs) have concluded that initiating EN within 24 hours results in decreased mortality and pneumonia, though overall

Table 1
Modified NUTRIC score

Variable	Range	Points
Age	<50	0
	50–74	1
	75 or greater	2
APACHE II	<15	0
	15–19	1
	20–28	2
	>28	3
SOFA	<6	0
	6–9	1
	10 or greater	2
Number of comorbidities	0–1	0
	2 or greater	1
Days from hospital to ICU admission	0	0
	1 or greater	1

mNUTRIC score 0 to 4 = low risk.
mNUTRIC score 5 to 9 = high risk.

trial quality was low and sample sizes were small.[12] The 2016 SCCM/ASPEN guidelines recommend that "early EN be initiated within 24 to 48 hours in the critically ill patient who is unable to maintain volitional intake."[7] Similarly, the ESPEN guidelines state that "early EN (within 48 h) in critically ill adult patients should be initiated rather than delaying

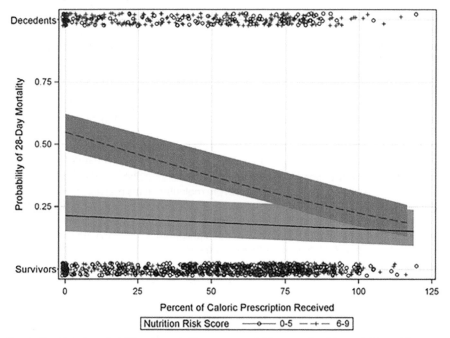

Fig. 1. Predicted probability of mortality versus nutrition received by nutrition risk score. (*From* Rahman A, Hasan RM, Agarwala R, Martin C, Day AG, Heyland DK. Identifying critically-ill patients who will benefit most from nutritional therapy: Further validation of the "modified NUTRIC" nutritional risk assessment tool. Clin Nutr. 2016;35(1):158–162.)

EN."[11] Thus, in the absence of absolute contraindications (such as GI discontinuity or bowel obstruction), EN should be initiated within 48 h after ICU admission. For burn patients, SCCM/ASPEN recommend initiating EN within 4 to 6 hours of injury, if possible and for trauma patients, EN is recommended to initiate within 24 to 48 hours injury, even in patients with open abdomen.[7]

Once initiating EN, there are no evidence-based recommendations on how quickly to advance tube feeds from "trophic" rate to full target rate, and the authors recommend following institutional and local practice. However, the recently published enteral versus parenteral early nutrition in ventilated adults with shock (NUTRIREA-2)[13] trial provides additional guidance. NUTRIREA-2 randomized critically ill ventilated adults receiving vasopressors to either early *aggressive* (ie, full target) EN or early PN. Subjects randomized to early EN had their EN advanced to goal on day 1; those randomized to PN transitioned to EN when hemodynamic stability was achieved or at 7 days. Although the trial was terminated for futility at its secondary planned interim analysis, the authors did report that those assigned to early aggressive EN had significantly higher rates of the secondary outcome of bowel ischemia (median time from initiation of nutritional support to bowel ischemia diagnosis was 4 days). Therefore, although it is safe to initiate trophic EN in the setting of vasopressor therapy, it is recommended based on best-level evidence to wait until the resolution of shock before attempting to advance EN to goal. In a follow-up trial (NUTRIREA-3),[14] the same French investigators compared low versus standard calorie and protein targets (6 kcal/kg per day and 0.2 - 0.4 g/kg per day protein vs 25 kcal/kg per day and 1.0 - 1.3 g/kg per day protein) during the first 7 ICU days in mechanically ventilated patients receiving vasopressor support. Subjects randomized to the low calorie/protein targets achieved earlier median time to readiness for ICU discharge and experienced fewer gastrointestinal complications such as vomiting, diarrhea, bowel ischemia, and liver dysfunction. Importantly, trauma patients comprised less than 2% of all NUTRIREA-3 subjects and the vast majority (>90%) of enrolled subjects did not have pre-existing malnutrition. However, extrapolating from best-level evidence, low calorie/protein targets while on vasopressors and mechanical ventilation during the first week of critical illness are preferred, especially in patients with low nutritional risk.

The more difficult challenge is deciding when to supplement EN with PN when EN is insufficient to meet nutritional requirements. Gastrointestinal dysfunction is very common in the ICU and patients are often unable to tolerate EN in the early acute phase of critical illness. Therefore, at some point, the clinician must decide whether or not to supplement inadequate EN with PN. The multicenter Early Parenteral Nutrition Completing Enteral Nutrition in Adult Critically Ill Patients (EPaNIC) trial was conducted.[15] EPaNIC enrolled patients at risk for severe malnutrition (as measured by the Nutrition Risk Screening (NRS) 2002 score) and randomized them to either early (within 48 h) or late (ICU day 8) initiation of PN if EN was insufficient to meet their nutritional targets.[3] One study protocol feature which must be highlighted is that the early PN group received intravenous 20% glucose infusion for the first 2 ICU days prior to initiating supplemental PN (SPN) on ICU day 3. It is also important to note several additional features of the study population: (1) only a minority of enrolled subjects fell into the highest nutritional risk category and the majority of subjects had a relatively normal body mass index (BMI); (2) greater than 60% of enrolled subjects were post-cardiac surgery; (3) and median ICU stay was only 3 and 4 days, respectively. While the 2 groups had similar ICU and hospital mortality rates at 3 months, the late PN initiation group had decreased infections, decrease duration of renal replacement therapy, decreased mechanical ventilator days, and shorter ICU and hospital stays. Although cursory interpretation of the EPaNIC trial would suggest overall harm of early PN initiation, one must remember that enrolled subjects were highly specialized (cardiac surgery), unlikely to be malnourished at baseline, unlikely to be severely ill, and that the unusual practice of 20% glucose infusion may have led to increased hyperglycemic episodes (as demonstrated by the nearly double insulin requirements) and may have harmed the early PN group. Therefore, these conclusions should be interpreted with caution.

Whereas the 2016 SCCM/ASPEN recommends to withhold PN for 7 days in low-nutritional risk (mNUTRIC <5) patients unable to eat or receive EN, for high-nutritional risk patients, they recommend initiating exclusive PN as soon as possible following ICU admission only when EN is not feasible; if the patient can receive any amount of EN, SCCM/ASPEN recommends to withhold SPN for 7 to 10 days *regardless of nutritional risk.*[7] In contrast, the ESPEN guidelines recommend SPN be initiated within 3 days in all patients regardless of nutritional risk.[11]

To summarize, in the absence of GI discontinuity or bowel obstruction, trophic EN should be started within the first 48 h after ICU admission. While the patient remains on vasopressors, a low calorie/protein target is recommended, but this should be advanced to goal after 7 days or after extubation and liberation from vasopressors. In well-nourished or low-nutritional risk patients, SPN to supplement inadequate EN should not be given during the first ICU week. In malnourished or high- nutritional risk patients, clinical judgment should be used to weigh the risks and benefits of early SPN compared to ongoing macronutrient deficit.

DOSE OF SUPPLEMENTAL NUTRITION—HOW MUCH SHOULD WE FEED?

The issue of how much nutrition (calories and protein) to prescribe a critically patient is the most controversial topic in this field. Multiple large scale randomized trials have been conducted in the past 20 years and we still lack clarity about the optimal macronutrient prescription. The first challenge is to determine the individual patient's metabolic requirements which can be measured using indirect calorimetry (IC) or estimated using mathematical equations. Because IC overcomes inaccuracies including (but not limited to) anasarca, ascites, obesity, amputation, both SCCM/ASPEN and ESPEN recommend the use of IC, if available, to determine the patient's metabolic requirements.[7,11]

Three major trials have investigated the use of IC to guide nutritional prescription in the ICU. The 2011 tight calorie control study (TICACOS) investigated whether repeated measurements of resting energy expenditure (REE) would result in improved hospital survival compared to a single initial weight-based formula estimation. The "tight calorie" group had their energy target determined by IC measurements every 48 h and the control group energy target was calculated as 25 kcal/kg/d based on pre-admission weight. SPN was used to meet energy targets in the tight calorie group. Surgical and trauma patients comprised nearly 50% of enrolled subjects in this single-center pilot study. The intervention group received an average of 2086 kcal and 76 g protein per day while the control group received 1480 kcal and 53 g protein. However, these totals do not account for non-nutritional caloric intake (for example from dextrose-containing carrier fluids for medications or propofol). Although it was a negative trial, there was a trend toward decreased hospital mortality in the intervention group (32.3% vs 47.7%, $P = .058$) and the negative result may have been a type 2 error due to small sample size. Additionally, there was an increase in infections in the intervention group, mainly ventilator-associated pneumonia and bacteremia, though the infection count tally began at 48 h after ICU admission, before nutritional intervention could have a plausible effect. Ultimately, this trial could not definitively prove the benefit of routine IC due to the confounding factor of supplemental PN in the intervention group, the potential of overfeeding due to unaccounted non-nutritional calories, and the small sample size.

Another trial, the "Swiss SPN study" enrolled ICU patients who were not meeting their nutritional needs on ICU day 3 and randomized them to either individually optimized energy provision (using SPN) or standard of care (25–30 kcal/kg/d ideal body weight).[16] The SPN group had their PN adjusted *twice a day* to target exactly 100% of measured REE. The primary endpoint was the incidence of nosocomial infection from day 8 to 28, a mechanistically plausible outcome of nutrition intervention. Trauma patients comprised 13% of enrolled subjects. The SPN group received approximately 20% to 40% of their energy on ICU days 4 through 7, with a mean cumulative calorie balance of 125 kcal compared to −2317 kcal deficit in the control group. Mean protein delivery was also significantly greater in the SPN group (1.2 g/kg/d vs 0.8 g/kg/d). In terms of the primary endpoint, fewer patients in the SPN group developed subsequent nosocomial infection compared to the standard of care group (27% vs 38%, $P = .03$) and there were more antibiotic-free days in the SPN group. There was no difference in mechanical ventilation, ICU stay, or mortality. Unlike the EPaNIC SPN trial, this Swiss SPN trial delayed SPN until ICU day 4, did not provide a large early glucose load, and included twice daily adjustment to avoid overfeeding. Furthermore, the patients were "sicker" as demonstrated by the longer ICU length of stay and mechanical ventilation duration. Unlike the TICACOS trial, the Swiss SPN was multicenter and selected a mechanistically plausible and clinically meaningful primary endpoint resulting in a "positive" conclusion. There were no obvious detrimental effects of SPN used in this fashion, but the effort required to perform twice daily IC and PN adjustment may be a major barrier to implementation.

The EAT-ICU trial was a single-center trial comparing early goal-directed nutrition (EGDN) guided by IC with SPN started on day 1 to standard care (25 kcal/kg/d).[17] Trauma patients comprised 9% of the study population. The primary endpoint was physical quality of life at 6 months. While in the first week after enrollment, the EGDN group had significantly higher amounts of calorie and protein intake, by the last trial day, the cumulative energy difference between groups was only 498 kcal and there was negligible protein difference between groups. EGDN had higher rates of hyperglycemia and higher insulin requirements, but there were no differences in any of the examined secondary outcomes. Taken together, the 3 recent trials comparing IC to standard of care are confounded by the concomitant use of SPN in the IC groups, selected different primary endpoints, and arrive at conflicting conclusions. Notably, all 3 trials targeted 100% of measured REE, though emerging data suggest that "full" energy delivery in the first week of critical illness may not be ideal.[14] Therefore, although IC can provide a more accurate understanding of the individual patient's metabolic requirements, clinicians are often confused about whether or not routine IC actually improves patient outcomes and whether or not to prescribe the full amount to match metabolic requirements.

While ASPEN and ESPEN recommend using IC to guide nutrition therapy in the ICU, the vast majority of clinicians lack access to IC. In a large survey of 7872 patients treated in 252 ICUs across 33 countries, indirect calorimetry was used in only 37 (0.5%) patients.[18] Therefore, predictive equations based on regression analyses such as the Harris Benedict, Schofield, Mifflin-St. Jeor, Ireton-Jones equations, or simple weight-based equations are most often employed to estimate energy (caloric) requirements. The regression-based equations incorporate combinations of anthropometric data such as age, height, sex, and additional factors such as activity level and ventilator dependency to estimate basal energy expenditure (BEE). Some intensivists also apply a stress factor to the calculated BEE due to the assumption that critically ill patients have higher metabolic rates. Weight-based equations, for example, 25 to 30 kcal/kg, are much simpler, but do not account for age, sex or stress-related influences on metabolic requirements. If IC is not available, ASPEN recommends "a published predictive equation or a simplistic weight-based equation (25–30 kcal/kg/day) be used to determine energy requirements."[7]

Once the REE or BEE has been determined via IC or calculated with an equation, the clinician must then decide whether or not to provide the full REE/BEE amount or some fraction of the REE/BEE, especially in the early phase of critical illness. Observational studies showing shorter mechanical ventilation and improved mortality in those receiving less nutrition[19–21] have prompted some to suggest that providing 100% of estimated metabolic requirements may actually be harmful.

Trophic Feeding

While there is no universally accepted definition, the term "trophic feeding" generally refers to a strategy of providing a small amount of EN (typically <20% of estimated nutritional requirements, or between 10–30 mL/h of standard concentration formula) in order to reap the non-nutritional benefits (**Fig. 2**) while avoiding some of the potential negative consequences of full feeding, mainly GI intolerance and aspiration. Trophic feeding strategy is not applied to PN; while PN may be provided at a reduced dose in the first few days to avoid precipitating refeeding syndrome, PN is usually advanced to goal if the electrolytes remain within normal limits.

The 2012 Initial Trophic versus Full Enteral Feeding in Patients with Acute Lung Injury (EDEN) trial randomized ventilated patients to trophic-feeding or full-feeding for the first 6 ICU days.[22] Trauma patients comprised only 4% of enrolled subjects. Those assigned to the full-feeding group initiated EN at a rate of 25 mL/h and advanced to goal rate as quickly as possible according to protocol. Goal energy was calculated as 25 to 30 kcal/kg of ideal body weight (IBW) and goal protein was

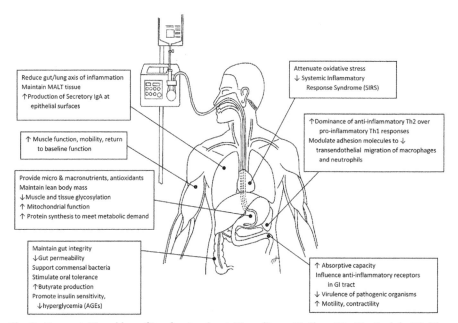

Fig. 2. Non-nutritional benefits of enteral nutrition. (*From* McClave SA, Martindale RG, Rice TW, Heyland DK. Feeding the critically ill patient. Crit Care Med. 2014;42(12):2600–2610.)

calculated as 1.2 to 1.6 g/kg. There was no report of nutritional risk, but the mean weight for the full-feeding group was 87 kg and the mean body mass index (BMI) was 30.4 kg/m^2. The trophic group received an average of 400 kcal/d (approximately 4.7 kcal/kg/d) and the full-feeding group received 1300 kcal/d (approximately 14.9 kcal/kg/d). The full-feeding group had significantly higher cumulative net fluid balance throughout the entire study. There was no difference in ventilator-free days or mortality, though GI intolerance was less common and fluid gain was less in the trophic group. The EDEN trial was considered a "negative" trial, as the trophic EN strategy was *not superior* to full EN strategy. However, beyond the paucity of trauma patients, several additional caveats deserve mention: (1) the enrolled subjects were about 10 years younger than typical ICU patients, (2) although no data on nutritional risk were presented, the weights and BMIs suggest that the enrolled patients were not malnourished, (3) mortality was lower (23%) than expected (40%) for the moderate acute respiratory distress syndrome severity, and the "full" feeding group did not receive the full amount (25–30 kcal/kg/d) of prescribed calories.

The 2015 Permissive Underfeeding or Standard Enteral Feeding in Critically Ill Adults (PermiT) trial randomized subjects to either permissive-underfeeding (40%–60% of calculated caloric requirements) or standard enteral feeding (70%–100%) for up to 14 days. Nonoperative trauma patients comprised 21% of enrolled subjects and 13% had traumatic brain injury. Caloric requirements were determined using the Penn State equation[23] for non-obese patients and the 1992 Ireton-Jones equation[24] for obese patients. Protein target was 1.2 to 1.5 g/kg/d for both groups and saline or water was administered to the permissive-underfeeding group to ensure equivalent fluid volumes in both groups. As in the EDEN trial, the average age was about 50 years and the average BMI was 29 kg/m^2 without comment about nutritional risk. Another similarity to the EDEN trial is that PermiT patients randomized to standard feeding only received about 71% of prescribed calories. Both permissive and standard feeding groups received only about 69% of their prescribed protein. There was no difference in 90-day mortality (primary outcome) or any of the secondary outcomes examined in this trial. Importantly, there were no differences in the rate of GI complications between groups, possibly related to equivalent fluid balances, as cumulative net fluid gain has been associated with GI tract dysfunction in the ICU.

The 2015 Intensive Nutrition in Acute Lung Injury (INTACT) trial similarly enrolled patients with acute lung injury and hypothesized that intensive medical nutrition therapy (IMNT) would result in fewer infections, shorter hospital and ICU stays, and lower mortality compared to standard nutrition support (SNSC).[25] Subjects assigned to the IMNT strategy were prescribed 30 kcal/kg of *actual body weight* and 1.5 g/kg protein. EN was initiated within 6 hours of hemodynamic stability and EN rate changes were made to compensate for feeding interruptions. Unlike many other ICU nutrition trials, the intervention strategy was carried forth beyond the ICU to hospital discharge. The trial was terminated early for safety because of increased mortality (40%) observed in the IMNT group compared to the SNSC group (16%). However, of the total 22 deaths in both arms, 18 were attributed to "terminal extubation," presumably after transition to comfort care. Although the investigators concluded that IMNT increases mortality, interpretation of the study should be tempered by the recognition that (1) studies with small sample sizes are at risk for type 1 error; (2) transitions to comfort care can confound ICU trials; and (3) nearly half of enrolled subjects had BMI > 30 and prescribing calories based on actual body weight in obese patients may risk overfeeding compared to metabolic requirements.

The EDEN and PermiT trials were unable to show any benefit associated with a strategy of trophic or permissive underfeeding, though they enrolled mainly younger patients who were presumably not at high nutritional risk and only a minority of subjects were surgical or trauma. Both trials struggled to deliver the full amount of prescribed calories to the control group subjects and both groups delivered less protein than what is currently recommended by ASPEN guidelines. The INTACT trial was a single-center RCT which was stopped early for safety and failed to demonstrate a survival benefit of aggressive EN intervention. Taken together, it is reasonable to infer that neither trophic or permissive underfeeding (for the first 7–14 days) nor aggressive full nutrition (carried forth through hospital discharge) is beneficial to low-risk patients.

Between the 2 extremes of prolonged trophic feeding and early aggressive (full) feeding, is a moderate strategy that is practiced by most clinicians. Large international surveys have consistently reported that most patients receive approximately 60% to 80% of prescribed nutrition based on targets calculated using simple weight-based equations or predictive equations.[18] Analysis of a large cohort (n = 7,872) of mechanically ventilated ICU patients revealed a U-shaped curve association between mortality and the percentage of caloric prescription received in the first 12 ICU days (**Fig. 3**).[18] These data suggest that delivering only about 80% of estimated energy requirements in the early phase of critical illness may be optimal. Interestingly, the association between mortality and protein was linear, suggesting that protein should probably be delivered at near 100% of estimated requirements. The most recent ESPEN guidelines recommend "hypocaloric nutrition (not exceeding 70% of energy expenditure) should be administered in the early phase of acute illness," and subsequently "after day 3, caloric delivery can be increased up to 80% to 100% of measured energy expenditure."[11] It is the authors' practice to begin trophic nutrition within 24 to 48 hours of

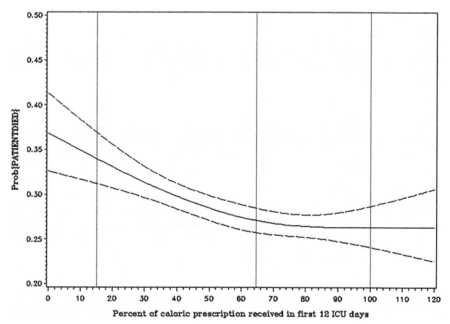

Fig. 3. Association between 1-day average percentage of prescribed calories received and 60-day hospital mortality. *(From* Heyland DK, Cahill N, Day AG. Optimal amount of calories for critically ill patients: depends on how you slice the cake! Crit Care Med. 2011;39(12):2619–2626.)

ICU admission, advance to goal rate as tolerated over the subsequent 1 to 2 days, and cease aggressive EN once the patient is no longer critically ill.

One special population requires mention: obese patients. It is recognized that in obesity, most excess body weight is in the form of adipose tissue which has low metabolic demands. Therefore, prescribing calories based on ideal body weight (IBW) will necessarily result in underestimation of metabolic requirements, while basing calculations on actual body weight (ABW) will necessarily result in overestimation. Therefore, current recommendations recommend a strategy of hypocaloric feeding (target 11–14 kcal/kg ABW) in order to more closely approximate actual metabolic requirements.

Protein

Until recently, clinicians were limited by the fact that EN formulas contained only a fixed amount of protein and therefore protein delivery was necessarily tethered to tube feeding delivery. At goal calorie prescriptions, most EN formulas provided only about 1 g/kg/d protein and some older versions of disease-specific formulas (ex: renal failure) had even lower protein content. With growing recognition of the importance of adequate protein delivery *separate from* calorie delivery, ICU clinicians have increasingly turned to modular protein supplements (ex: Beneprotein , Nestle Health Science, Bridgewater, NJ) that allow additional protein delivery. The 2016 SCCM/ASPEN guidelines recommend 1.2 to 2 g/kg (actual body weight) per day, and even higher amounts in burn (1.5–2 g/kg)[7] and ESPEN guidelines recommend 1.3 g/kg protein per day.[11] For trauma patients with a temporary abdominal closure ("open abdomen"), an additional 15 to 30 g protein should be provided for every liter of exudate drained from the dressing.[7] As mentioned earlier, obese patients should be prescribed a hypocaloric regimen, but with increased protein targets due to the recognition that the majority of obese patients also have relative sarcopenia and are at greater risk for muscle deterioration in critical illness: 2 g/kg IBW for patients with BMI 30 to 40 kg/m^2, and 2.5 g/kg IBW for those with BMI >40 kg/m^2.[7]

The EFFORT Protein trial by Heyland and colleagues[28] has recently challenged the idea that high protein delivery in critical illness is beneficial. This large pragmatic trial enrolled over 1300 patients and randomized them to either usual dose protein (<1.2 g/kg/day) or high-dose protein (>2.2 g/kg/day). Trauma patients comprised about 10% of enrolled subjects and the median mNUTRIC score was 5. The patients were all mechanically ventilated and about 40% were also requiring vasopressor support at study enrollment. Congruent with previous critical care nutrition trials, enrolled subjects did not receive their full prescribed amount: those in the high-dose group received a mean of 1.6 g/kg/day while those in the usual dose group received a mean of 0.9 g/kg/day. Both groups received about 14 kcal/kg/day of energy intake. At 60 days, there was no significant difference in the cumulative incidence of alive hospital discharge and no significant difference in mortality (a secondary endpoint). Importantly, subgroup analyses demonstrated that harm associated with higher protein provision to patients with acute kidney injury and higher initial organ failure scores. Therefore, clinicians should consider limiting protein delivery to 0.9 g/kg/d in these patients.

FEEDING ROUTE—HOW SHOULD WE FEED?

Nutritional supplementation can be delivered via enteral or parenteral route. If the patient is a candidate for either EN or PN, all professional societies are in agreement that in general the enteral route is preferred over parenteral route[7,11] due to lower cost and more physiologic feeding. Enteral nutrition also has numerous intangible non-nutritional benefits[26] and based on older literature, PN carries a stigma of being harmful to the patient. Indeed, 1 prominent thought leader proclaimed that the acronym TPN may represent "total poisonous nutrition."[27] However, it is also recognized that some of the detrimental effects of PN seen in previous decades may not have been related not to the PN *per se*, but rather due to the manner in which it was delivered. Permissive hyperglycemia, zealous overfeeding, and lax catheter care may have been responsible for the increase in morbidity, specifically infectious complications, associated with PN as it was delivered in older eras.

The 2014 CALORIES trial[29] was a large multicenter study that enrolled adult ICU patients who were eligible for both EN and PN. Subjects were randomized to 5 days of *exclusive* EN or PN until transition to oral feeding, ICU discharge, or death. Surgical patients comprised 14% of enrolled subjects. The vast majority (>90%) of subjects were assessed as "none" for degree of malnutrition. Calorie targets were set at 25 kcal/kg actual body weight and protein targets were set according to local practice. Insulin was administered to target moderate glycemic control (serum glucose < 180 mg/dL) and calories from non-nutritional sources (such as propofol and dextrose-containing carrier fluids) were included in calculations. Interestingly, both groups had difficulty delivering their prescribed calories, with <50% of subjects in both groups meeting their caloric targets. Protein delivery was similarly poor, with a median < 1 g/kg/d delivered. Ultimately, there was no difference between groups for the primary endpoint of death within 30 days (33.1% vs 34.2%, $P = .57$), though the PN group had significantly lower rates of hypoglycemia (3.7% vs 6.2%, $P = .006$) and vomiting (8.4% vs 16.2%, $P < .001$). Importantly, there were no differences in infectious complications. Thus, the CALORIES trial demonstrated that modern delivery of PN is safe, resulting in fewer episodes of hypoglycemia and vomiting, without any discernible increase in any adverse effects. The most recent 2022 updated ASPEN guidelines state that "because similar energy intake provided as PN is not superior to EN and no differences in harm were identified, we recommend that either PN or EN is acceptable."[30]

CONTROVERSIES IN ENTERAL NUTRITION

Because GI intolerance is very common in critically ill patients (higher in surgical compared to medical patients), several dilemmas may arise when attempting to provide enteral nutrition, namely gastric residual volume monitoring and post-pyloric feeding. Specific to trauma patients, inadequate EN due to repeated trips to the operating room present another problem.

Gastric Residual Volume Monitoring

The practice of gastric residual volume (GRV) measurements arose in the 1980s in the nursing literature and is predicated on chain assumptions that elevated GRV leads to increased risk of vomiting, vomiting leads to aspiration, aspiration leads to pneumonia, and pneumonia leads to worse outcomes. However, this chain of assumptions has never been definitively proven and GRV measurements have never been standardized nor validated, as the amount will be dependent upon tube size, tube tip position, patient body position, and frequency of monitoring. Furthermore, the definition of a "high" GRV varies across institutions, ranging from as low as "double the hourly feeding rate" to 500 mL. Regardless of definition, the traditional management has been to suspend EN if the GRV threshold is crossed. This can result in inadequate EN delivery and contribute to iatrogenic malnutrition. A multicenter randomized trial comparing "high" GRV thresholds of 200 mL versus 500 mL measured every 6 hours unsurprisingly reported higher rates of "high" GRV using the 200 mL definition (42.4% vs 26.8%, $P = .003$), but reported no differences in clinically relevant outcomes such as vomiting, distention, diarrhea, duration of mechanical ventilation, ICU length of stay, or pneumonia rates.[31] Trauma patients comprised <15% of the enrolled subjects. The 2013 NUTRIREA1 noninferiority trial compared a strategy of no GRV monitoring with a standard care group (GRV threshold 250 mL). In the intervention group, GI intolerance was diagnosed by regurgitation and vomiting. There was no significant difference in the primary endpoint, rate of ventilator-associated pneumonia (15.8% vs 16.7%), thus proving noninferiority, but there was a significantly higher rate of vomiting in the intervention group: 41.8% versus 26.5%. Importantly, medical patients comprised >90% of the study population. Based on this study, the 2016 SCCM/ASPEN guidelines suggest that "GRVs not be used as part of routine care to monitor ICU patients on EN," but then state that "for those ICUs where GRVs are still utilized, holding EN for GRVs <500 mL in the absences of other signs of intolerance should be avoided."[7] However, these recommendations may not apply to trauma patients, as the foundational evidence was in mainly medical patients. It is known that surgical patients have higher rates of GI intolerance,[32] and earlier identification of delayed gastric emptying may be beneficial if it prompts earlier initiation of prokinetic agents[33–36] and post-pyloric feeding (discussed below). It is the authors' practice to measure GRVs in surgical and trauma patients; for GRVs < 250 mL, the aspirated EN is returned to the patient and EN continued; for GRVs 250 to 500 mL, the aspirated EN is returned to the patient, prokinetic agents are initiated, and EN continued; and for GRVs >500 mL, prokinetic agents are initiated, the EN is suspended for 6 hours, and the GRV is rechecked in 6 hours. For 2 consecutive GRV measurements >500 mL, post-pyloric access is sought and PN is considered.

Post-Pyloric Feeding

Nasogastric (usually 14 Fr to 18 Fr Salem sump) tubes are often inserted in the ICU to provide EN and also decompress the stomach. Theoretically, feeding the stomach (vs duodenum or jejunum) may increase aspiration risk due to closer proximity to the pulmonary tree. However, it is widely accepted that most patients receiving EN will initially tolerate gastric feeding. Furthermore, obtaining post-pyloric enteral access may be challenging and resource intensive, requiring endoscopic or fluoroscopic placement if bedside insertion is unsuccessful; this may result in delay of initiation of EN. Assistive devices using cameras or magnets can increase bedside placement success, though at financial cost.[37] Although multiple randomized trials have been performed, most are decades old, enrolled heterogenous populations of patients, had small sample size, had low quality ratings, and did not distinguish between duodenal versus jejunal feeding. The vast majority did not routinely confirm that the feeding tube did not migrate (a common occurrence) after initial placement. Meta-analyses of these trials have demonstrated significant decrease in pneumonia in patients receiving post-pyloric feeding compared to gastric feeding, though no difference in mortality, duration of mechanical ventilation, or ICU length of stay. While

Table 2
Contraindications to PEG placement

Absolute	Relative
Hemodynamic instability	Abdominal wall abnormalities
Uncorrected severe coagulopathy	Carcinomatosis
Distal obstruction	Ascites
Pharyngeal or esophageal obstruction	Portal hypertension with gastric varices
	Prior gastric surgery

ESPEN does not provide a statement on pre-vs. post-pyloric feeding, SCCM/ASPEN recommend post-pyloric feeding for "patients deemed to be at high risk for aspiration" and abdominal/thoracic surgery or trauma is listed as an aspiration risk factor. Ultimately, the decision whether or not to pursue routine post-pyloric feeding in trauma patients requiring EN must consider nutritional risk, local bedside success rates, and potential delays in EN initiation.

Percutaneous gastrostomy tube placement is another route for EN delivery. They are generally indicated in patients with and at risk of severe malnutrition, and those patients who will not be able to have oral intake for long periods of time. Intensivists should have extensive discussion with caregivers when there is consideration of percutaneous endoscopic gastrostomy (peg) tube placement to ensure everyone understands the benefits and risks. There are several absolute contraindications to PEG tubes including but not limited to severe coagulopathy, distal obstruction, hemodynamic instability, etc. **Table 2** below shows both absolute and relative contraindications.

Peri-Operative Nutrition

In surgical and trauma patients, interruption of EN for frequent operative procedures can be a major reason for iatrogenic malnutrition.[38,39] Although patients requiring elective intubation for an operation should adhere to standard pre-operative fasting guidelines,[40] patients already intubated or with tracheostomy do not require anesthesia induction and are at very low risk of aspiration. Multiple studies have demonstrated the safety of continuing EN up until surgery[41–44] or even continuation during surgery[45,46] (mainly burn excisions). It is the authors' practice to continue EN up until the time of surgery in critically ill trauma patients if 3 conditions are met: (1) the patient already has a controlled airway (endotracheal tube or tracheostomy); (2) operation will be performed in the supine position; (3) operation does not involve the airway or gastrointestinal tract.

Another way to mitigate iatrogenic malnutrition due to EN cessation for operative procedures or extubation is to provide compensatory feeding. For example, if the EN was suspended for 6 hours, then the hourly rate can be increased for several hours once EN is resumed. By the end of the day, the patient will have received the full prescribed amount of EN. This strategy is also known as "volume-based feeding"[47–51] and is included in a bundle of interventions known as Enhanced Protein-Energy Provision via the Enteral Route (PEPuP).[52] In addition to volume-based feeding, the other components of the PEPuP protocol include (1) initiation of EN immediately at calculated goal rate (instead of gradually ramping up from a low initial starting rate); (2) semi-elemental formula (instead of standard polymeric formula); (3) prophylactic use of prokinetic agent; and (4) modular protein supplementation. The PEPuP protocol has been shown to be safe and significantly increases the protein and calorie intake,[53] though the benefit may be smaller in surgical patients.[54,55]

SUMMARY

In critically ill trauma patients, EN should be initiated within 24 to 48 hours of injury, starting at a trophic rate and increasing to goal rate after hemodynamic stability is achieved. The modified NUTRIC score can help identify patients who will benefit most from aggressive and early nutritional intervention. In the first week of critical illness, the patient should receive only 70% to 80% of estimated calories and protein should be targeted to 1.5 to 2 g/kg. PN can be provided safely without increased adverse events and can be provided either exclusively or as an adjunct to inadequate EN. Many patients can tolerate gastric feeding, though post-pyloric feeding has been shown to decrease pneumonia rates. Gastric residual volume monitoring has not been shown to decrease the rate of aspiration pneumonia. Peri-operative (and intra-operative) feeding has been shown to be safe in selected patients and volume-based feeding strategies may help reduce iatrogenic macronutrient deficits.

CLINICS CARE POINTS

- In critically ill trauma patients, EN should be initiated within 24 to 48 hours of injury.
- In the first week of critical illness, the patient should receive only 70% to 80% of estimated calories and protein should be targeted to 1.5 to 2 g/kg.
- PN can be provided safely without increased adverse events.
- Gastric residual volume monitoring has not been shown to decrease the rate of aspiration pneumonia.
- Peri-operative (and intra-operative) feeding has been shown to be safe in selected patients.

DISCLOSURE

The authors have nothing to disclose.

REFERENCES

1. Rivers E, Nguyen B, Havstad S, et al, Early Goal-Directed Therapy Collaborative Group. Early goal-directed therapy in the treatment of severe sepsis and septic shock. N Engl J Med 2001;345(19):1368–77.
2. Hebert PC, Wells G, Blajchman MA, et al. A multicenter, randomized, controlled clinical trial of transfusion requirements in critical care. transfusion requirements in critical care investigators, canadian critical care trials group. N Engl J Med 1999;340(6):409–17.
3. Acute Respiratory Distress Syndrome Network, Brower RG, Matthay MA, Morris A, et al. Ventilation with lower tidal volumes as compared with traditional tidal volumes for acute lung injury and the acute respiratory distress syndrome. the acute respiratory distress syndrome network. N Engl J Med 2000;342(18): 1301–8.
4. Pronovost P, Needham D, Berenholtz S, et al. An intervention to decrease catheter-related bloodstream infections in the ICU. N Engl J Med 2006;355(26): 2725–32.
5. Investigators N-SS, Finfer S, Chittock DR, et al. Intensive versus conventional glucose control in critically ill patients. N Engl J Med 2009;360(13):1283–97.
6. National Heart L, Blood Institute Acute Respiratory Distress Syndrome Clinical Trials N, Wiedemann HP, Wheeler AP, Bernard GR, et al. Comparison of two fluid-management strategies in acute lung injury. N Engl J Med 2006;354(24):2564–75.
7. Taylor BE, McClave SA, Martindale RG, et al. Guidelines for the Provision and Assessment of Nutrition Support Therapy in the Adult Critically Ill Patient: Society of Critical Care Medicine (SCCM) and American Society for Parenteral and Enteral Nutrition (A.S.P.E.N.). Crit Care Med 2016;44(2):390–438.
8. Yeh DD, Johnson E, Harrison T, et al. Serum Levels of Albumin and Prealbumin Do Not Correlate With Nutrient Delivery in Surgical Intensive Care Unit Patients. Nutr Clin Pract 2018;33(3):419–25.

9. Heyland DK, Dhaliwal R, Jiang X, et al. Identifying critically ill patients who benefit the most from nutrition therapy: the development and initial validation of a novel risk assessment tool. Crit Care 2011;15(6):R268.

10. Rahman A, Hasan RM, Agarwala R, et al. Identifying critically-ill patients who will benefit most from nutritional therapy: Further validation of the "modified NUTRIC" nutritional risk assessment tool. Clin Nutr 2016;35(1):158–62.

11. Singer P, Blaser AR, Berger MM, et al. ESPEN guideline on clinical nutrition in the intensive care unit. Clin Nutr 2019;38(1):48–79.

12. Doig GS, Heighes PT, Simpson F, et al. Early enteral nutrition, provided within 24 h of injury or intensive care unit admission, significantly reduces mortality in critically ill patients: a meta-analysis of randomised controlled trials. Intensive Care Med 2009;35(12):2018–27.

13. Reignier J, Boisrame-Helms J, Brisard L, et al. Enteral versus parenteral early nutrition in ventilated adults with shock: a randomised, controlled, multicentre, open-label, parallel-group study (NUTRIREA-2). Lancet 2017;391(10116):133–43.

14. Reignier J, Plantefeve G, Mira JP, et al. Low versus standard calorie and protein feeding in ventilated adults with shock: a randomised, controlled, multicentre, open-label, parallel-group trial (NUTRIREA-3). Lancet Respir Med 2023;11(7): 602–12.

15. Casaer MP, Mesotten D, Hermans G, et al. Early versus late parenteral nutrition in critically Ill adults. N Engl J Med 2011;365(6):506–17.

16. Heidegger CP, Berger MM, Graf S, et al. Optimisation of energy provision with supplemental parenteral nutrition in critically ill patients: a randomised controlled clinical trial. Lancet 2012;381(9864):385–93.

17. Allingstrup MJ, Kondrup J, Wiis J, et al. Early goal-directed nutrition versus standard of care in adult intensive care patients: the single-centre, randomised, outcome assessor-blinded EAT-ICU trial. Intensive Care Med 2017;43(11): 1637–47.

18. Heyland DK, Cahill N, Day AG. Optimal amount of calories for critically ill patients: depends on how you slice the cake. Crit Care Med 2011;39(12):2619–26.

19. Dickerson RN, Boschert KJ, Kudsk KA, et al. Hypocaloric enteral tube feeding in critically ill obese patients. Nutrition 2002;18(3):241–6.

20. Krishnan JA, Parce PB, Martinez A, et al. Caloric intake in medical ICU patients: consistency of care with guidelines and relationship to clinical outcomes. Chest 2003;124(1):297–305.

21. Arabi YM, Haddad SH, Tamim HM, et al. Near-target caloric intake in critically ill medical-surgical patients is associated with adverse outcomes. JPEN J Parenter Enteral Nutr 2010;34(3):280–8.

22. Rice TW, Wheeler AP, Thompson BT, et al. Initial trophic vs full enteral feeding in patients with acute lung injury: the EDEN randomized trial. JAMA 2012;307(8): 795–803.

23. Frankenfield D, Smith JS, Cooney RN. Validation of 2 approaches to predicting resting metabolic rate in critically ill patients. JPEN J Parenter Enteral Nutr 2004;28(4):259–64.

24. Ireton-Jones CS, Turner WW Jr, Liepa GU, et al. Equations for the estimation of energy expenditures in patients with burns with special reference to ventilatory status. J Burn Care Rehabil 1992;13(3):330–3.

25. Braunschweig CA, Sheean PM, Peterson SJ, et al. Intensive nutrition in acute lung injury: a clinical trial (INTACT). JPEN J Parenter Enteral Nutr 2015;39(1):13–20.

26. McClave SA, Martindale RG, Rice TW, et al. Feeding the critically ill patient. Crit Care Med 2014;42(12):2600–10.

27. Marik PE, Pinsky M. Death by parenteral nutrition. Intensive Care Med 2003;29(6): 867–9.
28. Heyland DK, Patel J, Compher C, et al. The effect of higher protein dosing in critically ill patients with high nutritional risk (EFFORT Protein): an international, multicentre, pragmatic, registry-based randomised trial. Lancet 2023;401(10376): 568–76.
29. Harvey SE, Parrott F, Harrison DA, et al. Trial of the route of early nutritional support in critically ill adults. N Engl J Med 2014;371(18):1673–84.
30. Compher C, Bingham AL, McCall M, et al. Guidelines for the provision of nutrition support therapy in the adult critically ill patient: the american society for parenteral and enteral nutrition. JPEN J Parenter Enteral Nutr 2022;46(1):12–41.
31. Montejo JC, Minambres E, Bordeje L, et al. Gastric residual volume during enteral nutrition in ICU patients: the REGANE study. Intensive Care Med 2010;36(8): 1386–93.
32. Heyland DK, Ortiz A, Stoppe C, et al. Incidence, risk factors, and clinical consequence of enteral feeding intolerance in the mechanically ventilated critically Ill: an analysis of a multicenter, multiyear database. Crit Care Med 2021;49(1):49–59.
33. Berne JD, Norwood SH, McAuley CE, et al. Erythromycin reduces delayed gastric emptying in critically ill trauma patients: a randomized, controlled trial. J Trauma 2002;53(3):422–5.
34. Dive A, Miesse C, Galanti L, et al. Effect of erythromycin on gastric motility in mechanically ventilated critically ill patients: a double-blind, randomized, placebo-controlled study. Crit Care Med 1995;23(8):1356–62.
35. Jooste CA, Mustoe J, Collee G. Metoclopramide improves gastric motility in critically ill patients. Intensive Care Med 1999;25(5):464–8.
36. Nguyen NQ, Chapman M, Fraser RJ, et al. Prokinetic therapy for feed intolerance in critical illness: one drug or two? Crit Care Med 2007;35(11):2561–7.
37. Wischmeyer PE, McMoon MM, Waldron NH, et al. Successful identification of anatomical markers and placement of feeding tubes in critically Ill Patients via camera-assisted technology with real-time video guidance. JPEN J Parenter Enteral Nutr 2019;43(1):118–25.
38. Peev MP, Yeh DD, Quraishi SA, et al. Causes and consequences of interrupted enteral nutrition: a prospective observational study in critically ill surgical patients. JPEN J Parenter Enteral Nutr 2015;39(1):21–7.
39. Passier RH, Davies AR, Ridley E, et al. Periprocedural cessation of nutrition in the intensive care unit: opportunities for improvement. Intensive Care Med 2013; 39(7):1221–6.
40. Practice guidelines for preoperative fasting and the use of pharmacologic agents to reduce the risk of pulmonary aspiration: application to healthy patients undergoing elective procedures: an updated report by the american society of anesthesiologists task force on preoperative fasting and the use of pharmacologic agents to reduce the risk of pulmonary aspiration. Anesthesiology 2017;126(3): 376–93.
41. Pousman RM, Pepper C, Pandharipande P, et al. Feasibility of implementing a reduced fasting protocol for critically ill trauma patients undergoing operative and nonoperative procedures. JPEN J Parenter Enteral Nutr 2009;33(2):176–80.
42. Moncure M, Samaha E, Moncure K, et al. Jejunostomy tube feedings should not be stopped in the perioperative patient. JPEN J Parenter Enteral Nutr 1999;23(6): 356–9.
43. McElroy LM, Codner PA, Brasel KJ. A pilot study to explore the safety of perioperative postpyloric enteral nutrition. Nutr Clin Pract 2012;27(6):777–80.

44. Parent BA, Mandell SP, Maier RV, et al. Safety of minimizing preoperative starvation in critically ill and intubated trauma patients. J Trauma Acute Care Surg 2016; 80(6):957–63.
45. Jenkins ME, Gottschlich MM, Warden GD. Enteral feeding during operative procedures in thermal injuries. J Burn Care Rehabil 1994;15(2):199–205.
46. Yeh DD, Cropano C, Quraishi SA, et al. Periprocedural nutrition in the intensive care unit: a pilot study. J Surg Res 2015;198(2):346–50.
47. Haskins IN, Baginsky M, Gamsky N, et al. Volume-based enteral nutrition support regimen improves caloric delivery but may not affect clinical outcomes in critically Ill patients. JPEN J Parenter Enteral Nutr 2017;41(4):607–11.
48. Holyk A, Belden V, Sirimaturos M, et al. Volume-based feeding enhances enteral delivery by maximizing the optimal rate of enteral feeding (FEED MORE). JPEN J Parenter Enteral Nutr 2020;44(6):1038–46.
49. Prest PJ, Justice J, Bell N, et al. A volume-based feeding protocol improves nutrient delivery and glycemic control in a surgical trauma intensive care unit. JPEN J Parenter Enteral Nutr 2019;44(5):880–8.
50. Sachdev G, Backes K, Thomas BW, et al. Volume-based protocol improves delivery of enteral nutrition in critically Ill trauma patients. JPEN J Parenter Enteral Nutr 2020;44(5):874–9.
51. Roberts S, Brody R, Rawal S, et al. Volume-based vs rate-based enteral nutrition in the intensive care unit: impact on nutrition delivery and glycemic control. JPEN J Parenter Enteral Nutr 2019;43(3):365–75.
52. Heyland DK, Cahill NE, Dhaliwal R, et al. Enhanced protein-energy provision via the enteral route in critically ill patients: a single center feasibility trial of the PEP uP protocol. Crit Care 2010;14(2):R78.
53. Heyland DK, Murch L, Cahill N, et al. Enhanced protein-energy provision via the enteral route feeding protocol in critically ill patients: results of a cluster randomized trial. Crit Care Med 2013;41(12):2743–53.
54. Declercq B, Deane AM, Wang M, et al. Enhanced Protein-Energy Provision via the Enteral Route Feeding (PEPuP) protocol in critically ill surgical patients: a multicentre prospective evaluation. Anaesth Intensive Care 2016;44(1):93–8.
55. Yeh DD, Ortiz LA, Lee JM, et al. PEP uP (Enhanced Protein-Energy Provision via the Enteral Route Feeding Protocol) in Surgical Patients-A Multicenter Pilot Randomized Controlled Trial. JPEN J Parenter Enteral Nutr 2020;44(2):197–204.

Management of the Geriatric Trauma Patient

Megan Elizabeth Lundy, MD, Bo Zhang, MD, Michael Ditillo, DO*

KEYWORDS

- Geriatric • Geriatric trauma • Frailty • Acute care surgery

KEY POINTS

- With the aging population, hospitals and trauma centers will see increasing numbers of geriatric trauma patients.
- Geriatric trauma patients are not just older adults but rather patients with unique changes in physiology that impact their response to injury.
- Physiologic changes combined with an increasing incidence of comorbidities that accompany aging portend worse outcomes after injury.
- A multidisciplinary and comprehensive approach is key to the treatment of geriatric trauma patients.

INTRODUCTION

The profound shift in global demographics toward an increasingly aged population presents an essential challenge to trauma surgery. Traditionally, "geriatric" has referred to people older than the age of 65. There likely is, however, some fluidity to this cutoff that has yet to be defined. It remains unclear at exactly what age physiologic changes occur and what impact external factors have on these patients. Regardless, over time, physiologic changes assuredly influence injury patterns, response to injury, and subsequent management.

Geriatric trauma—encompassing the evaluation, management, and rehabilitation of traumatic injuries in the elderly—has become a crucial focus of modern surgical care. This population's characteristic physiologic changes, combined with comorbid conditions and polypharmacy, produce a complex clinical tableau that necessitates a tailored approach to their care. This article explores the nuanced and intricate world of geriatric trauma, outlining key principles and strategies for providing optimal care, navigating the intersection of aging physiology with trauma pathophysiology,

University of Arizona Division of Trauma, Surgical Critical Care, Burns, and Acute Care Surgery, 1501 North Campbell Avenue, Tucson, AZ 85724, USA
* Corresponding author.
E-mail address: mfditillo@surgery.arizona.edu
Twitter: @MLundyMD (M.E.L.); @bo_zhang1 (B.Z.); @mikeditillo (M.D.)

Surg Clin N Am 104 (2024) 423–436
https://doi.org/10.1016/j.suc.2023.09.010
0039-6109/24/© 2023 Elsevier Inc. All rights reserved.

and enhancing outcomes in this rapidly growing, and often vulnerable, patient population. Our understanding of this essential aspect of trauma surgery begins with a solid understanding of the unique epidemiologic patterns, injury mechanisms, and pathophysiological responses seen in geriatric trauma patients.

CHANGES IN PHYSIOLOGY

Geriatric patients experience changes in all organ systems and commonly have more comorbidities compared to their younger counterparts. These changes are not uniform and are also affected by preexisting conditions. The response to injury and treatment is highly variable and therefore can be challenging for the clinician.[1] With each physiologic alteration, mechanism of injury, response to injury, and recovery from injury are impacted (**Table 1**).[2–4]

FRAILTY

Frailty is defined as a "state of low physiologic capacity and increased susceptibility to disability because of age-related loss of physical, cognitive, social, and psychological functioning."[5] It is important to recognize that not all geriatric patients are frail and not all frail patients are geriatric; however, the overlap of these two groups presents a special challenge for providers. Frailty should be immediately assessed on presentation. The Trauma-Specific Frailty Index created by Joseph and colleagues has been validated across multiple centers (**Fig. 1**).[6,7] It is recommended that all patients age 65 and more undergo this simple scoring system as it can be instrumental in guiding care throughout the hospital stay with the opportunity to also predict final disposition.[8]

To use this tool, it is recommended that the patient be interviewed within 24 hours of presentation. Any member of the trauma team may survey the patient and subsequently determine the score. Once the data are collected, the score is calculated by adding up the numbers as seen in **Fig. 1**. Once the gross score is obtained, it is divided by 15. The patients are considered non-frail with a score less than or equal to 0.12, pre-frail with a score of 0.13 to 0.25, and frail with a score greater than 0.25.[7]

Understanding frailty can assist with the management of the geriatric trauma patient at each stage after injury and help predict overall outcomes.[9] Assessment of frailty should ideally be established during the initial assessment of the patient after primary and secondary survey and the necessary adjunctive studies are completed. Recognition of frailty can impact the initial disposition. Although the patient may have injuries that would typically be managed on the floor, the diminished physiologic reserve may necessitate closer monitoring in the intensive care unit (ICU). If operative intervention is required, frailty should be considered when counseling patients. Although a decision on operative management may be unchanged, this will allow the physician to better advise the patient and recognize an increased risk of morbidity, mortality, and diminished functional status.

Early recognition of potential discharge disposition can allow for smooth transition to the next stage of care. Most acute care centers are limited in rehabilitation capabilities, and therapists are typically used for evaluation rather than ongoing therapy. Early assessment of frailty will trigger a timely recognition of ongoing therapy needs and allow the care team to identify those that would benefit most from a rehabilitation facility. Once initiated, this process can lead to decreases in length of stay. Frail patients are subject to worse in-hospital complications if their mobility and independence declines further, and therefore, rapid discharge planning may allow them to avoid a skilled nursing facility (SNF) stay.[8]

Table 1
Physiologic changes by system with the resultant impact

System	Change	Impact
Neurologic	Cerebral atrophy Altered HPA axis Altered feedback mechanism Decreased vision Decreased hearing Impaired balance	Delirium Altered perception and reporting of pain Increased risk of falls Increased susceptibility to psychotropic and pain medications
Cardiovascular	Replacement of cardiac muscle with fat/fibrous tissues Increased SVR CO augmented by ↑ ventricular filling (preload dependent)	Predisposition to arrhythmia Inability to mount tachycardic response Normal BP when severely injured Increased sensitivity to small changes in volume status
Pulmonary	Decreased chest wall compliance Weaker diaphragm Decreased inspiratory and expiratory strength Decreased mucociliary epithelial function Decreased response to foreign antigen increased oropharyngeal colonization with microorganisms[3]	Rapid respiratory decline with lesser insult Diminished respiratory effort Increased risk of aspiration and pneumonia
Gastrointestinal	Decreased hepatic clearance Decreased motility Decreased secretory capacity Decreased absorption	Reduced first-pass metabolism of drugs variable drug bioavailability Variable drug absorption Increased risk of malnutrition
Renal	Decreased GFR Glomerulosclerosis Replacement of glomerular tissue with fibrous tissue Smooth muscle atrophy of renal vasculature: "renovascular dysautonomia"[4]	Increased risk of acute kidney injury and decreased recovery Altered response to renally cleared medications
Body composition	Decreased bone density Increased fat:muscle ratio Decreased joint mobility	Increased risk of fracture Difficulty managing fractures surgically Increased volume of distribution of drugs

Abbreviations: CO, cardiac output; HPA, hypothalamic–pituitary–adrenal; SVR, systemic vascular resistance.

MECHANISMS OF INJURY

Falls are the most common cause of injury in patients older than 65, accounting for 58% of unintentional injuries sustained by this patient population.[10] Sensory impairments coupled with a desire to maintain independence by driving results in motor vehicle accidents as another major source of injury accounting for 12% of unintentional injuries.[10] Penetrating trauma decreases, but it should be noted that older White men are at high risk of injury from self-inflicted gunshot wounds.[11] As independence

Fifteen Variable Trauma Specific Frailty Index			
Comorbidities			
Cancer history	YES (1)	No (0)	
Coronary Heart Disease	MI (1)	CABG (0.75)	PCI (0.5)
	Medication (0.25)	None (0)	
Dementia	Severe (1)	Moderate (0.5)	Mild (0.25)
	No (0)		
Daily Activities			
Help with grooming	Yes (1)	No (0)	
Help managing money	Yes (1)	No (0)	
Help doing housework	Yes (1)	No (0)	
Help toileting	Yes (1)	No (0)	
Help walking	Wheelchair (1)	Walker (0.75)	Cane (0.5)
	No (0)		
Health Attitude			
Feel less useful	Most time (1)	Sometimes (0.5)	Never (0)
Feel sad	Most time (1)	Sometimes (0.5)	Never (0)
Feel effort to do everything	Most time (1)	Sometimes (0.5)	Never (0)
Falls	Within last month (1)	Present not in last month (0.5)	None (0)
Feel lonely	Most time (1)	Sometimes (0.5)	Never (0)
Function			
Sexual active	Yes (0)	No (1)	
Nutrition			
Albumin	<3 (1)	>3 (0)	

Fig. 1. Trauma-Specific Frailty Index. (*Courtesy of* Bellal Joseph, MD, FACS; University of Arizona, Tucson, AZ.)

wanes, elder abuse becomes more prevalent, especially if there is concomitant dementia.

Despite what may seem like a mild mechanism of injury, it is important to recognize that with increased number of comorbidities and decreased reserve, even a minor accident or injury can be life-threatening. This requires a stringent triage criterion for geriatric patients to rapidly identify injuries that would otherwise be trivial in a younger adult. Widely accepted trauma management pathways defined by specific institutions or governing societies account for differences in geriatric patients. These generally consider physiology rather than just mechanism. Although this may result in over triage, it is necessary because even small injuries can result in a greater impact on activities of daily living in the geriatric population incomparison to their younger counterparts.

APPROACH TO MANAGEMENT
Triage

For most trauma centers, adult activation criteria incorporate vital signs and mechanism of injury into triage criteria and subsequent level of activation. Geriatric patients' vital signs do not accurately represent their physiology.[12] This can result in under triage, especially in patients who have sustained a fall.[13] As detailed above, increased systemic vascular resistance may result in higher blood pressure, and replacement of cardiac muscle with fibrous tissue along with medications (beta blockers, calcium channel blockers, and so forth) limits the tachycardic response, which may lull one into a false sense of security. A geriatric patient may have normal vital signs even when impending deterioration is near. When their physiology deteriorates due to their injuries, resuscitation can become much more difficult.

It is critical to identify geriatric patients with survivable injuries and provide them with immediate and aggressive trauma care. It is equally important to recognize patients within this population where expansive treatments are futile, and an acceptable quality of life will not be achieved.[14]

Prehospital

The care of any trauma patient most commonly begins in the prehospital setting where decisions are made that can impact patient care, especially for that of a geriatric patient. There are guidelines established by the American College of Surgeons Committee on Trauma, which help prehospital providers determine where best to take their injured patient. This suggests that patients more than 55 years old, regardless of mechanism, should bypass local hospitals and go straight to a trauma center. Frequently, "normal" vital signs result in under-triage and delays in appropriate care.[15,16]

Initial Evaluation

Primary and secondary survey should follow the standard Advanced Trauma Life Support pathway with special recognition that a "normal" heart rate and blood pressure are very likely abnormal and a high index of suspicion for more severe injury should be ever present. Liberal adjunctive studies and imaging should be used, especially for those on anticoagulation or antiplatelet therapy.[17] It is important to recognize that occult injuries are more common in the elderly population.[18]

Admission

Given that injury severity is frequently underappreciated in this patient population, careful consideration should be made as to the level of admission if indicated. Although there are certainly risks to unnecessary ICU admission, most notably exacerbation of delirium, it may be best to have a lower threshold for admission to this level of care for a geriatric trauma patient.[19,20] Initial injuries may not seem as severe, but again, these patients are liable to rapidly decompensate.[21] Frequently, poorly controlled pre-existing conditions or an undiagnosed infection are contributing or exacerbating factors that results in their trauma.[22] These uncontrolled medical conditions often need the care of an intensivist. In isolated injuries with more urgent need for medical management, it remains unclear as to which team is best to admit patients. This is institution-dependent. Regardless, a multidisciplinary approach is needed.

Injury-Specific Management

Each injured system comes with unique challenges that are not typically found in younger counterparts.

Traumatic Brain Injury

Traumatic brain injury (TBI) is a significant cause of morbidity in the geriatric trauma population. Owing to the physiologic changes of the brain with aging, the risk of suffering a TBI even from minor injuries such as a fall is significantly higher.[23] With age, the dura becomes more adherent to the skull, and at the same time, brain volume decreases.[24] This stretches the bridging veins of the subdural space, causing them to be more prone to tearing and bleeding after even seemingly minor blunt trauma.[25] In addition, atherosclerotic disease of the cerebrovascular vessels, along with decreased free radical clearance, diminishes or delays recovery after a brain injury, risking a secondary insult.[25] Geriatric patients are also frequently on anticoagulation or antiplatelet therapy given their comorbidities, leading to a 4 to 5x increased risk of mortality compared with those who are not on these medications.[26] Indications for use frequently include atrial fibrillation, peripheral vascular disease, stents, prior strokes, or prior thromboembolism. After identifying a TBI in a patient on anticoagulation, reversal is frequently necessary but also carries the risk of worsening the original medical problem that the anticoagulation was treating and so it must be considered with care. It subsequently falls to the traumatologist to help the patient and/or family determine the risk–benefit ratio for the reversal, followed by the possible resumption of these medications. There are currently no standard guidelines as to when to safely resume anticoagulation or antiplatelet therapies and many determinations are institution-based or on a case-by-case basis. In addition, it is important to recognize even small decreases in Glasgow Coma Score (GCS) in the initial trauma survey for the elderly patient. A decline in GCS from 15 to 14 portends higher mortality in elderly patients than their younger counterparts.[27]

Thoracic Injury and Rib Fractures

Blunt thoracic injuries, frequently from even minor mechanisms such as ground-level falls, are common in the geriatric population. The altered physiology of the respiratory system, such as decreased compliance, relative muscle atrophy leading to weakness of the diaphragm and intrathoracic muscles, and diminished lung clearance means that there is poorer tolerance of any insult or injury. Morbidity increases with the presence of common concomitant injuries such as traumatic pulmonary contusions or flail chest; however, in the elderly, even isolated rib fractures carry a significant morbidity and mortality.[28] The mortality rate for patients more than 65 year with isolated rib fractures is about 22%, which is twice that of similarly injured young patients.[29] Mortality increases with each additional broken rib, with an odds ratio of death of 1.19 for each additional broken rib and overall, nearly 20% risk of death after three broken ribs.[29,30] As elderly patients are at particular risk for developing complications such as pneumonia, acute respiratory failure, hypoxemia, and atelectasis with the potential need for the ventilator or care in the ICU, attempts have been made to identify patients who would require early treatment or hospitalization. Identified risk factors for delayed adverse events include age greater than 85 years, pulmonary contusions, the presence of pneumothorax or hemothorax, or hypotension on arrival.[31] The development of a model to identify those who are at higher risk of having delayed adverse events that would require intubation or other advanced therapies is in progress; however, factors such as age, number of rib fractures, and the presence of cardiopulmonary disease, have been identified as risk factors for intubation or admission to the ICU. The advanced age of greater than 80 years, flail chest, tension pneumothoraxes, and blood loss places patients at a higher mortality risk.[32]

Musculoskeletal Injuries

Orthopedic injuries in the geriatric population carry a high morbidity burden. Osteoporosis is common with age, especially in women, which leads to significant fractures even in low-energy mechanisms of trauma. In addition, there are significant declines in muscular function with age even in healthy older adults, most notably in the lower extremities.[33] This finding is additionally compounded with visible diminishment in muscle size in those with limited mobility.[33] It is known that with age, muscles, especially the paraspinals, are progressively replaced by fatty tissue, a phenomenon that does not seem to correlate with either body weight or body mass index (BMI), and not deterred by exercise.[34] Together, the loss of muscle mass and function, known as sarcopenia, has an independent association with increased mortality in the geriatric population.[35]

Pelvic fractures carry increased morbidity and mortality in the elderly. Despite having similar or decreased injury severity compared to younger patients based on injury patterns alone, geriatric patients with pelvic trauma have a higher mortality rate as well as increased hospital length of stay, indicating that age itself was an independent predictor of death.[36] The most common type of pelvic fracture in geriatric trauma is a lateral compression fracture, which is often not amenable to surgical fixation.[36,37] Compared with similarly injured younger patients, geriatric pelvic trauma patients with lateral compression fractures are at eight times higher risk for bleeding, and therefore, awareness of potential ongoing blood loss that may require angioembolization, even without blush found on CT imaging, should be maintained.[38,39] Despite aggressive treatment, more than 70% of these patients are unable to return home and require nursing home care after hospital discharge.[39]

Extremity trauma in the elderly often occurs after minor injuries and falls, and a low index of suspicion should be kept. The presence of osteoporosis causes a higher severity of injury than would otherwise be seen. Insufficiency fractures, from either osteoporosis, medications such as steroids, rheumatoid arthritis, or chronic comorbidities that weaken bone, can occur after even minor trauma. In addition, pathologic fractures and periprosthetic fractures are more common and can complicate repair. Femur fractures carry particularly high morbidity due to significant mobility limitations.

Goals of therapy in musculoskeletal trauma are primarily pain control and physical rehabilitation, with or without operative repair, with the purpose of returning the patient to their prior functionality as much as possible. This often requires the assistance of trained physical therapists to evaluate the patient for need of new assistive devices, rearrangement of home-living situations, or an extended stay in a rehabilitation or nursing care facility if the burden of care is too much for patients and/or their family members. This change in lifestyle can be a difficult adjustment especially for the previously active patient and can be a source of psychological burden such as depression. A focus on maintaining activities of daily living and recognition of possible changes in the patient's psychological state can be useful. Dedicated geriatric teams to evaluate geriatric trauma patients are helpful in reducing polypharmacy and have been shown to improve hospital mortality.[40]

Spinal Trauma

Regarding spinal trauma, increases in spinal rigidity associated with age due to degenerative osseous changes, diffuse idiopathic skeletal hyperostosis, ankylosing spondylitis, or spondylitis deformans portend significant injuries even from minor mechanisms such as fall from seated height. This is especially prominent in the cervical region. With age, the C1–C2 region becomes the most mobile, compared with younger patients where the most mobile regions are C4–C7. Accordingly, the most common cervical spine fracture in geriatric patients is a Type II or Type III dens fracture. Clinical clearance in the elderly population must be carefully considered. The Canadian C-spine clearance criteria take into account patients' age greater than 65 year. The National Emergency X-radiography Utilization Study (NEXUS) C-spine clearance criteria do not take age into account; however, data showed that patients more than 65 year had C-spine injuries of 4.6%, twice that of non-geriatric patients, although when low-risk injuries were specified, the incidence of injury was more equal.[41] Retrospective trials on using modified NEXUS criteria for C-spine clearance in elderly trauma patients have shown some success, specifically those presenting with low-risk trauma, have a GCS of 15 on arrival, is otherwise fully alert and aware, and has only head or neck trauma as a possible distraction injury.[42] There is a suggestion that all patients more than 75 years old should undergo C-spine imaging as the incidence of high C-spine injuries increase in this more elderly geriatric population.[43] However, this remains an area of further study. Lower spine injuries are less common in the elderly than cervical spine injuries, however, the same risks for bony changes apply. Osteoporotic vertebral compression fractures are most common in the T12–L2 region, followed by the mid-thoracic spine.[44] Ankylosing spondylitis causes stiffening, which places these areas at higher risk for fracture patterns.

Abdominal Injuries

Although blunt abdominal injury occurs as frequently in the elderly as in younger patients, the mortality rate for the elderly is markedly increased. A retrospective study of blunt splenic injuries showed that older patients had a higher failure rate than younger patients for nonoperative management, with a subsequently higher mortality rate than those that were intervened on admission.[45] Factors that were associated with need for early intervention included an Injury Severity Score (ISS) greater than 20, grade III or above splenic injury; large volume hemoperitoneum, the presence of active extravasation on initial CT scan, or high-energy mechanisms of injury.[46] In addition, patients who have coexistent blunt splenic injury and liver cirrhosis also have a higher mortality rate with nonoperative management, even with a lower initial ISS.[47] However, nonoperative management for splenic injuries is still feasible for geriatric patients and successful in a majority of cases. Although at one point age was thought to be a contraindication to nonoperative blunt splenic injury management, more recent data have shown that this is not the case.[48] An Eastern Association for the Surgery of Trauma multicenter study showed that morbidity and mortality was increased in patients older than age 55 year and that failure of nonoperative treatment in this population, especially in women was associated with worse outcomes.[45] Individualized treatment must be used in the management of these patients.

Most blunt liver injuries can be managed nonoperatively, even with higher grades of injury.[21,49] This is feasible due to increased technology and ability of adjunctive procedures, such as angiographic embolization or endoscopic retrograde cholangiopancreatography (ERCP), to manage associated injuries or manage bleeding. Nonoperative management of blunt hepatic injuries is best performed in an environment that can perform close hemodynamic monitoring and has the availability of an operating room for urgent laparotomy.[50] Although the mortality in geriatric and younger populations is about the same for nonoperative management blunt liver trauma, it is markedly increased in those that require operative intervention. One retrospective study found that patients greater than age 65 year who needed operative intervention had a 122× increased risk of mortality compared with those who did not.[51]

ICU

Intensive care for geriatric trauma patients is different than that for younger patients. The geriatric population has much lower physiologic reserve, which limits their ability to withstand a traumatic insult due to a diminished ability to generate an appropriate hemodynamic response to injury. Cardiac index and oxygen delivery are diminished in the older population after trauma compared with their younger counterparts, even after resuscitation efforts, and this is attributed to decreased myocardial function even in patients without baseline heart failure.[52] This phenomenon may be compounded by the common use of beta-blockers, angiotension-converting enzyme (ACE) inhibitors, or calcium channel blockers that also affect cardiac output. The early use of inotropy, along with serial monitoring of cardiac output, either via noninvasive or invasive methods, may be of use in resuscitative efforts.[14] Although routine use of pulmonary artery catheters has gone away in noncardiac ICUs, its use might be considered in the select geriatric trauma patient.[52] Normal vital signs should be taken with a grain of salt. Occult hypoperfusion, which is a state of decreased oxygen delivery despite the appearance of normal hemodynamics, may be present in at least 40% of geriatric patients, including up to a third of those with otherwise normal vitals.[53] Patients in this group do require additional support, however, and typically have lengths of stay in the ICU more on par with patients who present with clear shock on admission.[53] The presence on initial laboratory work of an abnormal base deficit (>−2) or elevated lactic acid (<2.2) can be a clue to identifying this group of patients.[53]

Chronic comorbid conditions that can significantly affect patient physiology are common in the geriatric population. In particular, renal function is often diminished, despite normal creatinine. Using creatinine as a marker for renal function may not be accurate, as oftentimes the elderly have diminished muscle mass causing decreases in baseline creatinine. Estimated glomerular filtration rate (GFR) may be a better tool. Nearly all trauma patients with few exceptions undergo contrast imaging as part of the initial trauma assessment, and although there will always be concern for potential contrast nephropathy, studies have shown that it is generally safe to use for geriatric traumas without any difference in the development of post-contrast acute kidney injury.[54] In addition, older patients are commonly on medications, such as beta-blockers or calcium channel blockers that can mask abnormal vital signs and cause underrecognition of early shock. Timely medication reconciliation and appropriate resumption of chronic medications is of paramount importance, with recognition of diminished renal or hepatic clearance and appropriate medication dose reduction. Finally, elderly patients remain at risk for multi-organ system failure after a traumatic stress event, and a continued close monitoring and supportive care is necessary for these patients throughout their ICU stay.

Special Considerations in Symptom Management

There is a fine balance when treating pain in the geriatric population. Pain is frequently undertreated in this patient population because physicians are afraid to over medicate or induce delirium but sometimes fail to recognize that pain itself is deliriogenic. Inadequate treatment of pain is also associated with depression, anxiety, sleep disturbances, and mood changes.[55] In addition, the current aging population may have concerns regarding addiction to opioids.

The first step in the management of acute pain is to educate the patient and family on what to expect with regard to severity of pain considering the traumatic injury sustained and how we approach management. The assessment of pain is difficult as perception of pain is different between individuals, and ability to communicate pain level may be affected by confusion, memory loss, and dementia.[55] This can result in inappropriate reporting of pain control metrics. Therefore, it is important to recognize other signs of suboptimal pain control such as limited movement even while in bed, worsening delirium, poor inspiratory effort, increasing atelectasis on chest x-ray, grimacing, and/or moaning.

Many geriatric trauma patients may have chronic pain from prior trauma, arthritis, or other medical conditions. It is important to continue their current outpatient regimen with the understanding that this will treat baseline pain, but there may be a need to increase or add alternate agents for acute pain treatment.

A multimodal approach to pain treatment is standard of care with the aim of maximizing pain control while minimizing side effects of each drug class. Dose adjustments must be made recognizing the altered pharmacodynamics of geriatric trauma patients. Scheduled nonsteroidal anti-inflammatory medications are a key component of the baseline regimen. Opiates are frequently necessary in the management of acute pain. Consideration of low-dose scheduled opiates can be helpful as many geriatric patients will not ask for their "as needed" medications. If enteral access is not well established, alternative routes such as rectal or transdermal can be considered.

Regional blocks are an excellent adjunct for pain control as they minimize the psychotropic side effects of many pain medications.

Nonmedicinal pain management has been shown to help with pain control in the geriatric population such as physical therapy, osteopathic manipulation, acupuncture, biofeedback, cognitive behavioral therapy, and psychotherapy.[55] Although these may be more difficult to do in the acute post-injury phase, they may be helpful down the line.

UNIQUE CONSIDERATIONS
Geriatric Trauma Centers

The official designation of a "Geriatric Trauma Center" has yet to be established but should be a future goal. Further research is needed to determine the optimal location for the care of geriatric trauma patients. Should they be taken to level I or level II trauma centers? Should they be admitted to a medicine/geriatric service or is trauma the best team? Should there be a designated geriatric trauma unit? Current evidence is mixed and likely dependent on statewide trauma systems and different hospitals. Within centers, studies have shown that the creation of a dedicated geriatric trauma unit could be beneficial.[56,57]

Multidisciplinary Geriatric Care

Regardless of the admission unit or team, care of the geriatric trauma patient requires multidisciplinary care and flexibility. Early involvement of geriatrics and/or medicine, depending on the hospital's availability, may help identify and manage underlying medical conditions that triggered the traumatic event or will complicate their inpatient care. Whether it is an adjustment of preexisting polypharmacy or in-hospital medication regimens, assessment of mobility, or identifying a patient's goals of care, geriatricians can provide an alternative perspective that augments the trauma team's care of the patient.

Immediate consultation of physical and occupation therapy is key once acute traumatic injuries are managed. Early engagement of therapists and social workers expedites disposition for geriatric trauma patients who more frequently require placement in facilities such as skilled nursing facility (SNF), long-term acute care hospital (LTACH), or inpatient rehabilitation (IPR) compared with their younger counterparts. The rapid facilitation of placement optimizes patient outcomes by avoiding prolonged length of stay in the acute setting where rehabilitation is minimal, and risk of in-hospital iatrogenic complications increases.

Frequently, geriatric patients have outlined advance directives or living wills, which can be helpful in guiding care and counseling family about treatments that are in line with patients' previously established goals.[58] When this is less clear, depending on the comfort level of the trauma physician, consultation of palliative care can be highly beneficial.

If frailty has been identified in the patient, this can also help guide discussions about goals of care. Recognizing that frailty increases odds of death from a major complication, also known as failure-to-rescue, frailty status provides powerful information when counseling these patients.[59]

Geriatric psychiatric needs are frequently underrecognized and/or undertreated. Suicide rates in this population are high.[60,61] Unfortunately, there is a paucity of geriatric psychiatry units in the country and those that exist are frequently at capacity.

Given the rising incidence of geriatric trauma, resident education is of paramount importance. Training in the management of geriatric patients in the postoperative, post-injury, and critical care settings are key to the future of successful systems that support these patients.

SUMMARY

Geriatric trauma is of paramount importance due to the rapidly aging global population. Elderly trauma patients often present complex challenges, including preexisting chronic conditions, altered physiology, polypharmacy, and increased susceptibility to injury. The management of geriatric trauma necessitates a multidisciplinary approach, considering not only immediate surgical intervention but also rehabilitation and psychosocial aspects. Understanding geriatric trauma's distinctiveness is vital to improving outcomes, reducing morbidity and mortality rates, and enhancing the quality of life for our aging population.

CLINICS CARE POINTS

- Geriatric patients are not just old adults. They have unique physiology that predisposes them to different trauma mechanisms and outcomes. Understanding these physiologic differences is key to management of the critically ill or injured geriatric patient.

- Frailty adds another dimension to the management of geriatric patients. A systemic scoring system helps to identify frail geriatric patients who may benefit from comprehensive assessment to review and intervene on medications, mobility, functional status, and goals of care.

- Pain management of the injured geriatric patient is arguably the most complex component of their care with opportunities to both greatly help and greatly harm them. Multimodal pain control with conscientious use of medications that balances risks and benefits is key. Conversely, understanding that the perception of pain and subsequent reporting may be skewed resulting in undertreatment of pain, and therefore worsening the delirium we are trying to avoid.

- Establish goals of care for all geriatric patients to ensure you are caring for them in a way that is in line with their values.

DISCLOSURE

The authors have nothing to disclose.

REFERENCES

1. Mangoni AA, Jackson SH. Age-related changes in pharmacokinetics and pharmacodynamics: basic principles and practical applications. Br J Clin Pharmacol 2004;57(1):6–14.
2. Brooks SE, Peetz AB. Evidence-Based Care of Geriatric Trauma Patients. Surg Clin North Am 2017;97(5):1157–74.
3. Janssens JP. Aging of the respiratory system: impact on pulmonary function tests and adaptation to exertion. Clin Chest Med 2005;26(3):469–84, vi-vii.
4. Baldea AJ. Effect of aging on renal function plus monitoring and support. Surg Clin North Am 2015;95(1):71–83.
5. Fried LP, Tangen CM, Walston J, et al. Frailty in older adults: evidence for a phenotype. Journals of Gerontology Series A: Biological Sciences and Medical Sciences 2001;56(3):M146–57.

6. Joseph B, Pandit V, Zangbar B, et al. Validating trauma-specific frailty index for geriatric trauma patients: a prospective analysis. J Am Coll Surg 2014;219(1): 10–7.e1.

7. Joseph B, Saljuqi AT, Amos JD, et al. Prospective validation and application of the Trauma-Specific Frailty Index: Results of an American Association for the Surgery of Trauma multi-institutional observational trial. J Trauma Acute Care Surg 2023; 94(1):36–44.

8. Joseph B, Pandit V, Rhee P, et al. Predicting hospital discharge disposition in geriatric trauma patients: is frailty the answer? J Trauma Acute Care Surg 2014;76(1): 196–200.

9. Joseph B, Pandit V, Zangbar B, et al. Superiority of frailty over age in predicting outcomes among geriatric trauma patients: a prospective analysis. JAMA Surgery 2014;149(8):766–72.

10. Centers for Disease Control and Prevention. Web-based Injury Statistics Query and Reporting System (WISQARS) Online. (2003), https://wisqars.cdc.gov/data/lcd/drill-down?causeLabel=Unintentional%20Injury&agegrp=65%2B. Accessed 06 19, 2023.

11. Lustenberger T, Inaba K, Schnüriger B, et al. Gunshot injuries in the elderly: patterns and outcomes. A national trauma databank analysis. World J Surg 2011; 35(3):528–34.

12. Heffernan DS, Thakkar RK, Monaghan SF, et al. Normal presenting vital signs are unreliable in geriatric blunt trauma victims. J Trauma 2010;69(4):813–20.

13. Kodadek LM, Selvarajah S, Velopulos CG, et al. Undertriage of older trauma patients: is this a national phenomenon? J Surg Res 2015;199(1):220–9.

14. Jacobs DG, Plaisier BR, Barie PS, et al. Practice Management Guidelines for Geriatric Trauma: The EAST Practice Management Guidelines Work Group. J Trauma Acute Care Surg 2003;54(2):391–416.

15. Ma MH, MacKenzie EJ, Alcorta R, et al. Compliance with prehospital triage protocols for major trauma patients. J Trauma 1999;46(1):168–75.

16. Phillips S, Rond PC 3rd, Kelly SM, et al. The failure of triage criteria to identify geriatric patients with trauma: results from the Florida Trauma Triage Study. J Trauma 1996;40(2):278–83.

17. Trauma ACoSCo. ACS TQIP geriatric trauma management guidelines. 2015.

18. Rathlev NK, Medzon R, Lowery D, et al. Intracranial pathology in elders with blunt head trauma. Acad Emerg Med 2006;13(3):302–7.

19. Scalea TM, Simon HM, Duncan AO, et al. Geriatric blunt multiple trauma: improved survival with early invasive monitoring. J Trauma 1990;30(2):129–34 ; discussion 134.

20. Pandharipande PP, Girard TD, Jackson JC, et al. Long-term cognitive impairment after critical illness. N Engl J Med 2013;369(14):1306–16.

21. Demetriades D, Karaiskakis M, Velmahos G, et al. Effect on outcome of early intensive management of geriatric trauma patients. Br J Surg 2002;89(10):1319–22.

22. Blair A, Manian FA. Coexisting Systemic Infections (CSIs) in Patients Presenting With a Fall: Tripped by Objects or Pathogens? Open Forum Infect Dis 2015; 2(suppl_1). https://doi.org/10.1093/ofid/ofv133.530.

23. Mack LR, Chan SB, Silva JC, et al. The use of head computed tomography in elderly patients sustaining minor head trauma. J Emerg Med 2003;24(2):157–62.

24. DeCarli C, Massaro J, Harvey D, et al. Measures of brain morphology and infarction in the framingham heart study: establishing what is normal. Neurobiol Aging 2005;26(4):491–510.

25. Thompson HJ, McCormick WC, Kagan SH. Traumatic brain injury in older adults: epidemiology, outcomes, and future implications. J Am Geriatr Soc 2006;54(10): 1590–5.

26. Mina AA, Knipfer JF, Park DY, et al. Intracranial complications of preinjury anticoagulation in trauma patients with head injury. J Trauma Acute Care Surg 2002; 53(4):668–72.

27. Caterino JM, Raubenolt A, Cudnik MT. Modification of Glasgow Coma Scale criteria for injured elders. Acad Emerg Med 2011;18(10):1014–21.

28. Holcomb JB, McMullin NR, Kozar RA, et al. Morbidity from rib fractures increases after age 45. J Am Coll Surg 2003;196(4):549–55.

29. Stawicki SP, Grossman MD, Hoey BA, et al. Rib fractures in the elderly: a marker of injury severity. J Am Geriatr Soc 2004;52(5):805–8.

30. Bulger EM, Arneson MA, Mock CN, Jurkovich GJ. Rib fractures in the elderly. J Trauma 2000;48(6):1040–6.

31. Lotfipour S, Kaku SK, Vaca FE, et al. Factors associated with complications in older adults with isolated blunt chest trauma. West J Emerg Med 2009;10(2):79.

32. Sikander N, Ahmad T, Shaikh KA Sr, et al. Analysis of injury patterns and outcomes of blunt thoracic trauma in elderly patients. Cureus 2020;12(8).

33. Reid KF, Pasha E, Doros G, et al. Longitudinal decline of lower extremity muscle power in healthy and mobility-limited older adults: influence of muscle mass, strength, composition, neuromuscular activation and single fiber contractile properties. Eur J Appl Physiol 2014;114:29–39.

34. Dahlqvist JR, Vissing CR, Hedermann G, et al. Fat Replacement of Paraspinal Muscles with Aging in Healthy Adults. Med Sci Sports Exerc 2017;49(3):595–601.

35. Landi F, Cruz-Jentoft AJ, Liperoti R, et al. Sarcopenia and mortality risk in frail older persons aged 80 years and older: results from ilSIRENTE study. Age Ageing 2013; 42(2):203–9.

36. O'brien DP, Luchette FA, Pereira SJ, et al. Pelvic fracture in the elderly is associated with increased mortality. Surgery 2002;132(4):710–5.

37. Henry SM, Pollak AN, Jones AL, et al. Pelvic fracture in geriatric patients: a distinct clinical entity. J Trauma Acute Care Surg 2002;53(1):15–20.

38. Velmahos GC, Toutouzas KG, Vassiliu P, et al. A prospective study on the safety and efficacy of angiographic embolization for pelvic and visceral injuries. J Trauma Acute Care Surg 2002;53(2):303–8.

39. Dechert TA, Duane TM, Frykberg BP, et al. Elderly patients with pelvic fracture: interventions and outcomes. Am Surg 2009;75(4):291–5.

40. Fallon WF Jr, Rader E, Zyzanski S, et al. Geriatric outcomes are improved by a geriatric trauma consultation service. J Trauma Acute Care Surg 2006;61(5): 1040–6.

41. Touger M, Gennis P, Nathanson N, et al. Validity of a decision rule to reduce cervical spine radiography in elderly patients with blunt trauma. Ann Emerg Med 2002;40(3):287–93.

42. Tran J, Jeanmonod D, Agresti D, et al. Prospective validation of modified NEXUS cervical spine injury criteria in low-risk elderly fall patients. West J Emerg Med 2016;17(3):252.

43. Lomoschitz F, Blackmore C, Mirza S, et al. Cervical spine injuries in patients 65 years old and older: epidemiologic analysis regarding the effects of age and injury mechanism on distribution, type, and stability of injuries. Am J Roentgenol 2002;178(3):573–7.

44. Kim DH, Vaccaro AR. Osteoporotic compression fractures of the spine; current options and considerations for treatment. Spine J 2006;6(5):479–87.

45. Harbrecht BG, Peitzman AB, Rivera L, et al. Contribution of age and gender to outcome of blunt splenic injury in adults: multicenter study of the eastern association for the surgery of trauma. J Trauma Acute Care Surg 2001;51(5):887–95.

46. Tsugawa K, Koyanagi N, Hashizume M, et al. New insight for management of blunt splenic trauma: significant differences between young and elderly. Hepato-Gastroenterology 2002;49(46):1144–9.

47. Fang J-F, Chen R-J, Lin B-C, et al. Liver cirrhosis: an unfavorable factor for nonoperative management of blunt splenic injury. J Trauma Acute Care Surg 2003; 54(6):1131–6.

48. Myers JG, Dent DL, Stewart RM, et al. Blunt splenic injuries: dedicated trauma surgeons can achieve a high rate of nonoperative success in patients of all ages. J Trauma Acute Care Surg 2000;48(5):801–6.

49. Sherman HF, Savage BA, Jones LM, et al. Nonoperative management of blunt hepatic injuries: safe at any grade? J Trauma 1994;37(4):616–21.

50. Stassen NA, Bhullar I, Cheng JD, et al. Nonoperative management of blunt hepatic injury: an Eastern Association for the Surgery of Trauma practice management guideline. J Trauma Acute Care Surg 2012;73(5):S288–93.

51. Gorman E, Bukur M, Frangos S, et al. Increasing age is associated with worse outcomes in elderly patients with severe liver injury. Am J Surg 2020;220(5): 1308–11.

52. McKinley BA, Marvin RG, Cocanour CS, et al. Blunt trauma resuscitation: the old can respond. Arch Surg 2000;135(6):688–95.

53. Martin JT, Alkhoury F, O'Connor JA, et al. 'Normal'vital signs belie occult hypoperfusion in geriatric trauma patients. Am Surg 2010;76(1):65–9.

54. McGillicuddy EA, Schuster KM, Kaplan LJ, et al. Contrast-induced nephropathy in elderly trauma patients. J Trauma Acute Care Surg 2010;68(2):294–7.

55. Borsheski R, Johnson QL. Pain management in the geriatric population. Mo Med 2014;111(6):508–11.

56. Mangram AJ, Mitchell CD, Shifflette VK, et al. Geriatric trauma service: a one-year experience. J Trauma Acute Care Surg 2012;72(1):119–22.

57. Mangram AJ, Shifflette VK, Mitchell CD, et al. The creation of a geriatric trauma unit "G-60". Am Surg 2011;77(9):1144–6.

58. Stevens CL, Torke AM. Geriatric Trauma: A Clinical and Ethical Review. J Trauma Nurs 2016;23(1):36–41, quiz E3-4.

59. Joseph B, Phelan H, Hassan A, et al. The impact of frailty on failure-to-rescue in geriatric trauma patients: A prospective study. J Trauma Acute Care Surg 2016; 81(6):1150–5.

60. Heisel MJ, Conwell Y, Pisani AR, et al. Concordance of self-and proxy-reported suicide ideation in depressed adults 50 years of age or older. Can J Psychiatr 2011;56(4):219–26.

61. Heisel MJ. Suicide and its prevention among older adults. Can J Psychiatr 2006; 51(3):143–54.

The Role of Minimally Invasive Surgeries in Trauma

Atif Jastaniah, MD, MHSc, FRCSC*,
Jeremey Grushka, MD, MSc, MPH, FRCSC

KEYWORDS

- MIS • DL • Laparoscopy • Trauma • Thoracoscopy • VATS • TDI
- Diaphragmatic injury

KEY POINTS

- Minimally invasive surgery (MIS) in trauma has become increasingly beneficial, offering advantages such as less surgical trauma, shorter hospital stays, reduced pain, and faster recovery.
- Laparoscopy and video-assisted thoracoscopic surgery (VATS) play vital roles in trauma, serving as means for screening, diagnosis, and treatment, with high accuracy in detecting injuries and reducing unnecessary open surgeries.
- Laparoscopy is commonly used in penetrating abdominal injuries to detect peritoneal violation, allowing for expedited management and reduced hospital stays.
- Systematic reviews and meta-analyses show high sensitivity and specificity of laparoscopy in trauma, leading to a significant reduction in nontherapeutic laparotomies.
- Laparoscopy is also effective in diagnosing and treating diaphragmatic, hepatic, splenic, omental, and mesenteric injuries in cases of blunt abdominal trauma.
- Laparoscopy can be applied in cases of failed conservative management for solid organ injuries and can be beneficial in treating complications after nonoperative management for hepatic and pancreatic trauma.
- VATS is effective in diagnosing and treating traumatic diaphragmatic injuries, persistent posttraumatic pneumothoraces, retained hemothorax, and controlling thoracic bleeding in hemodynamically stable patients.
- MIS should not be performed on patients who are hemodynamically unstable or have severe traumatic brain injury, along with other specific contraindications.

INTRODUCTION

Advances in trauma and prehospital care have resulted in a change in the pattern of fatalities, with most deaths occurring within the first few hours of the initial impact.

Division of General Surgery, Department of Surgery, McGill University, 1650 Cedar Avenue, L9-521, Montreal, QC H3G1A4, Canada
* Corresponding author.
E-mail address: atif.jastaniah@gmail.com

Surg Clin N Am 104 (2024) 437–449
https://doi.org/10.1016/j.suc.2023.10.003
0039-6109/24/© 2023 Elsevier Inc. All rights reserved.

However, the chances of survival for those who do survive have increased, and late deaths have become less common.[1] Over the years, the care of injured patients has improved significantly due to advancements in resuscitation methods, imaging technologies, surgical equipment, and the introduction of new devices such as resuscitative endovascular balloon occlusion of the aorta, which have enabled patients with trauma to survive the initial impact.[1] As a result, we now face different injury patterns, each with its unique set of challenges requiring a shift in how we approach these new challenges and the push to adapt to new technologies.

Minimally invasive surgery (MIS) approaches in trauma have existed for a while. However, they have become more mainstream in recent years. Reports in the early 1920s described some form of minimally invasive approach to examine the peritoneum.[2] During the second half of the twentieth century, the use of laparoscopy in patients with trauma began to gain popularity. Early reports on laparoscopy mainly focused on its diagnostic role. Laparoscopy was only used for diagnosis, and open laparotomy was performed for cases requiring further procedures such as achieving hemostasis or bowel resection.[3-6] Several reports showing its effectiveness in evaluating hemoperitoneum in patients with traumatic abdominal injuries were published.[4,5,7,8] Since then, there have been several studies on the physiologic changes, clinical outcomes, and complications associated with MIS, as well as advances in optics, instrumentation, and surgical training, leading to its widespread acceptance across all surgical specialties for elective and emergency procedures.[3,9,10]

MIS offers several advantages over traditional open surgery. These include less surgical trauma during the procedure, shorter hospital stays, reduced postoperative pain, faster functional recovery, and better cosmetic results.[3,7,9,11,12] In particular, MIS is beneficial for trauma patients because it offers a clear view of the thoracic cavity, peritoneal space, and anterior abdominal wall and can potentially provide therapeutic intervention while minimizing unnecessary nontherapeutic procedures.[4,8] In the past, MIS in trauma was only used for more stable patients to diagnose peritoneal violation in penetrating injury and diagnosing and treating thoracic and diaphragmatic injury. However, with the shift to more conservative treatment initially, and the limitation of imaging modalities despite their advances, minimally invasive approaches have become more beneficial and widely used.[3,4]

LAPAROSCOPY

The primary objective of MIS in cases of abdominal trauma is to diagnose injuries and avoid unnecessary laparotomies.[7,13] Laparoscopy, which can be used for both blunt and penetrating trauma cases, serves as a means of screening, diagnosis, and treatment. **Box 1** shows reported indications for laparoscopy in trauma.[4,5,8,9,14-17]

Screening laparoscopy will identify peritoneal violation and signs of visceral injury leading to further intervention. Meanwhile, diagnostic laparoscopy (DL) must be as effective as other diagnostic methods, such as computed tomography (CT), if not better in detecting all injuries.[3,8] The initial laparoscopic examination will categorize the patient into patients without intra-abdominal injuries, those with nonoperative injuries, and those who require further therapeutic intervention laparoscopically or via a laparotomy.[8] For therapeutic laparoscopy to be successful, it must not only detect but also repair all injuries. Many successful therapeutic laparoscopic operations for acute trauma have been reported.[4,5,8,14,18]

Negative and nontherapeutic exploratory laparotomies for trauma remain high at 30%. These laparotomies can lead to high morbidity rates of up to 41%. They are also associated with increased health-care costs and length of hospital stay.[19,20]

Box 1
Indications of Laparoscopy in Trauma

- Determination of peritoneal violation in penetrating abdominal injuries.

- Unclear abdomen (eg, unexplained free fluid without parenchymal injury)

- Unexaminable abdomen with positive CT findings (eg, mesenteric hematoma, and bowel wall thickening)

- Peritonitis

- Free air

- Penetrating injury to the thoracoabdominal region to rule out diaphragmatic injury

- Repair of a diaphragmatic injury

- Penetrating injury with evisceration

- Failure of NOM of solid organ injury

- Management of complications after NOM of solid organ injury

- Intraperitoneal bladder rupture

- Management of rectal injury

- Hernia repair after penetrating or blunt abdominal injury

NOM, Nonoperative management.

Laparoscopy in abdominal injury plays an essential role in minimizing unnecessary laparotomies. It has been reported that DL reduced the rate of nontherapeutic laparotomy by up to 73%.[7,11,21] At the same time, the goal of laparoscopy is to identify all injuries as safely as the gold standard approach of laparotomy. Missed injuries are potentially disastrous, and DL has proven helpful in diagnosing intraperitoneal pathologic condition in trauma. Laparoscopy has demonstrated a specificity of 98% to 100% compared with exploratory laparotomy.[5,7,9,11,12]

Laparoscopy in Penetrating Abdominal Injuries

One of the most common indications for laparoscopy in trauma is in the event of penetrating injury. Earlier reports used laparoscopy for screening and diagnosis. With the advancement in technology and improvement in skills, using it as a therapeutic tool has increased.[5,11,13,15,16,22–24] Laparoscopy is commonly used in patients with low-velocity injuries to detect a peritoneal violation. This approach allows expedited management and reduces hospital stays.[8,14,19] Experts continue to debate the appropriate course of action following the documentation of a violation. The decision heavily relies on the surgeon's experience and comfort level. There is concern that small injuries may go unnoticed, and the gastrointestinal tract may not be thoroughly examined, particularly the lesser sac or retroperitoneal region.[4,7,9] If a surgeon lacks confidence and suspects potential missed injuries, it is crucial to maintain a low threshold to convert to laparotomy.

Many systematic reviews and meta-analyses have been done to analyze the accuracy of laparoscopic surgery in penetrating injuries. A systematic review by Hajibandeh and colleagues included 9 articles and found that the sensitivity ranges from 92% to 100% and specificity from 74% to 100% for laparoscopic procedures in trauma.[11] These ranges were better compared with those in an earlier review by O'Malley and colleagues. In their review, they analyzed 51 research articles on the use of laparoscopy in penetrating abdominal trauma. The results showed a sensitivity range of 66.7% to 100%, a specificity range of 33.3% to 100%, and an accuracy range of 50% to 100%.[5] These high sensitivities and specificity allowed the surgeons to avoid unnecessary laparotomies with their associated morbidity. Using laparoscopy in a systematic and standardized approach to evaluate intra-abdominal injuries can reduce the rate of nontherapeutic laparotomies by 73%.[11,21]

The other important role of MIS in penetrating injury is to diagnose and treat diaphragmatic injuries, especially in the context of left-sided thoracoabdominal injuries, which will be discussed later in the article.

Laparoscopy in Blunt Abdominal Injuries

Role of laparoscopy in the unclear abdomen

After experiencing blunt abdominal trauma, urgent laparotomy is necessary if there is hemodynamic instability and a positive result from focused assessment with sonography in trauma. DL is a helpful tool for hemodynamically stable patients who do not require immediate exploratory laparotomy and whose imaging findings are unclear (such as free fluid without solid organ injury, mesenteric fat stranding, bowel wall thickening, and distended bowel loops) or whose clinical status is unclear.[3,4,14,17,25] DL provides excellent visualization of the peritoneal cavity, identification of intraperitoneal injuries, and assessment of free intraperitoneal fluid. This enables a precise diagnosis for therapeutic intervention, either minimally invasive or via an exploratory laparotomy.[9,14,17,18]

In a meta-analysis by Ki and colleagues, the incidence of laparoscopy missing injuries in blunt abdominal trauma was only 0.003, with a minimal rate of conversion to laparotomy and nontherapeutic laparotomy.[7] Another review conducted by Nicolau demonstrated the high accuracy of laparoscopy in detecting diaphragmatic, hepatic, splenic, omental, and mesenteric injuries, with rate of 98% to 100%, sensitivity ranging from 94.1% to 100%, and specificity between 91% and 100%.[17] In terms of identifying small bowel injuries based on indirect indications, DL is more efficient than a CT scan. The sensitivity of CT scans for intestinal injury diagnosis ranges from 82% to 95%, with a specificity of 98%.[17] These statistics have convinced surgeons to incorporate laparoscopy as a diagnostic tool, resulting in a decrease of up to 78% in the occurrence of nontherapeutic laparotomy in cases of blunt abdominal trauma.[7,26] With advancements in laparoscopic skills, surgeons have started using laparoscopy as a therapeutic tool once injuries have been identified, leading to a decrease in laparotomies and shorter hospital stays. This includes various laparoscopic procedures such as bowel resection and repair, bladder repair, splenectomy, distal pancreatectomy, diaphragm repair, and bleeding control.[7,12,14]

Other indications in blunt abdominal injuries

In cases where conservative management for solid organ injury succeeded but the patient remains symptomatic, laparoscopy can be applied. This technique is especially useful if there is pain secondary to hemoperitoneum and an operation is necessary for washout and/or splenectomy.[4,25] Additionally, laparoscopy can be used when a finding on a CT scan lends itself to serial abdominal examinations but the patient is not reliable or able to participate.[4,25]

Furthermore, laparoscopy has proven useful in treating complications after nonoperative management (NOM) for hepatic trauma when interventions such as percutaneous drainage fail. Successful laparoscopic management of infected perihepatic collections and treatment of bile peritonitis after severe hepatic trauma initially treated by NOM have been described and recommended.[4,25] These interventions are usually necessary 3 to 5 days after injury. Eastern Association for the Surgery of Trauma (EAST) guidelines on NOM for blunt hepatic trauma consider laparoscopy as an adjunct to nonoperative management of hepatic injuries.[27] Laparoscopy can also be useful to debride subsequent necrosis after NOM for pancreatic injuries. Minimally invasive and nonoperative approaches have been described for pancreatic duct injuries in stable patients.[4,25]

VIDEO-ASSISTED THORACOSCOPIC SURGERY

Thoracic trauma is responsible for about 25% of trauma-related deaths, especially for those who die at the scene due to injuries to the heart and major blood vessels. Around 80% to 85% of chest injuries can be treated with resuscitation and tube thoracostomy alone. However, the remaining 15% to 20% of patients require operative interventions.[28]

Video-assisted thoracoscopic surgery (VATS) is becoming a popular diagnostic and therapeutic modality in thoracic trauma. It is indicated for the diagnosis and repair of diaphragmatic injuries, management of persistent pneumothorax, retained hemothorax, empyema, control of bleeding in hemodynamically stable patients, and management of thoracic duct injuries (**Box 2**).[29–32] Compared with thoracotomy, VATS has fewer postoperative complications, better postoperative pain control, fewer wound and pulmonary complications, shorter chest tube duration, and a faster return to regular activities.[29,33]

Traumatic Diaphragmatic Injury

Diagnosing injuries to the diaphragm caused by trauma poses a challenge. The rate of traumatic diaphragmatic injury (TDI) varies in different studies due to difficulties in detecting them on imaging. In fact, up to 77% of patients with penetrating thoracoabdominal trauma may have normal chest radiographs. According to the largest review published in 2012, which included 833,309 cases from the American College of Surgeons National Trauma Data Bank, the TDI rate was 0.46%.[34,35] However, other reports have suggested rates as high as 8%.[36,37] Among these injuries, two-thirds result from penetrating mechanisms. Diaphragmatic injuries are most commonly diagnosed on the left side, accounting for 75% of cases. Right-sided injuries are less common, with rates reported at 35% to 49%. Nevertheless, diagnosing right-sided injuries is more challenging because they are covered by the liver, and their true incidence is likely higher than reported.[34–36] This article will focus on penetrating TDI because blunt mechanisms are usually associated with other injuries and hemodynamic instability that require urgent intervention.

Box 2
Indications of Video-Assisted Thoracoscopic Surgery in Trauma

- Penetrating injury to the thoracoabdominal region to rule out traumatic diaphragmatic injury (TDI)
- Repair of a TDI
- Evacuation of retained hemothorax
- Persistent posttraumatic pneumothoraces or bronchopleural fistula
- Management of empyema
- Bleeding control in hemodynamically stable patients
- Management of thoracic duct injuries

Penetrating TDI can be missed if there is no other indication for surgery in isolated thoracoabdominal wounds. This can be dangerous because missed diaphragmatic injuries can lead to herniation and strangulation of organs through the diaphragmatic defect.[36,38,39] Surgeons should, therefore, consider using DL or VATS to diagnose these injuries, particularly with left-sided thoracoabdominal penetrating wounds, even if there are no other indications for intervention.[34] Additionally, with the rapid advances in minimally invasive techniques and instrumentation, most of these injuries can be safely and effectively repaired laparoscopically or by VATS with a significantly better postoperative course compared with open approaches.[3,29,33]

Most published reports advocate for the abdominal approach because it allows for the identification and repair of associated intra-abdominal injuries and most surgeons are familiar with the technique and anatomy compared with VATS.[34] DL has shown a specificity of 100%, a sensitivity of 87.5%, and a negative predictive value of 96.8% in assessing the diaphragm after penetrating injury.[40,41] However, VATS has demonstrated that it can detect TDI with 100% sensitivity and specificity.[32,42] Additionally, thoracoscopy is better than DL for posterior or right-sided diaphragmatic injuries.[32,34,37] Furthermore, it is particularly useful for dealing with associated thoracic injuries and in patients with challenging laparoscopic access due to multiple previous laparotomies.[37]

In the acute setting for thoracoabdominal injuries, if a thoracic approach is selected and there is no clear indication for urgent operation, it is recommended to delay undergoing VATS for at least 24 hours. This is done to ensure that there is no intra-abdominal injury that requires an intervention.[3,34,36] In our institution, we established a pathway for patients with low-velocity penetrating injury to the left thoracoabdominal area (**Fig. 1**).

Evacuation of Hemothorax

Another use of VATS in trauma involves treating with retained hemothorax.[29–32] *Retained hemothorax* is defined as blood occupying at least one-third of the pleural space, which cannot be drained by thoracostomy after 72 hours or clots of at least 500 mL volume.[43] Hemothoraces can sometimes liquefy and be drained through a thoracostomy tube. However, if they persist, they can form a fibrothorax and cause complications such as entrapped lungs, volume loss of functioning lungs, and respiratory insufficiency. Traditional treatment of persistent hemothorax is to place additional chest tubes but this procedure's failure rate is as high as 40%.[30,32] A systematic review by Billeter and colleagues showed that VATS has an 87% success rate in evacuating retained hemothorax with an 11% conversion rate to thoracotomy.[31] EAST guidelines recommend the usage of early VATS instead of inserting another chest tube after failure of the initial drainage attempt.[44]

The optimal timing for VATS in posttraumatic retained hemothorax is uncertain. A recent review in 2020 showed that earlier intervention (within 1–3 days) is more successful and has better outcomes than a later intervention (after 7 days). The use of early VATS also drastically reduces hospital length of stay and costs.[45] Delaying VATS for more than 5 days posttrauma results in significantly higher rates of both empyema and thoracotomy.[30,44] Independent predictors of successful VATS as definitive treatment include the absence of an associated diaphragm injury, use of periprocedural antibiotics for thoracostomy placement, and volume of residual hemothorax 900 cc or less.[30]

Other Thoracic Indications

Persistent posttraumatic pneumothoraces occur in approximately 10% of patients.[32,46] They are typically treated with prolonged chest tube drainage, which can

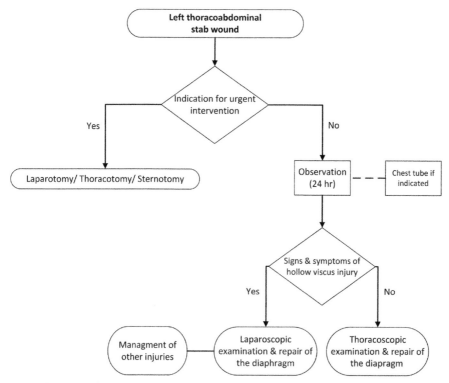

Fig. 1. Flow chart for the management of left thoracoabdominal stab wounds.

be painful and increase potential morbidity and length of hospital stay.[32] The use of VATS to treat recurrent and persistent pneumothorax is well established. It allows for direct visualization and repair of the air leak via stapling, sealant, or pleurodesis.[31,47–49]

VATS is also indicated in stable patients with ongoing thoracic bleeding after chest tube insertion.[29] The main source of persistent bleeding after tube thoracostomy is usually ongoing bleeding from intercostal vessels resulting from chest wall trauma and rib fractures. Other possible sources of bleeding include injuries to the pulmonary parenchyma or pulmonary vascular system.[29,31] VATS plays a role in diagnosis and treatment. According to a report by Villavicencio and colleagues, VATS was successful in controlling hemorrhage in 82% of patients with nonhemodynamically significant intrathoracic hemorrhage.[29]

CONTRAINDICATIONS

Advancements in MIS have allowed surgeons to push the boundaries of trauma patient care. However, it is essential to consider that patients with trauma have unique pathophysiology and injury patterns, setting them apart from other patients. Some reports suggest that laparoscopy might be feasible in unstable patients with trauma[50]; however, experts and evidence firmly uphold that hemodynamic instability is an absolute contraindication to MIS in trauma.[27,40,51]

Moreover, it is crucial to be cautious with patients with severe traumatic brain injury (TBI) because laparoscopy is an absolute contraindication in such cases. Studies have demonstrated that pneumoperitoneum can increase intracranial pressure and worsen the existing brain injury.[52] In light of this, a thoughtful approach and careful consideration of individual patient conditions are necessary to ensure the best possible outcomes in MIS for patients with trauma. **Table 1** summarizes the contraindications to laparoscopy in trauma.[3,4,17]

Apart from the contraindications mentioned earlier, additional specific contraindications should be considered for VATS. These include suspected cardiac injury, a need to perform laparotomy, as well as the inability of the patient to tolerate either single lung ventilation or the lateral decubitus position, which is necessary to carry out the procedure.[32]

COMPLICATIONS

When using laparoscopy in patients with trauma, there are potential complications that are similar to those seen in elective surgeries. These complications may include wound infections, hernias, and iatrogenic injuries.[4,13] One specific complication that trauma patients with diaphragmatic injury may experience is tension pneumothorax caused by positive pressure pneumoperitoneum, which requires immediate tube thoracostomy.[4,8] To reduce this risk, alternative methods such as VATS (which does not require gas), lower insufflation pressure, or prophylactic insertion of a needle thoracostomy or chest tube should be considered.[32] The presence of intra-abdominal venous injuries may lead to gas embolism.[4,8] Moreover, pneumoperitoneum may cause hemodynamic compromise due to reduced venous return and may lead to increased intracranial pressure in patients with existing brain injuries.[4,52] In general, the reported complication rate for laparoscopy in patients with trauma is less than 1%.[5,8,11]

CONCERNS AND CONTROVERSIES

The use of laparoscopy in trauma has raised concerns about missing injuries, particularly evident in early reports, with high rates of missed injuries ranging from 41% to 77% during abdominal exploration with laparoscopy.[8,11] However, these rates were influenced by factors such as the surgeon's experience, comfort with laparoscopy, and availability of technological resources. Recent reports indicate a significant improvement, with missed injury rates reduced to less than 1% when using DL.[7,9,11] Ultimately, the success of laparoscopy as a diagnostic tool largely hinges on the surgeon's skill and expertise. Surgeons who perform at least 20 laparoscopic procedures per month for acute care surgery are more likely to safely and accurately conduct DL for abdominal stab wounds.[53] Nevertheless, if a surgeon lacks the necessary technical skill or a suspected injury to the hollow viscus cannot be thoroughly evaluated laparoscopically, immediate conversion to laparotomy is necessary.

In the past, laparoscopy was primarily recommended for screening and diagnosis. Once peritoneal violation in penetrating injury had been established, converting to

Table 1 Contraindications to laparoscopy in trauma	
Absolute	**Relative**
Hemodynamic instability	Difficult access to the abdomen due to adhesions or bowel distension
Immediate life-threatening injuries	Advance Pregnancy
Severe TBI	Severe cardiac and pulmonary dysfunction
	Multisystem injuries

laparotomy was the standard of care.[8] However, advancements in proficiency have challenged this approach, leading to successful therapeutic interventions using laparoscopy.[9,15,22] Since 2000, a significant amount of published research has advocated for the therapeutic utility of laparoscopy in both blunt and penetrating trauma, compared with the limited literature before that.[54] Laparoscopic interventions have been successfully performed on various organs, including the diaphragm, stomach, small intestine, colon, bladder, pancreas, and spleen. Notably, numerous reports demonstrate high success rates in addressing bowel perforations through laparoscopic-assisted procedures, achieving hemostasis, and managing injuries to solid organs and the mesentery.[3,4,17] This expanding body of evidence supports the broader application of laparoscopy in trauma settings.

There are additional issues associated with using MIS in trauma cases. These include the logistical challenges associated with preparing an operating room for MIS procedures, gaining access to an anatomic cavity, longer surgery times, and delays in achieving source control and hemostasis. These factors may potentially exacerbate temperature shifts and coagulopathy, further complicating the management of patients with trauma.[3,4]

FUTURE DIRECTIONS

The role of laparoscopy in trauma is constantly evolving and will continue to be significant. However, the success of using MIS in trauma surgery relies on the surgeon's level of expertise. As trauma surgeons become more comfortable with MIS, participate in acute care surgery, and use technological advancements, they will be better equipped to use and evaluate MIS as a valuable therapeutic option for patients requiring intervention.

With the continuous advancement of diagnostic imaging modalities, the role of laparoscopy in injury screening and diagnosis may diminish. However, this will encourage the surgical community to explore innovative approaches to use MIS in the care of injured patients.

SUMMARY

MIS has seen increasing benefits and widespread adoption in trauma cases, providing a clear view of affected areas and enabling effective interventions, ultimately reducing unnecessary nontherapeutic procedures. The main goal of MIS in trauma is to accurately diagnose injuries and avoid unnecessary open surgeries, leading to reduced morbidity, shorter hospital stays, and lower costs. Laparoscopy and VATS can play a major role in screening, diagnosis, and treatment in both blunt and penetrating trauma cases.

Although MIS offers promise in trauma care, there are valid concerns regarding missed injuries and potential complications, emphasizing the significance of surgeon expertise and careful patient selection. As technology and surgical skills advance, the role of laparoscopy in trauma is expected to continue evolving, likely leading to its expanded application in the future.

CLINICS CARE POINTS

- MIS in trauma has become increasingly beneficial, offering advantages such as less surgical trauma, shorter hospital stays, reduced pain, and faster recovery.

- Laparoscopy and VATS play vital roles in trauma, serving as means for screening, diagnosis, and treatment, with high accuracy in detecting injuries and reducing unnecessary open surgeries.
- Laparoscopy is commonly used in penetrating abdominal injuries to detect peritoneal violation, allowing for expedited management and reduced hospital stays.
- Systematic reviews and meta-analyses show high sensitivity and specificity of laparoscopy in trauma, leading to a significant reduction in nontherapeutic laparotomies.
- Laparoscopy is also effective in diagnosing and treating diaphragmatic, hepatic, splenic, omental, and mesenteric injuries in cases of blunt abdominal trauma.
- Laparoscopy can be applied in cases of failed conservative management for solid organ injuries and can be beneficial in treating complications after nonoperative management for hepatic and pancreatic trauma.
- VATS is effective in diagnosing and treating TDI, persistent posttraumatic pneumothoraces, retained hemothorax, and controlling thoracic bleeding in hemodynamically stable patients.
- MIS should not be performed on patients who are hemodynamically unstable or have severe TBI, along with other specific contraindications.

DISCLOSURE

The authors have nothing to disclose.

REFERENCES

1. Gunst M, Ghaemmaghami V, Gruszecki A, et al. Changing epidemiology of trauma deaths leads to a bimodal distribution. Baylor University Medical Center Proceedings 2010;23(4):349–54.
2. Short AR. The uses of coelioscopy. Br Med J 1925;2(3371):254–5.
3. Grushka J, Ginzburg E. Through the 10-mm looking glass: Advances in minimally invasive surgery in trauma. Scand J Surg 2014;103(2):143–8.
4. Di Saverio S, Birindelli A, Podda M, et al. Trauma laparoscopy and the six w 's: Why, where, who, when, what, and how? J Trauma Acute Care Surg 2019;86: 344–67.
5. O'Malley E, Boyle E, O'Callaghan A, et al. Role of laparoscopy in penetrating abdominal trauma: A systematic review. World J Surg 2013;37(1):113–22.
6. Matsevych O, Koto M, Balabyeki M, et al. Trauma laparoscopy: when to start and when to convert? Surg Endosc 2018;32(3):1344–52.
7. Ki YJ, Jo YG, Park YC, et al. The efficacy and safety of laparoscopy for blunt abdominal trauma: A systematic review and meta-analysis. J Clin Med 2021; 10(9). https://doi.org/10.3390/jcm10091853.
8. Villavicencio RT, Aucar JA. Analysis of laparoscopy in trauma. J Am Coll Surg 1999;189(1):11–20.
9. Cirocchi R, Birindelli A, Inaba K, et al. Laparoscopy for trauma and the changes in its use from 1990 to 2016: a current systematic review and meta-analysis. Surg Laparosc Endosc Percutaneous Tech 2018;28(1):1–12.
10. Chol YB, Lim KS. Therapeutic laparoscopy for abdominal trauma. Surg Endosc 2003;17(3):421–7.
11. Hajibandeh S, Hajibandeh S, Gumber AO, et al. Laparoscopy versus laparotomy for the management of penetrating abdominal trauma: A systematic review and meta-analysis. Int J Surg 2016;34:127–36.

12. Li Y, Xiang Y, Wu N, et al. A Comparison of laparoscopy and laparotomy for the management of abdominal trauma: a systematic review and meta-analysis. World J Surg 2015;39(12):2862–71.

13. Zantut LF, Ivatury RR, Smith RS, et al. Diagnostic and therapeutic laparoscopy for penetrating abdominal trauma: a multicenter experience. J Trauma 1997;42(5):825–9, discussion 829-31.

14. Ozkan OV, Justin V, Fingerhut A, et al. Laparoscopy in abdominal trauma. Current Trauma Reports 2016;2(4):238–46.

15. Bain K, Meytes V, Chang GC, et al. Laparoscopy in penetrating abdominal trauma is a safe and effective alternative to laparotomy. Surg Endosc 2019;33(5):1618–25.

16. Cocco AM, Bhagvan S, Bouffler C, et al. Diagnostic laparoscopy in penetrating abdominal trauma. ANZ J Surg 2019;89(4):353–6.

17. Nicolau AE. Is Laparoscopy still needed in blunt abdominal trauma. Chirurgia (Romania) 2011;108(1):59–66.

18. Zafar SN, Onwugbufor MT, Hughes K, et al. Laparoscopic surgery for trauma: The realm of therapeutic management. Am J Surg 2015;209(4):627–32.

19. Marks JM, Youngelman DF, Berk T. Cost analysis of diagnostic laparoscopy vs laparotomy in the evaluation of penetrating abdominal trauma. Surg Endosc 1997;11(3):272–6.

20. Renz BM, Feliciano DV. Unnecessary laparotomies for trauma: a prospective study of morbidity. J Trauma 1995;38(3):350–6.

21. Kawahara NT, Alster C, Fujimura I, et al. Standard examination system for laparoscopy in penetrating abdominal trauma. J Trauma Inj Infect Crit Care 2009;67(3):589–95.

22. Felipe Cabrera Vargas L, Mendoza Zuchini A, Pedraza Ciro M, et al. Therapeutic Laparoscopy for Penetrating Abdominal Trauma in Stable Patients. J Am Coll Surg 2020;231(4):e254.

23. Chestovich PJ, Browder TD, Morrissey SL, et al. Minimally invasive is maximally effective: Diagnostic and therapeutic laparoscopy for penetrating abdominal injuries. J Trauma Acute Care Surg 2015;78(6):1076–85.

24. Uranues S, Popa DE, Diaconescu B, et al. Laparoscopy in penetrating abdominal trauma. World J Surg 2015;39(6):1381–8.

25. Justin V, Fingerhut A, Uranues S. Laparoscopy in Blunt Abdominal Trauma: for Whom? When?and Why? Current Trauma Reports 2017;3(1):43–50.

26. Mitsuhide K, Junichi S, Atsushi N, et al. Computed tomographic scanning and selective laparoscopy in the diagnosis of blunt bowel injury: a prospective study. J Trauma 2005;58(4):696–701, discussion 701-3.

27. Stassen NA, Bhullar I, Cheng JD, et al. Nonoperative management of blunt hepatic injury: an Eastern Association for the Surgery of Trauma practice management guideline. J Trauma Acute Care Surg 2012;73(5 Suppl 4):S288–93.

28. Richardson JD, Miller FB, Carrillo EH, et al. Complex thoracic injuries. Surg Clin North Am. Aug 1996;76(4):725–48.

29. Villavicencio RT, Aucar JA, Wall MJ. Analysis of thoracoscopy in trauma. Surg Endosc 1999;13(1):3–9.

30. DuBose J, Inaba K, Demetriades D, et al. Management of post-traumatic retained hemothorax: A prospective, observational, multicenter AAST study. J Trauma Acute Care Surg 2012;72(1):11–24.

31. Billeter AT, Druen D, Franklin GA, et al. Video-assisted thoracoscopy as an important tool for trauma surgeons: A systematic review. Langenbeck's Arch Surg 2013;398(4):515–23.

32. Ahmed N, Jones D. Video-assisted thoracic surgery: State of the art in trauma care. Injury 2004;35(5):479–89.

33. Wu N, Wu L, Qiu C, et al. A comparison of video-assisted thoracoscopic surgery with open thoracotomy for the management of chest trauma: a systematic review and meta-analysis. World J Surg 2015;39(4):940–52.

34. McDonald AA, Robinson BRH, Alarcon L, et al. Evaluation and management of traumatic diaphragmatic injuries: A Practice Management Guideline from the Eastern Association for the Surgery of Trauma. J Trauma Acute Care Surg 2018; 85(1):198–207.

35. Fair KA, Gordon NT, Barbosa RR, et al. Traumatic diaphragmatic injury in the American College of Surgeons National Trauma Data Bank: a new examination of a rare diagnosis. Am J Surg 2015;209(5):864–8, discussion 868-9.

36. DeBarros M, Martin MJ. Penetrating Traumatic Diaphragm Injuries. Current Trauma Reports 2015;1(2):92–101.

37. Freeman RK, Al-Dossari G, Hutcheson KA, et al. Indications for using video-assisted thoracoscopic surgery to diagnose diaphragmatic injuries after penetrating chest trauma. Ann Thorac Surg 2001;72(2):342–7.

38. Murray JA, Weng J, Velmahos GC, et al. Abdominal approach to chronic diaphragmatic hernias: is it safe? Am Surg 2004;70(10):897–900.

39. Turhan K, Makay O, Cakan A, et al. Traumatic diaphragmatic rupture: look to see. Eur J Cardio Thorac Surg 2008;33(6):1082–5.

40. Como JJ, Bokhari F, Chiu WC, et al. Practice management guidelines for selective nonoperative management of penetrating abdominal trauma. J Trauma Inj Infect Crit Care 2010;68(3):721–33.

41. Ahmed N, Whelan J, Brownlee J, et al. The contribution of laparoscopy in evaluation of penetrating abdominal wounds. J Am Coll Surg 2005;201(2):213–6.

42. Spann JC, Nwariaku FE, Wait M. Evaluation of video-assisted thoracoscopic surgery in the diagnosis of diaphragmatic injuries. Am J Surg 1995;170(6):628–31.

43. Zeiler J, Idell S, Norwood S, et al. Hemothorax: A Review of the Literature. Clin Pulm Med 2020;27(1):1–12.

44. Mowery NT, Gunter OL, Collier BR, et al. Practice management guidelines for management of hemothorax and occult pneumothorax. J Trauma 2011;70(2): 510–8.

45. Ziapour B, Mostafidi E, Sadeghi-Bazargani H, et al. Timing to perform VATS for traumatic-retained hemothorax (a systematic review and meta-analysis). Eur J Trauma Emerg Surg 2020;46(2):337–46.

46. Reddy VS. Minimally Invasive Techniques in Thoracic Trauma. Semin Thorac Cardiovasc Surg 2008;20(1):72–7.

47. Carrillo EH, Schmacht DC, Gable DR, et al. Thoracoscopy in the management of posttraumatic persistent pneumothorax. J Am Coll Surg 1998;186(6):636–9, discussion 639-40.

48. Carrillo EH, Kozloff M, Saridakis A, et al. Thoracoscopic application of a topical sealant for the management of persistent posttraumatic pneumothorax. J Trauma 2006;60(1):111–4.

49. Liu DW, Liu HP, Lin PJ, et al. Video-assisted thoracic surgery in treatment of chest trauma. J Trauma 1997;42(4):670–4.

50. Cherkasov M, Sitnikov V, Sarkisyan B, et al. Laparoscopy versus laparotomy in management of abdominal trauma. Surg Endosc 2008;22(1):228–31.

51. Ball CG, Karmali S, Rajani RR. Laparoscopy in trauma: An evolution in progress. Injury 2009;40(1):7–10.

52. Mobbs RJ, Yang MO. The dangers of diagnostic laparoscopy in the head injured patient. J Clin Neurosci 2002;9(5):592–3.
53. Lin HF, Chen YD, Chen SC. Value of diagnostic and therapeutic laparoscopy for patients with blunt abdominal trauma: A 10-year medical center experience. PLoS One 2018;13(2):1–14.
54. Coleman L, Gilna G, Portenier D, et al. Trauma laparoscopy from 1925 to 2017: Publication history and study demographics of an evolving modality. J Trauma Acute Care Surg 2018;84(4):664–9.

Teaching Before, During, and After a Surgical Resuscitation

Paul J. Schenarts, MD*, Alec J. Scarborough, MD,
Ren J. Abraham, MD, George Philip, MD

KEYWORDS

• Teaching • Learning • Trauma • Resuscitation • Education

KEY POINTS

- The US population is aging at an unprecedented rate and with this comes increased complexity of resuscitation, surgical procedures, and perioperative management necessitating the need for trainees to prepare.
- Educating and learning in a surgical crisis can be difficult due to the lack of repeated exposure to these scenarios. Furthermore, when these scenarios do occur, cognitive overload or excessive stress can hamper learning during the crisis.
- Antiquated ways of teaching such as through textbooks and lectures may not adequately prepare trainees for managing these patients; therefore, modern techniques such as simulation and education by the attending surgeon must occur.
- A surgical crisis is unpredictable, and exposure is inconsistent throughout residency programs. Therefore, preparation and practice are necessary.

INTRODUCTION

This article focuses on educating medical students, residents, and fellows in the management of traumatically injured patients. Because resuscitation of trauma patients may be required at any point during their hospital course and the approaches used in managing trauma patients should be applied to all surgical patients in crisis, the term surgical resuscitation is used throughout this article. The road map for educating learners about surgical resuscitation begins with a discussion of the current and future burden of surgical emergencies. Next, an overview of the biopsychology of learning, including the impact of stress on learning, memory, and the development of clinical reasoning skills, is presented. Having established the importance and educational foundation of learning, this article sequentially provides a detailed review of educational methods used before, during, and after the resuscitation.

Department of Surgery, School of Medicine, Creighton University, Omaha, NE, USA
* Corresponding author. Education Building, Suite 501 77 Mercy Road, Omaha, NE 68124-2368.
E-mail address: paulschenarts@creighton.edu

Surg Clin N Am 104 (2024) 451–471
https://doi.org/10.1016/j.suc.2023.10.004
0039-6109/24/© 2023 Elsevier Inc. All rights reserved.

surgical.theclinics.com

Why Trainees Need More Education on Management of Surgical Emergencies

Although some surgical patients present in extremis, all surgical patients are at risk of developing a crisis at any point during their perioperative course or in the operating room. Surgical crises occur in approximately 1.5% of operations, impacting up to 3 million people worldwide.[1,2] Organ dysfunction constituting a need for resuscitation, including cardiac arrests, strokes, and respiratory failure after noncardiac surgery, has remained stubbornly persistent at about 2%.[3] For those patients requiring an emergency operation, there is a sevenfold increase in morbidity and mortality compared with elective operations.[4]

According to the US Census, by 2035, 77 million people will be older than age 65 years, outnumbering the number of children in the United States.[5] This elderly population will account for a significantly greater proportion of surgical patients.[6] With increasing age, there is also a predictable decline physiologic reserve as well as the development of anatomic abnormalities, such as cancer or heart disease. These changes will result in a greater need for emergency surgery, further increasing the potential for an operative or perioperative crisis.[7]

Similar trends have also been documented in trauma patients. According to the National Trauma Data Bank, mortality after injury increases after the age of 50 years and 34% of trauma patients are aged 55 years or older.[8] As a result of an aging population, it is anticipated that surgical residents will be caring for sicker patients, with more confounding medical conditions and performing more complex interventions.[9]

Arguably most surgical residents obtain most of their education in management of surgical resuscitations on the acute care surgery or trauma surgery services. However, only 9.5% of trauma patients have sustained moderate injuries (Injury Severity Score [ISS] 16 to 24) and only 7.8% serious injuries (ISS > 24).[8] Complicating this infrequency in managing complicated trauma patients, there is significant variability in resident training in trauma, burns, and surgical critical care across the United States.[10] A recent study by Jordan and colleagues[11] found that only 50% of residents completed a formal surgical critical care rotation, 9% had no formal surgical critical care experience, and only 78% were satisfied with their critical care training.

Making matters worse, there has been an increase in nonoperative management of critically ill and injured surgical patients[12,13] and an overall decrease in clinical experiences due to duty hour limits.[14] The current state of resident education in management of surgical patients in crisis is lacking, inconsistent, and at a time when the need for these skills is anticipated to increase.

BASIC BIOPHYSIOLOGY OF LEARNING

Given the unique aspects of learning to manage the complexities of a surgical resuscitation, it is important to have a basic understanding of how learning occurs and the impact that stress has on this process. At its core, learning is a biological process of acquiring new knowledge by forming associations between different environmental stimuli that cause an anatomic rewiring of our plastic or dynamic nervous system.[15] With repeated exposure to these stimuli, there is activation of post-synaptic N-methyl-D-aspartate receptors that promote synthesis of new proteins, which cause a strengthening of the neuronal cytoskeleton, thereby solidifying memories into a physical manifestation of learning.[16–18] Additional protein synthesis, genetic expression to construct new synapses and new, enlarged dendritic spines, leads to a further consolidation of this anatomic relationship.[19,20] On the contrary, the lack of repeated exposure to these stimuli results in reversal of these processes, and synaptic connections are weakened and then lost.[16–18]

Learning motor skills is also dependent on increasing synaptic efficacy but involves activation of Purkinje neurons, which depress transmission at the synapse. This depression is persistent and is considered the cellular basis of motor learning.[21,22] Although neuronal plasticity and establishing anatomic connections are responsible for an individual's intellectual and motor skills development, much of early surgical learning is observational. Adult brains have special mirror neurons that allow humans to visually compare what we are seeing to a remembered action in our memory.[23] This is the physiologic basis for learning through watching.

This is only a brief, superficial overview of the biology of learning. An in-depth review of the biology and psychology of surgical learning was published in a recent edition of Surgical Clinics of North America.[15]

FUNCTION OF MEMORY DURING A RESUSCITATION

To effectively manage any resuscitation, a surgeon must be able to differentiate important information from the irrelevant. New information enters our cognition via the sensory memory. Unless these visual and auditory stimuli specifically catch our attention, say through the recognition of a pattern, they are immediately forgotten.[24] It is sensory memory that allows us to "screen in" and "screen out" relevant information.[25]

Once information is considered important it enters our working memory, which allows us to hold and manipulate information for seconds to minutes while we achieve a task. Working memory has a very limited capacity and is only able to hold 7 ± 2 elements of information at a time.[24] During a resuscitation, the sheer volume of inputs or distractions may overwhelm the learner's working memory and they may be unable to complete a task.

Working memory is also the conduit for experiences to enter long-term memory, where it may be held indefinitely and drawn on for future use.[24,26] Given the limitations of working memory, it is physiologically unlikely that a resident will walk away from a single resuscitation having established a large set of memories that can be applied in the future.

THE LEARNER'S BRAIN DURING A RESUSCITATION
Cognitive Overload

Learning is impaired when new information or the requirement to perform a new task exceeds the capacity of the working memory, which can only hold approximately seven elements of information.[15] There are three types of cognitive load that affect learning. Intrinsic load is the cognitive demand of the task and is directly related to the complexity of the task. Extraneous load refers to the cognitive load placed on the learner by factors not related to the task, such as distractions or excessive noise. The germane load is the amount of effort or concentration the learner devotes to the task. If intrinsic and/or extrinsic load is greater than the germane load, learning does not occur.[27–29]

Impact of Stress on the Biophysiology of Memory and Learning

The Yerkes–Dodson law[30,31] describes the optimal amount of stress for the peak performance of a task. Both too little stress and too much stress impair performance and learning. Stress that induces a low amplitude production of glucocorticoids is associated with improved memory, whereas the excessive amplitude significantly impairs it.[32] The neural cell adhesion molecule which is, in part, responsible for the neuron–neuron connections required for memory consolidation or learning[33] is induced by stress.[34]

The timing of the stress also has implications for surgical educators. If the stress occurs at the beginning or end of the learning experience, before memory consolidation can occur, performance is improved. However, if the stress of learning occurs far before the learning experience or after consolidation, there is a negative effect.[22]

The degree of stress a learner experiences is based on an individual's perception. This may be why clinical studies on the relationship between acute stress and medical performance have yielded ambiguous results.[35–38]

DEVELOPMENT OF CLINICAL REASONING

The science and the art of clinical reasoning is fundamental to surgical care, particularly in times of crisis. There is no consensus, however, as to how this problem-solving occurs. One view, made popular by the Nobel Prize winner Daniel Kahneman in his book *"Thinking Fast and Slow"*[39] articulates the work of Evans,[40] Sloman,[41] and Stanovich and West.[42] In layman's terms, problem-solving involves two independent systems of processing information. System 1 is a rapid, unconscious, intuitive, and automatic process, whereas System 2 is a slow, deliberate, and analytical process.[39–42] This two-system view has made its way into the medical education literature.[43–46] The application is that clinical problem-solving can occur either analytically by a process involving a feature-by-feature comparison of patient information with probable clinical conditions or, alternatively, through a nonanalytic process of intuition, gut feelings, scripts, schemas, or memories of previous patients.[47] Although the two-system view is attractive in its simplicity, others[47,48] have argued that clinical reasoning occurs across a cognitive continuum, in which one pole is intuition and pattern recognition and the opposite is the analytical pole, where algorithms and calculations are found.

Although this is an interesting intellectual debate, decision-making during a crisis is likely a combination of both systems in concert[49] or moving back and forth across this continuum. Regardless of your view, preparation of learners to manage surgical resuscitation must begin well before the arrival of the situation.

EDUCATING RESIDENTS BEFORE THE RESUSCITATION

The occurrence of surgical crises is unpredictable, so residents typically prepare for these events by developing a fund of factual knowledge, hoping they can draw on this information when the need arises. This is clearly a System 1, or analytical pole endeavor.[39–43,47,48] The development of System 2, or the intuitive pole of the continuum, most likely occurs while engaged in the crisis and will be discussed in the next section.

Surgical residents have near-immediate access to a massive, often overwhelming amounts of information. To assist in forming foundational knowledge, the teaching surgeon must be knowledgeable about various learning activities used to educate the modern surgical resident.

Self-Directed Learning Activities

Textbooks and other reading materials
Textbooks, either printed on paper or in an electronic format, have long been the mainstay of medical education. They are often considered a source of indisputable and sacred knowledge.[50] According to 2015 study[51] of 15 US general surgery residencies, surgical textbooks were the most commonly used resource to prepare for clinical duties and were used consistently throughout the academic year. It should be noted that it is difficult to completely divorce learning for clinical duties from examination

preparation. Although much of the literature on surgical resident reading habits are focused on examination preparation,[52–54] it is logical to assume that there is some degree of bleed over of knowledge gained to improve patient care. It is also interesting to note that Generation Z learners seems to be more interested in learning to gain knowledge and skills to be used in the future, rather than to achieve a particular score on an examination.[55]

Although textbooks have historically been a foundational source of information, their future role may be diminishing. It is likely that medical students carry their study habits into residency. A recent study[52] found that nearly 60% of medical students never use textbooks, instead favoring the use of review books and Internet sources. Correspondingly, Egle and colleagues[56] found surgical residents are abandoning textbooks in favor of Web-based resources. Similar changes in the use of textbooks by the next generation have also been cited in the nonsurgical literature.[57,58]

Textbooks have other issues which may limit use in the future. They are expensive, having increased in price between 1982 and 2015, by 697%, compared with only 244% for all consumer items over the same period.[59] The rapidity of medical advances may also be rendering textbooks unreliable for providing up to date information.[50,60] Recently, the European Society for Vascular Surgery has introduced a novel concept that integrates standard textbook chapters that are frequently updated with new information with videos, lectures, podcasts, and training courses.[60]

Journal clubs are also considered a form of individual study, which then morphs into a larger group activity. Frequently, a review of these articles is focused on evolving areas of clinical care, new research, and the discussion of how to critically evaluate scientific literature. Although these reviews may augment the resident's understanding, they typically are not used to improve understanding of foundational topics.

E-learning and videos

Today residents have immediate access to a wide variety of electronic educational resources. Many of these resources, including clinical practice guidelines produced by specialty associations, such as the Eastern Association for the Surgery of Trauma,[61] the American Association for the Surgery of Trauma,[62] and the Society for Critical Care Medicine,[63] are available at no cost. Others such as flashcards and examination preparation programs[64–66] may be expensive.

The Web-based video platform YouTube[67] has become a primary educational source for learning procedures.[68,69] Although watching performance of a procedure may be more engaging than reviewing a static atlas of pictures, more entertaining, brief (averaging 8 minutes) and free, the quality of these videos is uneven and not regulated.[70] Facebook and other platforms are also used for case discussions and peer-to-peer teaching among learners.[68,71] Some Web-based sources have evolved into a comprehensive set of surgical educational offerings including podcasts, videos, and examination preparation, all of which are well vetted and high quality.[72]

Large Group Learning Activities

Conferences and lectures

Didactic conferences focusing on core curriculum and Grand Rounds are another cornerstone of surgical resident education. These are frequently linked to required readings. Although there are a multitude of investigations into the role of didactics in improving examination scores,[73] excluding morbidity and mortality conference which will be discussed in another section of this article; there is essentially no literature on the direct relationship of resident conferences with decision-making and clinic outcomes.

Although the benefit of resident conferences is assumed, there are several concerns regarding the utility of conferences to improve resident performance during a resuscitation. Surgeon performance during a crisis is grounded and organized according to logical, scientific, and outcomes-based algorithms; however, it is impossible to teach the intuition or pattern recognition most frequently used in the management of a crisis. Even if intuition or snap judgments could be taught in this format, they are of mixed accuracy in a clinical setting,[74,75] so of limited preparatory value.

Another problem area is that lectures and conferences are typically large group learning sessions, with a wide target audience. Resident appropriate learning is frequently diluted by the content being aimed too low or too high for most participants; this leads to an overall poor expansion of knowledge.[76] The organization of conferences is frequently based on faculty availability rather than an organized, logical sequence or according to a formal teaching plan.

Finally, pure, comprehensive lectures are not an effective means of teaching adult learners. To effectively educate adults, the teacher must actively engage the audience by focusing on past experiences of the learners, be of practical and relevant significance, problem-centered and task-oriented. Gantwerker and Lee[77] have published an excellent and pragmatic review of adult learning principles within a surgical context.

Crew Resource Management

Before being able to teach what to do, the surgeon must be able to effectively lead the management of a resuscitation.[78,79] In the 1970s, the aviation industry first noted that in high-stress situations, errors were not the result of lack of knowledge or skills but rather failures of communication, leadership, and teamwork.[80] As a result of these findings, Cockpit and Crew Resource Management training were developed.[80] In 1992, Howard and colleagues[81] applied this approach to the management of medical crises. Since then, this training has been renamed to Crew or Crisis Resource Management (CRM) and has been taught to nurses,[82] medical students,[83] residents,[84,85] and physicians in a wide variety of specialties in multiple countries.[84–87] Although CRM can be taught to individual cohorts, its real strength is in teaching this strategy to interprofessional and interdisciplinary teams.[88–90] CRM has been tailored to trauma resuscitations[87,88] and found to improve communication, team behavior,[88] and clinical outcomes.[91]

Simulation

A full description of how surgical simulation augments clinical education is beyond the scope of this article. Interested readers are referred to *Fundamentals of Surgical Simulation: Principles and Practices*[92] or other textbooks devoted to clinical simulation for more in-depth information.

Simulation has been used to teach basic surgical skills for more than 2500 years[93] and continues to be an excellent method to teach trauma skills without any risk to patients.[94,95]

More recently, simulation has been used to integrate skills training with CRM. Burden's 2020 publication[96] provides an excellent review of combining these two educational methods. One particular advantage of this approach is the integration of different teams, each using their own skills and expertise to solve complex problems. This technique has been used with anesthesiologists and neurosurgeons confronting an unexpected cerebrovascular bleed,[97] otolaryngology and anesthesiology residents handling a cavernous carotid artery injury,[98] multidisciplinary teams during obstetric emergencies,[99] urologic operative emergencies,[100] and trauma team organization.[101] Many surgical resuscitations occur outside the emergency department or the operating room. Johanning and colleagues[102] have developed the postoperative rescue course, which combines skills training and CRM in more typical postoperative settings.

The importance of stress in learning has been outlined earlier in this article. Although simulation does not involve any risk to patients, the levels of stress encountered by learners during simulation are similar to those encountered in emergency departments,[103] critical care units,[104] and operating rooms.[105]

National certification courses

Several national organizations have developed standardized educational programs that have married algorithmic decision-making, technical skills, and simulation with testing. These courses provide both a common language and an effective approach that have been applied around the world.[106–108]

- Advanced Cardiac Life Support:[109]

  The Advanced Cardiac Life Support course provides training for managing cardiopulmonary arrest and other cardiovascular emergencies. Physicians learn to use basic life support skills inclusive of effective chest compressions and use of an automated external defibrillator. Skills are also enhanced in management of airways, acute coronary syndrome, and stroke. Through simulations, physicians develop effective communication skills to lead or participate in a resuscitation team.

- Advanced Trauma Life Support:[110]

  The Advanced Trauma Life Support course consists of a standardized approach to assessment and management of a trauma patient. Physicians learn and practice primary and secondary patient assessment. The course also focuses on identifying management priorities in emergent and acute life-threatening conditions. Practical skills developed through the course enable physicians to assess and treat patients who present with multiple injuries.

- Pediatric Advanced Life Support:[111]

  The Pediatric Advanced Life Support course prepares physicians to recognize and respond to cardiopulmonary arrest, shock, and respiratory emergencies in infants and children. The course teaches how to identify pediatric patients who require immediate intervention and reviews early treatment and management protocols. Physicians enhance their individual and team-based skills through simulated patient cases.

- Advanced Burn Life Support (ABLS):[112]

  The Advanced Burn Life Support course trains physicians in the emergency management of burn patients particularly within the critical 24-hour period following injury. Physicians learn to evaluate and define injury severity along with airway management and fluid resuscitation. Through lectures, case studies, and simulations, physicians learn to identify patients that require transfer to a burn center as well as other disaster management protocols.

- Advanced Trauma Operative Management:[113]

  The Advanced Trauma Operative Management course focuses on instructing surgeons on proper operative techniques for management of chest and abdominal penetrating injuries. The course is designed for surgical residents, trauma fellows, and other surgeons who do not commonly treat penetrating injuries. Surgeons learn to develop a plan to manage and repair traumatic injuries. Through the performance of presented operative procedures, surgeons increase their skills and confidence to treat these injuries.

- Advanced Surgical Skills for Exposure in Trauma:[114]
    - The Advanced Surgical Skills for Exposure in Trauma course prepares surgeons with the knowledge and technical skills to perform surgical exposure of anatomic structures that may be injured in trauma. The course is also designed for surgical residents, trauma fellows, and surgeons interested in anatomic exposures. Before the course, surgeons review anatomic exposures in the five areas of the neck, chest, abdomen and pelvis, and upper and lower extremities. During the cadaver-based portion of the course, surgeons practice and demonstrate exposures in each of the five anatomic areas. With a low participant to instructor ratio, each participant receives effective training and evaluation in anatomic exposures required in management of traumatic injuries.
- Fundamentals of Critical Care Support:[115]
    - The Fundamentals of Critical Care Support course is designed to train physicians, especially non-intensivists, in the initial management of critically ill patients within the first 24 hours or until the appropriate critical care specialist can be consulted. The course teaches physicians the essentials of assessment of the critically ill patient, diagnostic test selection, response to acute changes in the unstable patient, and management of life-threatening conditions. Physicians benefit from lectures on a range of critical care topics, along with case-based skills stations and pre- and post-tests to evaluate comprehension and practical skills.

Small-Group Learning Activities

War games

Many trauma and general surgery services have a daily "Morning Report" which is a combination of patient handoff and didactic and/or Socratic education.[116–118] Although some have questioned the educational validity of this traditional format due to the heterogenous goals, methods used, and difficulty measuring outcomes,[119] others have found this ability to "War Game" potential clinical scenarios a highly valuable educational tool.[120–122] The war game approach can also be used to educate residents on how to handle anticipated complications or loop closure for issues identified by the performance improvement committee. In addition to the educational benefits,[121,122] morning report has also been found to decrease trauma patient's length of hospital stay[123] and hospital costs.[124]

Other educational activities

Several other educational activities have been used to prepare residents for the complexities of trauma resuscitation. Active engagement of the learner is a core principle of adult learning but may be difficult to achieve. Leveraging the competitiveness of surgeons by using games has been demonstrated to be an effective strategy.[125–127] The use of trivial pursuit games has been used improve performance in both the prehospital setting,[128] emergency department,[129] and neonatal intensive care unit.[130] Other effective educational gaming strategies include surgical jeopardy[131] as well as a wide variety of serious video games, which teach clinical decision-making, technical skills, and non-technical skills.[132]

EDUCATING RESIDENTS DURING THE RESUSCITATION

During resuscitation, the attending surgeon faces two conflicting obligations. The first obligation is care of the patient, and the second is care for future patients through education of the resident or fellow. Which obligation deserves primary focus depends on the stability of the patient, the abilities of the learner, and the tolerances of the attending. Duty hour limits and other regulatory changes have decreased the clinical exposure of residents to complex trauma and emergency general surgery patients.[10,12,133] It could, therefore, be argued that current residents require greater focus on education during resuscitation than previous generations.

Pragmatic Methods to Teach While Actively Resuscitating a Critically Ill Patient

Taking time to teach and provide autonomy in the current clinical environment, with its focus on efficiency, revenue productivity, and low tolerance of complications, is difficult in all patient care settings. This difficulty is further amplified in the trauma bay, operating room, and surgical intensive care unit, where the most critically ill patients reside.

Chinai and colleagues[134] have reviewed seven different teaching models used in the emergency setting, whereas Irby and Wilkerson[135] provide a similar review of techniques used when time is limited in internal medicine settings. Although the methods described in both papers would apply to surgical learners, none are well-suited for teaching during resuscitations.

There are some general strategies that surgeons can use to improve the quality of the education they provide during any surgical crisis.

Speak your thoughts

During resuscitation, the surgeon does not have time to provide a comprehensive review of the factors influencing critical decisions. However, simply verbalizing what you are thinking is a very effective and efficient way to educate. This strategy also has the advantage of informing others involved with the resuscitation of what the leadership is thinking, so they can better anticipate the needs of the patient. This strategy may be used in other settings but is particularly effective when a crisis occurs without warning or with a rapidly dying patient.[136]

Rapid needs assessment

Determining what the resident needs to learn is the first step in any educational experience. Developing this need assessment is a combined effort between the attending and the resident. In the moments before the arrival of the patient or when heading into the operating room, simply asking the resident what they want to gain from this single experience, is an easy and rapid way to identify the learning needs of the resident. Depending on the situation, this need may be performance of a specific procedure or as broad as directing the resuscitation. The attending may also identify a specific educational gap and focus the resident in that direction.

Beyond filling in gaps in a resident's education, incorporating a needs assessment as a first step has two other advantages. First, this approach allows the learner to deliberately practice in an area in which they feel weak. This not only improves resident confidence, but deliberate practice is also required to develop expertise.[137–140] Another advantage is that if the resident and attending agree in advance what the resident will do, then the attending has granted permission to the resident to manage aspects of the resuscitation or operation. This has the potential to improve relationships between residents and attendings as well as increase efficiency. When combined with the strategy of verbalizing your thoughts, the resident gets a great learning experience, whereas the patient gets safe and rapid care.

Targeted teaching

Although the resident has perceptions of their learning needs, it is also important to remember that residents are poor judges of their own abilities.[141,142] Therefore, the attending surgeon may have a better insight into what areas the resident needs to concentrate. One well-studied method for targeted teaching is the "One-Minute Preceptor" model.[143,144] This model involves five steps: (1) get a commitment about what the learner thinks is going on, (2) quickly probe the reasons for this belief, (3) teach a general principle, (4) provide positive feedback, and (5) correct errors by making suggestions. Research on this method has yielded positive results by learners as well as teachers and has been demonstrated to improve performance.[143,144]

Role modeling as an educational tool

Attending surgeons who role model the nontechnical skills of effective communication, emotional intelligence, and leadership, significantly improve their effectiveness in teaching.[145–148] Data suggest that learning these nontechnical skills early in residency will pay dividends later in their career.[149] As discussed in the previous section on CRM, developing these skills is associated with improved patient outcomes.

In addition to positive teaching behaviors, attending surgeons should also role model their critical thinking and decision-making skills. There is a significant disparity between what a resident considers is important during an operation and what the attending considers important. A study by Pugh and colleagues[150] found that in the operating room, attending surgeons are focused on the natural history of disease, patient outcomes, and procedure choice while residents prioritize type of suture and instrument usage. Divorcing the technical aspects of operations from the patient outcome may be a consequence of decreased resident exposure to operations and the need to capitalize on technical learning while in the operating room.

EDUCATING RESIDENTS AFTER THE RESUSCITATION
Feedback

Feedback has been traditionally described as information that allows learners to compare their actual performance with that of a standard to which they aspire *and* that enables them to take action to remedy the gap between the two.[151,152] Feedback is typically immediate and formative, rather than summative, and tends to be provided by an expert.[153] When approached as a "coach," who shares mutual goals with the learner, the educational impact is significant.[154] Feedback is fundamentally different from debriefing, which requires the learner to self-reflect and is a more bidirectional discussion than feedback.[154]

Debriefing

The process of self and interprofessional group reflection of performance, facilitated by post-resuscitation debriefing, is a fundamental component to experiential learning.[155,156] Active reflection aids in the refinement of mental models and correction of flawed thinking for application for future resuscitations.[157,158] Debriefing has also been shown to improve procedural learning.[139,140] Knowledge gained during debriefings has been shown to improve competency in both similar and unrelated situations.[159]

Repeated exposure to traumatically injured patients is known to take a mental toll on physicians.[160] When residents are involved, they are also subject to mental stress, which will negatively impact future learning.[161–163] Attending trauma surgeons are also not immune to the psychological impact of repeated exposure to severely injured patients.[164–166] Debriefing has been found to improve compassion fatigue and promote resiliency after resuscitation.[167]

Although the benefits of debriefing are well-established, debriefing after critical cases occurs only a fraction of the time.[168] Barriers to using debriefing after trauma include: competing end of resuscitation duties, lack of time, lack of an appropriate environment, and lack of interest.[169] One strategy to overcome these barriers is to use team members, rather than attending surgeons, to lead the debriefing.[170] This approach is not only effective but it has also been associated with an impression of increased psychological safety and improved learning environment.[171]

Debriefing models

- The "Hot" Debrief

A hot debrief occurs within minutes of the resuscitation and involves participants directly involved with the resuscitation.[172–174] In a study comparing hot debriefing with video review, it was found to be 87% accurate.[175] Although hot debriefing is effective, it is important that the attending surgeons and resuscitation team are emotionally ready to enter a productive bidirectional discussion.

- "Cold" Debriefing

Cold debriefing occurs days to weeks after the resuscitation and may involve participants who were not involved in the resuscitation. It allows for greater time for reflection but may also be subject to recall bias.[172] Examples of cold debriefing would include morning report, morbidity and mortality conference, and performance improvement review. Inclusion of participants who were not directly involved in the resuscitation and who were not influenced by the "fog of war" may add new perspectives and alternative approaches to be considered in the future.

- After Action Review

The US Army has used the After Action Review (AAR) method for over 4 decades.[176] This method has also been used outside of the military.[157] When applied to the health care setting, the key steps in an AAR are (1) define the rules, (2) explain the learning objectives, (3) present benchmarks used for performance, (4) review what was supposed to happen, (5) identify what actually happened, (6) discuss why it happened, and (7) formalize the learning by summarizing what went well, what could have been better, and what will be done differently next time.[157]

- The ABCDE Method

The ABCDE method was specifically developed for the emergency department setting and to focus on the resuscitation goals rather than fault finding.[177] This method consists of A - Avoid Shaming/Personal Opinions, B - Build a Rapport, C - Choose a Communication Approach, D - Develop a Debriefing Content, and E - Ensure the Ergonomics of Debriefing. This approach is described in detail by Rajendran and colleagues[177] and is based on avoiding shaming, building rapport, communication, debriefing the details of what happened and the ergonomics of the debriefing (which includes the location of the debrief, participants, and audiovisual equipment).

- Video Review

Video review of trauma resuscitations has a long history of being an effective educational tool. Concerns about medicolegal ramifications and patient privacy lead to decreased usage of this tool. However, the use of video review is undergoing a resurgence.[178–180]

Summary

The education of trainees for preparation during a surgical crisis is pivotal. With an aging population, the complex nature of the disease process will only be further exacerbated requiring more resources than ever before. Teaching during a surgical resuscitation can be difficult due to the infrequency of these events. Furthermore, when these events do occur, the trainee can experience cognitive overload and an overwhelming amount of stress, thereby impairing the learning process. In addition, the emergent nature of these scenarios can make it difficult for the surgical educator to adequately teach. Repeated exposure through simulation, role play, and "war games" are great adjuncts to teaching and preparation before crisis. Surgical educators can further enhance the knowledge of their trainees during these scenarios by using tactics such as talking out loud, targeted teaching, and debriefing. With this, surgical trainees will be equipped to handle the ever-evolving complexity of surgical care.

DISCLOSURE

No author has any disclosures related to this article.

REFERENCES

1. Arriaga AF, Gawande AA, Raemer DB, et al. Pilot testing of a model for insurer-driven, large-scale multicenter simulation training for operating room teams. Ann Surg 2014;259(3):403–10.
2. Ziewacz JE, Arriaga AF, Bader AM, et al. Crisis checklists for the operating room: development and pilot testing. J Am Coll Surg 2011;213(2):212–7.
3. Thiele RH, Theodore DJ, Gan TJ. Outcome of Organ Dysfunction in the Perioperative Period. Anesth Analg 2021;133(2):393–405.
4. Shah AA, Haider AH, Zogg CK, et al. National estimates of predictors of outcomes for emergency general surgery. J Trauma Acute Care Surg 2015;78:482–90.
5. United States Census Bureau. "The graying of America: more older adults than kids by 2035". https://www.census.gov/library/stories/2018/03/graying- america.html Accessed August 17, 2023.
6. Halaweish I, Alam HB. Changing demographics of the American population. Surg Clin North Am 2015;95:1–10.
7. Deiner S, Westlake B, Dutton RP. Patterns of surgical care and complications in elderly adults. J Am Geriatr Soc 2014;62:829–35.
8. American College of Surgeons, National Trauma Data Base, 2016 Annual Report. https://www.facs.org/media/ez1hpdcu.ntdb-annual-report-2016.pdf Accessed August 17,2023.
9. Dawson S. Procedural simulation: a primer. J Vasc Intervent Radiol 2006;17(2 Pt 1):205–13.
10. Napolitano LM, Biester TW, Jurkovich GJ, et al, Members of the Trauma, Burns and Critical Care Board of the American Board of Surgery. Members of the Trauma, Burns and Critical Care Board of the American Board of Surgery. General surgery resident rotations in surgical critical care, trauma, and burns: what is optimal for residency training? Am J Surg 2016;212(4):629–37.
11. Jordan RM, Ullrich LA, Decapua-Guarino A, et al. Trends in Surgical Critical Care Training Among General Surgery Residents: Pursuing an Ideal Curriculum. Am Surg 2020;86(9):1119–23.
12. Drake FT, Van Eaton EG, Huntington CR, et al. ACGME case logs: Surgery resident experience in operative trauma for two decades. J Trauma Acute Care Surg 2012;73(6):1500–6.

13. Nordin AB, Wach MM, Jalal K, et al. General surgery resident operative experiences in solid organ injury: an examination of case logs. Am Surg 2023;89(4): 858–64.

14. Awan M, Zagales I, McKenney M, et al. ACGME 2011 duty hours restrictions and their effects on surgical residency training and patients outcomes: a systematic review. J Surg Educ 2021;78(6):e35–46.

15. Schenarts PJ, Schenkel RE, Sullivan ME. The biology and psychology of surgical learning. Surg Clin North Am 2021;101(4):541–54.

16. Miller G. How are memories stored and retrieved? Science 2005;309(5731):92.

17. Martin SJ, Grimwood PD, Morris RG. Synaptic plasticity and memory: an evaluation of the hypothesis. Annu Rev Neurosci 2000;23:649–711.

18. Martin SJ, Morris RG. New life in an old idea: the synaptic plasticity and memory hypothesis revisited. Hippocampus 2002;12(5):609–36.

19. Kandel ER, Dudai Y, Mayford MR. The molecular and systems biology of memory. Cell 2014;157(1):163–86.

20. Kandel ER. The molecular biology of memory storage: a dialog between genes and synapses. Biosci Rep 2001;21(5):565–611.

21. Ito M, Sakurai M, Tongroach P. Climbing fibre induced depression of both mossy fibre responsiveness and glutamate sensitivity of cerebellar Purkinje cells. J Physiol 1982;324:113–34.

22. Okano H, Hirano T, Balaban E. Learning and memory. Proc Natl Acad Sci U S A 2000;97(23):12403–4.

23. Collins JW. The neuroscience of learning. J Neurosci Nurs 2007;39(5):305–10.

24. Purves D, Augustine GJ, Fitzpatric D, et al. Neuroscience. 6th edition. New York: Oxford University Press; 2018.

25. Mayer RE. Applying the science of learning to medical education. Med Educ 2010;44(6):543–9.

26. Gagne ED, Yekovich CW, Yekovich FR. The cognitive psychology of school learning. 2nd edition. New York, NY: Harper Collins College Publishers; 1993.

27. van Merriënboer JJ, Sweller J. Cognitive load theory in health professional education: design principles and strategies. Med Educ 2010;44(1):85–93.

28. Young JQ, Van Merrienboer J, Durning S, et al. Cognitive Load Theory: implications for medical education: AMEE Guide No. 86. Med Teach 2014;36(5): 371–84.

29. Szulewski A, Howes D, van Merriënboer JJG, et al. From Theory to Practice: The Application of Cognitive Load Theory to the Practice of Medicine. Acad Med 2021;96(1):24–30.

30. Cohen RA. In: DeLuca J, Caplan B, editors. Yerkes-dodson law. Encyclopedia of clinical neuropsychology kreutzer JS. New York, NY: Springer; 2011.

31. Salehi B, Cordero MI, Sandi C. Learning under stress: the inverted-U-shape function revisited. Learn Mem 2010;17(10):522–30.

32. Sandi C. The role and mechanisms of action of glucocorticoid involvement in memory storage. Neural Plast 1998;6(3):41–52.

33. Togashi H, Sakisaka T, Takai Y. Cell adhesion molecules in the central nervous system. Cell Adh Migr 2009;3(1):29–35.

34. Bisaz R, Conboy L, Sandi C. Learning under stress: a role for the neural cell adhesion molecule NCAM. Neurobiol Learn Mem 2009;91(4):333–42.

35. LeBlanc VR. The effects of acute stress on performance: implications for health professions education. Acad Med 2009;84(10 Suppl):S25–33.

36. Harvey A, Nathens AB, Bandiera G, et al. Threat and challenge: cognitive appraisal and stress responses in simulated trauma resuscitations. Med Educ 2010;44(6):587–94.

37. LeBlanc V, Woodrow SI, Sidhu R, et al. Examination stress leads to improvements on fundamental technical skills for surgery. Am J Surg 2008;196(1):114–9.

38. Hunziker S, Semmer NK, Tschan F, et al. Dynamics and association of different acute stress markers with performance during a simulated resuscitation. Resuscitation 2012;83(5):572–8.

39. Kahneman D. Thinking, fast and slow. London UK: Penguin Books, Ltd; 2011.

40. Evans JS. Dual-processing accounts of reasoning, judgment, and social cognition. Annu Rev Psychol 2008;59:255–78.

41. Sloman SA. The empirical case for two systems of reasoning. Psychol Bull 1996;119(1):3–22.

42. Stanovich KE, West RF. Individual differences in reasoning: implications for the rationality debate? Behav Brain Sci 2000;23(5):645–65.

43. Ark TK, Brooks LR, Eva KW. The benefits of flexibility: the pedagogical value of instructions to adopt multifaceted diagnostic reasoning strategies. Med Educ 2007;41(3):281–7.

44. Croskerry P. Critical thinking and decision making: avoiding the perils of thin-slicing. Ann Emerg Med 2006;48(6):720–2.

45. Eva KW, Hatala RM, Leblanc VR, et al. Teaching from the clinical reasoning literature: combined reasoning strategies help novice diagnosticians overcome misleading information. Med Educ 2007;41(12):1152–8.

46. Norman G. Dual processing and diagnostic errors. Adv Health Sci Educ Theory Pract 2009;14(Suppl 1):37–49.

47. Custers EJ. Medical education and cognitive continuum theory: an alternative perspective on medical problem solving and clinical reasoning. Acad Med 2013;88(8):1074–80.

48. Osman M. An evaluation of dual-process theories of reasoning. Psychon Bull Rev 2004;11(6):988–1010.

49. van Merrienboer JG. Teaching based on thinking fast and slow. Acad Med 2014;89(1):8.

50. Tez M, Yildiz B. How Reliable Are Medical Textbooks? J Grad Med Educ 2017;9(4):550.

51. Kim JJ, Kim DY, Kaji AH, et al. Reading Habits of General Surgery Residents and Association With American Board of Surgery In- Training Examination Performance. JAMA Surg 2015;150(9):882–9.

52. Taylor JA, Shaw CM, Tan SA, et al. Are the kids alright? Review books and the internet as the most common study resources for the general surgery clerkship. Am J Surg 2018;215(1):191–5.

53. Ferguson CM, Warshaw AL. Failure of a Web-based educational tool to improve residents' scores on the American Board of Surgery In-Training Examination. Arch Surg 2006;141(4):414–6.

54. Glass NE, Kulaylat AN, Zheng F, et al. A national survey of educational resources utilized by the Resident and Associate Society of the American College of Surgeons membership. Am J Surg 2015;209(1):59–64.

55. Schenarts PJ. Now Arriving: Surgical Trainees From Generation Z. J Surg Educ 2020;77(2):246–53.

56. Egle JP, Smeenge DM, Kassem KM, et al. The Internet School of Medicine: use of electronic resources by medical trainees and the reliability of those resources. J Surg Educ 2015;72(2):316–20.

57. Twenge JM. Generational changes and their impact in the classroom: teaching Generation Me. Med Educ 2009;43(5):398–405.

58. Shappell E, Ahn J. A Needs Assessment for a Longitudinal Emergency Medicine. Intern Curriculum. West J Emerg Med. 2017;18(1):31–4.

59. George S, Aylward J, Wood J. The textbook: An endangered species. Med Teach 2018;40(2):214.

60. Björck M, Debus SE, Earnshaw JJ. The Vascular Textbook is Dead: Long Live Virtual Vascular. Eur J Vasc Endovasc Surg 2020;60(4):499.

61. Eastern Association for the Surgery of Trauma, Practice Management Guidelines. https://www.east.org/education-resources/practice-management- guidelines Accessed August 17, 2023.

62. American Association for the Surgery of Trauma, Practice Management Guidelines. https://www.aast.org/resourses/guidelines. Accessed August 17, 2023.

63. Society for Critical Care Medicine, Guidelines, https://www.sccm.org/Clinical-Resources/Guidelines/Guidelines Accessed August 17, 2023.

64. Quizlet. General Surgery Board Review Series, Flashcards. https://quizlet.com/ 25289066/general-surgery-board-review-series-flash-cards. Accessed August 17, 2023.

65. Brainscape, Study Surgery. https://www.brainscape.com/subjects/surgery. Accessed August 17, 2023.

66. The Pass Machine, General Surgery Board Review Course. https://www.thepass machine.com/general-surgery-board-review- courses/?creative=&keyword=''' general%20surgery%20board&matchtype=p&netw ork=o&device=c&msclki-d=837e510e6b9e174d2b0535dcffe23828&utm_source=b ing&utm_medium=cp c&utm_campaign=General%20Surgery09-20- 22&utm_term=general%20sur-gery%20board&utm_content=General%20Surgery %20Board%20Review%20 Course. Accessed August 17, 2023.

67. YouTube. https://www.youtube.com Accessed August 17, 2023.

68. Sterling M, Leung P, Wright D, et al. The Use of Social Media in Graduate Medical Education: A Systematic Review. Acad Med 2017;92(7):1043–56.

69. Rapp AK, Healy MG, Charlton ME, et al. YouTube is the Most Frequently Used Educational Video Source for Surgical Preparation. J Surg Educ 2016;73(6):1072–6.

70. Gupta T, Haidery TH, Sharma R, et al. How Reliable Are YouTube Videos for General Surgery Residents Learning? Cureus 2023;15(2):e34718.

71. Ponsky TA, Rothenberg SS. Modern, multi-media, advances in surgical information. Semin Pediatr Surg 2015;24(3):124–9.

72. Behind The Knife: The Premier Surgery Podcast | Surgical Education. https://behindtheknife.org Accessed August 17, 2023.

73. Kim RH, Tan TW. Interventions that affect resident performance on the American Board of Surgery In-Training Examination: a systematic review. J Surg Educ 2015;72(3):418–29.

74. Norman GR, Eva KW. Diagnostic error and clinical reasoning. Med Educ 2010;44(1):94–100.

75. Croskerry P. From mindless to mindful practice–cognitive bias and clinical decision making. N Engl J Med 2013;368(26):2445–8.

76. Farrohki ET, Jensen AR, Brock DM, et al. Expanding resident conferences while tailoring them to level of training: a longitudinal study. J Surg Educ 2008;65(2): 84–90.

77. Gantwerker EA, Lee GS. Principles of Adult Learning: Tips for the Pediatric Otolaryngologist. Otolaryngol Clin North Am 2022;55(6):1311–20.

78. O'Dea A, O'Connor P, Keogh I. A meta-analysis of the effectiveness of crew resource management training in acute care domains. Postgrad Med J 2014; 90(1070):699–708.

79. Hoff WS, Reilly PM, Rotondo MF, et al. The importance of the command-physician in trauma resuscitation. J Trauma 1997;43(5):772–7.

80. Helmreich RL. Managing human error in aviation. Sci Am 1997;276(5):62–7.

81. Howard SK, Gaba DM, Fish KJ, et al. Anesthesia crisis resource management training: teaching anesthesiologists to handle critical incidents. Aviat Space Environ Med 1992;63(9):763–70.

82. Sculli GL, Fore AM, Neily J, et al. The case for training Veterans Administration frontline nurses in crew resource management. J Nurs Adm 2011;41(12):524–30.

83. Hänsel M, Winkelmann AM, Hardt F, et al. Impact of simulator training and crew resource management training on final-year medical students' performance in sepsis resuscitation: a randomized trial. Minerva Anestesiol 2012;78(8):901–9.

84. Mannella P, Palla G, Cuttano A, et al. Effect of high-fidelity shoulder dystocia simulation on emergency obstetric skills and crew resource management skills among residents. Int J Gynaecol Obstet 2016;135(3):338–42.

85. Parsons JR, Crichlow A, Ponnuru S, et al. Filling the Gap: Simulation-based Crisis Resource Management Training for Emergency Medicine Residents. West J Emerg Med 2018;19(1):205–10.

86. Truta TS, Boeriu CM, Lazarovici M, et al. Improving Clinical Performance of an Interprofessional Emergency Medical Team Through a One-day Crisis Resource Management Training. J Crit Care Med (Targu Mures). 2018;4(4):126–36.

87. Ashcroft J, Wilkinson A, Khan M. A Systematic Review of Trauma Crew Resource Management Training: What Can the United States and the United Kingdom Learn From Each Other? J Surg Educ 2021;78(1):245–64.

88. Hughes KM, Benenson RS, Krichten AE, et al. A crew resource management program tailored to trauma resuscitation improves team behavior and communication. J Am Coll Surg 2014;219(3):545–51.

89. Jankouskas TS, Haidet KK, Hupcey JE, et al. Targeted crisis resource management training improves performance among randomized nursing and medical students. Simul Healthc 2011;6(6):316–26.

90. Fung L, Boet S, Bould MD, et al. Impact of crisis resource management simulation-based training for interprofessional and interdisciplinary teams: A systematic review. J Interprof Care 2015;29(5):433–44.

91. Boet S, Bould MD, Fung L, et al. Transfer of learning and patient outcome in simulated crisis resource management: a systematic review. Can J Anaesth 2014;61(6):571–82.

92. Gallenger AG, O'Sullivan GC, editors. Fundamentals of surgical simulation. London, UK: Springer; 2012.

93. Owen H. Early use of simulation in medical education. Simul Healthc 2012;7(2): 102–16.

94. Quick JA. Simulation Training in Trauma. Mo Med 2018;115(5):447–50.

95. Larraga-García B, Quintana-Díaz M, Gutiérrez Á. Simulation-Based Education in Trauma Management: A Scoping Review. Int J Environ Res Public Health 2022; 19(20):13546.

96. Burden AR. High-Fidelity Simulation Education and Crisis Resource Management. Anesthesiol Clin 2020;38(4):745–59.

97. Ciporen J, Gillham H, Noles M, et al. Crisis Management Simulation: Establishing a Dual Neurosurgery and Anesthesia Training Experience. J Neurosurg Anesthesiol 2018;30(1):65–70.

98. Calcagno HE, Lucke-Wold B, Noles M, et al. Integrated Otolaryngology and Anesthesia Simulation Model for Crisis Management of Cavernous Carotid Artery Injury. Arch Neurol Neuro Disord 2018;1(1):30–41.

99. Robertson B, Schumacher L, Gosman G, et al. Simulation-based crisis team training for multidisciplinary obstetric providers. Simul Healthc 2009 Summer; 4(2):77–83.

100. Goldenberg MG, Fok KH, Ordon M, et al. Simulation-Based Laparoscopic Surgery Crisis Resource Management Training-Predicting Technical and Nontechnical Skills. J Surg Educ 2018;75(4):1113–9.

101. Marr M, Hemmert K, Nguyen AH, et al. Team play in surgical education: a simulation-based study. J Surg Educ 2012;69(1):63–9.

102. VISN 23 conducts Post-Operative Rescue Course – VHA SimLEARN. https://www.simlearn.va.gov. Accessed August 17, 2023.

103. Daglius Dias R, Scalabrini Neto A. Stress levels during emergency care: A comparison between reality and simulated scenarios. J Crit Care 2016;33:8–13.

104. Bauer C, Rimmelé T, Duclos A, et al. Anxiety and stress among anaesthesiology and critical care residents during high-fidelity simulation sessions. Anaesth Crit Care Pain Med 2016;35(6):407–16.

105. Stecz P, Makara-Studzińska M, Białka S, et al. Stress responses in high-fidelity simulation among anesthesiology students. Sci Rep 2021;11(1):17073.

106. Mohammad A, Branicki F, Abu-Zidan FM. Educational and clinical impact of Advanced Trauma Life Support (ATLS) courses: a systematic review. World J Surg 2014;38(2):322–9.

107. Scharplatz D, Sutter PM. Fünf Jahre ATLS-Kurse in der Schweiz [5 years ATLS (Advanced Trauma Life Support) courses in Switzerland]. Swiss Surg 2003;9(6): 263–7.

108. Luedi MM, Wölfl CC, Wieferich K, et al. Teaching Advanced Trauma Life Support (ATLS): A nationwide retrospective analysis of 8202 lessons taught in Germany. J Surg Educ 2017;74(1):161–6.

109. Advanced cardiovascular life support: provider manual. Dallas, TX: American Heart Association; 2020.

110. Advanced trauma life support: student course manual. 10th edition. Chicago, IL: American College of Surgeons; 2018.

111. Pediatric advanced life support: provider manual. Dallas, TX: American Heart Association.; 2020.

112. Advanced burn life support course: provider manual. Chicago, IL: American Burn Association; 2018.

113. Advanced trauma operative management. 2nd edition. Chicago, IL: American College of Surgeons; 2010.

114. Advanced surgical skills for exposure in trauma: exposure techniques when time matters. Chicago, IL: American College of Surgeons; 2010.

115. Fundamentals of critical care support. 6th edition. IL: Society of Critical Care Medicine, Mount Prospect; 2016.

116. Pringle PL, Collins C, Santry HP. Utilization of morning report by acute care surgery teams: results from a qualitative study. Am J Surg 2013;206(5):647–54.

117. Stephen AH, Connolly MD, Harrington DT, et al. Trauma morning report is the ideal environment to teach and evaluate resident communication and sign-outs in the 80 hour work week. Injury 2017;48(9):2003–9.

118. Stiles BM, Reece TB, Hedrick TL, et al. General surgery morning report: a competency-based conference that enhances patient care and resident education. Curr Surg 2006;63(6):385–90.

119. McNeill M, Ali SK, Banks DE, et al. Morning report: can an established medical education tradition be validated? J Grad Med Educ 2013;5(3):374–84.

120. Schenarts PJ, Fuglestad MA. In: Williams AD, Green JY, Mann BD, editors. Medical student and resident survival at morning report. Surgery morning report: beyond the pearls. St Louis, MO: Elsevier; 2019.

121. Hedrick TL, Young JS. The use of "war games" to enhance high-risk clinical decision-making in students and residents. Am J Surg 2008;195(6):843–9.

122. Young JS, Dubose JE, Hedrick TL, et al. The use of "war games" to evaluate performance of students and residents in basic clinical scenarios: a disturbing analysis. J Trauma 2007;63(3):556–64.

123. Wolfe JD, Gardner JR, Beck WC, et al. Morning report decreases length of stay in trauma patients. Trauma Surg Acute Care Open 2018;3(1):e000185.

124. Boushehri E, Khamseh ME, Farshchi A, et al. Effects of morning report case presentation on length of stay and hospitalisation costs. Med Educ 2013;47(7):711–6.

125. Henry JM. Gaming: a teaching strategy to enhance adult learning. J Contin Educ Nurs 1997;28(5):231–4.

126. Garris R, Ahlers R, Driskell JE. Games, motivation, and learning: A research and practice model. Simulat Gaming 2002;33(4):441–67.

127. Akl EA, Sackett KM, Erdley WS, et al. Educational games for health professionals. Cochrane Database Syst Rev 2013;1:CD006411.

128. Trival Pursuit Emergency Medical Services Edition https://boardgamegeek.com/boardgame/196321/trivial-pursuit-emergency-   medical-services-edition. Accessed August 17, 2023.

129. Schmitz BD, MacLean SL, Shidler HM. An emergency pursuit game: a method for teaching emergency decision-making skills. J Contin Educ Nurs 1991;22(4):152–8.

130. Gordon DW, Brown HN. Fun and games in reviewing neonatal emergency care. Neonatal Netw 1995;14(3):45–9.

131. Hancock KJ, Klimberg VS, Williams TP, et al. Surgical Jeopardy: Play to Learn. J Surg Res 2021;257:9–14.

132. Graafland M, Schraagen JM, Schijven MP. Systematic review of serious games for medical education and surgical skills training. Br J Surg 2012;99(10):1322–30.

133. Feanny MA, Scott BG, Mattox KL, et al. Impact of the 80-hour work week on resident emergency operative experience. Am J Surg 2005;190(6):947–9.

134. Chinai SA, Guth T, Lovell E, et al. Taking Advantage of the Teachable Moment: A Review of Learner-Centered Clinical Teaching Models. West J Emerg Med 2018;19(1):28–34.

135. Irby DM, Wilkerson L. Teaching when time is limited. BMJ 2008;336(7640):384–7.

136. Schlitzkus LL, Waibel BH, Schenarts PJ. How to Teach Surgical Residents during Damage Control Surgery. Curr Surg Rep 2018;6:16.

137. Sadideen H, Alvand A, Saadeddin M, et al. Surgical experts: born or made? Int J Surg 2013;11(9):773–8.

138. Schaverien MV. Development of expertise in surgical training. J Surg Educ 2010;67(1):37–43.
139. Ericsson KA. Deliberate practice and the acquisition and maintenance of expert performance in medicine and related domains. Acad Med 2004;79(10 Suppl): S70–81.
140. Ericsson KA. Deliberate practice and acquisition of expert performance: a general overview. Acad Emerg Med 2008;15(11):988–94.
141. Gordon MJ. A review of the validity and accuracy of self-assessments in health professions training. Acad Med 1991;66(12):762–9.
142. Thinggaard E, Zetner DB, Fabrin A, et al. A Study of Surgical Residents' Self-Assessment of Open Surgery Skills Using Gap Analysis. Simul Healthc 2022; 18(5):305–11.
143. Aagaard E, Teherani A, Irby DM. Effectiveness of the one-minute preceptor model for diagnosing the patient and the learner: proof of concept. Acad Med 2004;79(1):42–9.
144. Teherani A, O'Sullivan P, Aagaard EM, et al. Student perceptions of the one minute preceptor and traditional preceptor models. Med Teach 2007;29(4):323–7.
145. Cox SS, Swanson MS. Identification of teaching excellence in operating room and clinical settings. Am J Surg 2002;183:251–5.
146. Butvidas LD, Anderson CI, Balogh D, et al. Disparities between resident and attending surgeon perceptions of intraoperative teaching. Am J Surg 2011; 201(3):385–9.
147. Vikis EA, Mihalynuk TV, Pratt DD, et al. Teaching and learning in the operating room is a two-way street: resident perceptions. Am J Surg 2008;195(5):594–8.
148. Claridge JA, Calland JF, Chandrasekhara V, et al. Comparing resident measurements to attending surgeon self- perceptions of surgical educators. Am J Surg 2003;185:323–7.
149. Doumouras AG, Engels PT. Early crisis nontechnical skill teaching in residency leads to long-term skill retention and improved performance during crises: a prospective, nonrandomized controlled study. Surgery 2017;162(1):174–81.
150. Pugh CM, DaRosa DA, Glenn D, et al. A comparison of faculty and resident perception of resident learning needs in the operating room. J Surg Educ 2007;64(5):250–5.
151. Sadler DR. Formative assessment and the design of instructional systems. Instr Sci 1989;18:119–44.
152. van de Ridder JM, Stokking KM, McGaghie WC, et al. What is feedback in clinical education? Med Educ 2008;42(2):189–97.
153. Voyer S, Hatala R. Debriefing and feedback: two sides of the same coin? Simul Healthc 2015;10(2):67–8.
154. Atkinson A, Watling CJ, Brand PLP. Feedback and coaching. Eur J Pediatr 2022; 181(2):441–6.
155. Kolb DA. Experiential learning. Upper Saddle River, NJ: Prentice Hall; 1984.
156. Salik I, Paige JT. Debriefing the Interprofessional Team in Medical Simulation.. In: Das JM, editor. *StatPearls [internet]*. Treasure island, FL: StatPearls Publishing; 2023.
157. Sawyer TL, Deering S. Adaptation of the US Army's After-Action Review for simulation debriefing in healthcare. Simul Healthc 2013;8(6):388–97.
158. Rudolph JW, Simon R, Raemer DB, et al. Debriefing as formative assessment: closing performance gaps in medical education. Acad Emerg Med 2008 Nov; 15(11):1010–6.

159. Rivière E, Jaffrelot M, Jouquan J, et al. Debriefing for the Transfer of Learning: The Importance of Context. Acad Med 2019;94(6):796–803.

160. Jahnke SA, Poston WS, Haddock CK, et al. Firefighting and mental health: Experiences of repeated exposure to trauma. Work 2016;53(4):737–44.

161. Thompson CV, Naumann DN, Fellows JL, et al. Post- traumatic stress disorder amongst surgical trainees: An unrecognized risk? Surgeon 2017;15(3):123–30.

162. Scott Z, O'Curry S, Mastroyannopoulou K. The impact and experience of debriefing for clinical staff following traumatic events in clinical settings: A systematic review. J Trauma Stress 2022;35(1):278–87.

163. Lowe SR, Walsh K, Uddin M, et al. Bidirectional relationships between trauma exposure and posttraumatic stress: a longitudinal study of Detroit residents. J Abnorm Psychol 2014;123(3):533–44.

164. Flannery RB. Psychological Trauma and the Trauma Surgeon. Psychiatr Q 2022; 93(1):27–33.

165. Warren AM, Jones AL, Shafi S, et al. Does caring for trauma patients lead to psychological stress in surgeons? J Trauma Acute Care Surg 2013;75(1): 179–84.

166. Kent Johnathan MD, Thornton Maura MD, Fong Allan MS, Hall Erin MD, MPH; Fitzgibbons, Shimae MD, MEd, Sava, Jack MD. Acute provider stress in high stakes medical care: Implications for trauma surgeons. J Trauma Acute Care Surg 2020;88(3):440–5.

167. Schmidt M, Haglund K. Debrief in Emergency Departments to Improve Compassion Fatigue and Promote Resiliency. J Trauma Nurs 2017;24(5):317–22.

168. Arriaga AF, Szyld D, Pian-Smith MCM. Real-Time Debriefing After Critical Events: Exploring the Gap Between Principle and Reality. Anesthesiol Clin 2020;38(4): 801–20.

169. Nathwani JN, Glarner CE, Law KE, et al. Integrating Postoperative Feedback Into Workflow: Perceived Practices and Barriers. J Surg Educ 2017;74(3):406–14.

170. Boet S, Bould MD, Sharma B, et al. Within-team debriefing versus instructor-led debriefing for simulation-based education: a randomized controlled trial. Ann Surg 2013;258(1):53–8.

171. Houzé-Cerfon CH, Boet S, Saint-Jean M, et al. Effect of combined individual-collective debriefing of participants in interprofessional simulation courses on crisis resource management: a randomized controlled multicenter trial. Emergencias 2020;32(2):111–7.

172. Couper K, Perkins GD. Debriefing after resuscitation. Curr Opin Crit Care 2013; 19(3):188–94.

173. Mullan PC, Wuestner E, Kerr TD, et al. Implementation of an in situ qualitative debriefing tool for resuscitations. Resuscitation 2013;84(7):946–51.

174. Gilmartin S, Martin L, Kenny S, et al. Promoting hot debriefing in an emergency department. BMJ Open Qual 2020;9(3):e000913.

175. Mullan PC, Cochrane NH, Chamberlain JM, et al. Accuracy of Postresuscitation Team Debriefings in a Pediatric Emergency Department. Ann Emerg Med 2017; 70(3):311–9.

176. Bosley JJ, Onoszko P, Kner C, et al. Tactical engagement simulation training techniques: two training programs for the conduct of after action review (ARI research product 79-2). Alexandria, VA: US Army research Institute for the Behavioral and Social Sciences; 1979 (AD A073 724).

177. Rajendran G, Mahalingam S, K A, et al. The ABCDE (Avoid Shaming/Personal Opinions, Build a Rapport, Choose a Communication Approach, Develop a Debriefing Content, Ensure the Ergonomics of Debriefing) Approach: A Simplified

Model for Debriefing During Simulation in Emergency Medicine. Cureus 2023; 15(2):e34569.

178. Oakley E, Stocker S, Staubli G, et al. Using video recording to identify management errors in pediatric trauma resuscitation. Pediatrics 2006;117(3):658–64.

179. Lowe DJ, Dewar A, Lloyd A, et al. Optimizing clinical performance during resuscitation using video evaluation. Postgrad Med J 2017;93(1102):449–53.

180. Vella MA, Dumas RP, Holena DN. Supporting the Educational, Research, and Clinical Care Goals of the Academic Trauma Center: Video Review for Trauma Resuscitation. JAMA Surg 2019;154(3):257–8.

Printed and bound by CPI Group (UK) Ltd, Croydon, CR0 4YY

03/10/2024

01040473-0006